Serono Symposia, USA
Norwell, Massachusetts

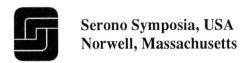

Serono Symposia, USA
Norwell, Massachusetts

Geula Gibori
Editor

Signaling Mechanisms and Gene Expression in the Ovary

With 207 Figures

Springer-Verlag
New York   Berlin   Heidelberg   London
Paris   Tokyo   Hong Kong   Barcelona

Geula Gibori, Ph.D.
Department of Physiology and Biophysics
College of Medicine
University of Illinois
Chicago, IL 60680
USA

Proceedings of the Eighth Ovarian Workshop on Regulatory Processes and Gene Expression in the Ovary, sponsored by Serono Symposia, USA, held July 12 to 14, 1990, in Maryville, Tennessee.

For information on previous volumes, please contact Serono Symposia, USA.

Printed on acid-free paper.

Production and typesetting services by Technical Texts, Scituate, Massachusetts.
Printed and bound by Edwards Brothers, Inc., Ann Arbor, Michigan.

Printed in the United States of America.

9 8 7 6 5 4 3 2 1

ISBN 0-387-97653-1 Springer-Verlag New York Berlin Heidelberg
ISBN 3-540-97653-1 Springer-Verlag Berlin Heidelberg New York

PROCEEDINGS OF THE EIGHTH OVARIAN WORKSHOP ON REGULATORY PROCESSES AND GENE EXPRESSION IN THE OVARY

Ovarian Workshop Board

Preface

Since its inception in 1976, the overall goal of the Ovarian Workshop has been to bring together biologists from various disciplines so that they may collectively achieve a better understanding of the latest developments and define important problems in ovarian physiology. The Ovarian Workshop, which was pioneered by Dr. A. Rees Midgley, has developed into a major biennial meeting for investigators in the ovarian field.

Largely as a consequence of advances in technology, especially in molecular biology, progress in the area of gene expression and signal transduction has been rapid. The Eighth Ovarian Workshop focused on two major topics: (1) the expression of hormonally and nonhormonally controlled genes involved in the functional and morphological differentiation of the cells forming the ovary and (2) the signaling mechanisms by which endogenous and exogenous hormones and cytokines affect ovarian differentiation and steroidogenesis.

The Eighth Ovarian Workshop, held on the campus of Maryville College in Maryville, Tennessee, July 12 to 14, 1990, was again generously funded and coordinated by Serono Symposia, USA. I would especially like to thank Dr. Lisa Kern of Serono for her expert help in organizing this meeting.

The board of directors of the Eighth Ovarian Workshop consisted of Drs. Eli Adashi, JoAnne Fortune, Anne Hirshfield, Aaron Hsueh, Julia Lobotsky, Gordon Niswender, David W. Schomberg, Richard Stouffer, and Jerry Strauss. Their valuable advice and the important roles they played in the planning of the scientific program are gratefully acknowledged.

GEULA GIBORI

Contents

Part III.   Hormonal Control and Gene Expression in the Ovary

Part IV.   Relevance of Resident Ovarian White Blood Cells

Part V.   Submitted Manuscripts

Contributors

ELI Y. ADASHI, Department of Obstetrics and Gynecology, University of Maryland School of Medicine, Baltimore, Maryland, USA.

CHRIS ALBANESE, Thyroid Unit, Massachusetts General Hospital, Boston, Massachusetts, USA.

CONSTANCE T. ALBARRACIN, Department of Physiology and Biophysics, College of Medicine, University of Illinois, Chicago, Illinois, USA.

JUAN G. ALVAREZ, Department of Obstetrics and Gynecology, University of Pennsylvania, Philadelphia, Pennsylvania, USA.

CRISTIANA L. ANDREANI, Department of Obstetrics and Gynecology, University of Maryland School of Medicine, Baltimore, Maryland, USA.

AKIRA ARIMURA, U.S.–Japan Biomedical Research Laboratories, Tulane University Hebert Center, Belle Chasse, and Departments of Medicine, Anatomy, and Physiology, Tulane University School of Medicine, New Orleans, Louisiana, USA.

D.T. ARMSTRONG, Departments of Physiology and Obstetrics and Gynecology, University of Western Ontario, London, Ontario, Canada.

C. AZOULAY-BARJONET, Inserm CJF 89-08, CHR La Grave, Toulouse Cedex, France.

P. BAGAVANDOSS, Departments of Physiology, Internal Medicine, and Pathology, The University of Michigan, Ann Arbor, Michigan, USA.

JANICE M. BAHR, Department of Animal Sciences, University of Illinois, Urbana, Illinois, USA.

B. GEORGE BARISAS, Departments of Physiology and Chemistry, Colorado State University, Fort Collins, Colorado, USA.

D. BARZILAI, Faculty of Medicine, Technion–Israel Institute of Technology, Haifa, Israel.

A. BÉLANGER, Laboratoire d'Endocrinologie Moléculaire du Centre Hospitalier de L'Université Laval, Quebec, Canada.

S. BILODEAU, Départment de Zootechnie, CHUL Research Centre and Université Laval, Quebec, Canada.

OREST W. BLASCHUK, Departments of Physiology and Urology, McGill University, Montreal, Quebec, Canada.

NATHALIE BRETON, Medical Research Council Group in Molecular Endocrinology, CHUL Research Center and Laval University, Quebec, Canada.

I. BUSSENOT, Inserm CJF 89-08, CHR La Grave, Toulouse Cedex, France.

IAN P. CALLARD, Mount Desert Island Biological Laboratory, Salsbury Cove, Maine, and Department of Biology, Boston University, Boston, Massachusetts, USA.

ELLEN M. CARNEY, Department of Cell, Molecular, and Structural Biology, Northwestern University Medical School, Chicago, Illinois, USA.

P. JORGE CHEDRESE, Reproductive Biology Research Unit, University of Saskatchewan, Saskatoon, Canada, and Departamento de Produccion Animal, Instituto Nacional de Tecnologia Agropecuaria (INTA), Balcarce, Argentina.

J.Y. CHOU, HGB NICHD, Bethesda, Maryland, USA.

T.K. CLINTON, Department of Physiology, University of Kansas Medical Center, Kansas City, Kansas, USA.

B.S. COOPER, U.S. Department of Agriculture, Agricultural Research Service, Beltsville Agricultural Research Center, Reproduction Laboratory, Beltsville, Maryland, USA.

JACQUES COUËT, Medical Research Council Group in Molecular Endocrinology, CHUL Research Center and Laval University, Quebec, Canada.

RICHARD E. CUTLER, JR., Department of Cell, Molecular, and Structural Biology, Northwestern University Medical School, Chicago, Illinois, USA.

JOHN S. DAVIS, Women's Research Institute, University of Kansas School of Medicine, Wichita, and Department of Veterans Affairs Medical Center, Wichita, Kansas, USA.

M. YUSOFF DAWOOD, Department of Obstetrics, Gynecology, and Reproductive Sciences, University of Texas Medical School, Houston, Texas, USA.

BEVERLY C. DELIDOW, Department of Obstetrics and Gynecology, University of Connecticut Health Center, Farmington, Connecticut, USA.

P. DEMENT-LIEBENOW, Department of Biological Sciences, Northern Illinois University, DeKalb, Illinois, USA.

MICHELLE DEMETER, Cecil H. and Ida Green Center for Reproductive Biology Sciences, and Departments of Biochemistry and Obstetrics and Gynecology, University of Texas Southwestern Medical Center, Dallas, Texas, USA.

DEBRA S. DRUST, Thyroid Unit, Massachusetts General Hospital, Boston, Massachusetts, USA.

ERIC DUPONT, Medical Research Council Group in Molecular Endocrinology, CHUL Research Center and Laval University, Quebec, Canada.

JOANNA C. DYKEMA, Department of Biochemistry, Molecular Biology, and Cell Biology, Northwestern University, Evanston, Illinois, USA.

H. ENGELHARDT, Department of Physiology, University of Western Ontario, London, Ontario, Canada.

KATHLEEN M. EYSTER, Department of Physiology and Pharmacology, University of South Dakota, Vermillion, South Dakota, USA.

RIAZ FAROOKHI, Departments of Physiology and Urology, McGill University, Montreal, Quebec, Canada.

LISA A. FILETI, Mount Desert Island Biological Laboratory, Salsbury Cove, Maine, and Department of Biology, Boston University, Boston, Massachusetts, USA.

J. JOE FORD, U.S. Department of Agriculture, Agricultural Research Service, U.S. Meat Animal Research Center, Clay Center, Nebraska, USA.

M.A. FORTIER, Laboratoire d'Ontogénie et de Reproduction, CHUL Research Centre and Université Laval, Quebec, Canada.

J.E. FORTUNE, Department and Section of Physiology, Cornell University, Ithaca, New York, USA.

G.S. GETZ, Department of Pathology, The University of Chicago, Chicago, Illinois, USA.

GEULA GIBORI, Department of Physiology and Biophysics, College of Medicine, University of Illinois, Chicago, Illinois, USA.

N. GLEICHER, Department of Obstetrics and Gynecology, Mount Sinai Medical Center, Chicago, Illinois, USA.

E.L. GONG, The Lawrence Berkeley Laboratory, Berkeley, California, USA.

R.E. GORE-LANGTON, Departments of Physiology and Obstetrics and Gynecology, University of Western Ontario, and John P. Robarts Research Institute, London, Ontario, Canada.

PAUL E. GOTTSCHALL, U.S.–Japan Biomedical Research Laboratories, Tulane University Hebert Center, Belle Chasse, and Departments of Medicine, Anatomy, and Physiology, Tulane University School of Medicine, New Orleans, Louisiana, USA.

J.M. GRIZZLE, U.S. Department of Agriculture, Agricultural Research Service, Roman L. Hruska U.S. Meat Animal Research Center, Clay Center, Nebraska, USA.

H.D. GUTHRIE, U.S. Department of Agriculture, Agricultural Research Service, Beltsville Agricultural Research Center, Reproduction Laboratory, Beltsville, Maryland, USA.

L. HARLOW, Department of Obstetrics and Gynecology, Mount Sinai Medical Center, Chicago, Illinois, USA.

S. HARRIS-HOOKER, Departments of Medicine and Pathology, Morehouse School of Medicine, Atlanta, Georgia, USA.

LARS HEDIN, Department of Physiology, University of Göteborg, Göteborg, Sweden.

JAMES R. HERMAN, Departments of Physiology and Chemistry, Colorado State University, Fort Collins, Colorado, USA.

S.G. HILLIER, Reproductive Endocrinology Laboratory, University of Edinburgh Centre for Reproductive Biology, Edinburgh, Scotland.

P.B. HOYER, Department of Physiology, University of Arizona, Tucson, Arizona, USA.

C.J. HUBBARD, Department of Biological Sciences, Northern Illinois University, DeKalb, Illinois, USA.

MARY HUNZICKER-DUNN, Department of Cell, Molecular, and Structural Biology, Northwestern University Medical School, Chicago, Illinois, USA.

ARYE HURWITZ, Department of Obstetrics and Gynecology, University of Maryland School of Medicine, Baltimore, Maryland, USA.

RICHARD IVELL, Institute of Hormone and Fertility Research, Hamburg, Germany.

VICTORIA JACKIW, Department of Cell, Molecular, and Structural Biology, Northwestern University Medical School, Chicago, Illinois, USA.

J. LARRY JAMESON, Thyroid Unit, Massachusetts General Hospital, Boston, Massachusetts, USA.

PATRICIA A. JOHNSON, Department of Poultry and Avian Sciences, Cornell University, Ithaca, New York, USA.

LEE-CHUAN KAO, Department of Obstetrics and Gynecology, University of Pennsylvania, Philadelphia, Pennsylvania, USA.

THOMAS W.H. KAY, Thyroid Unit, Massachusetts General Hospital, Boston, Massachusetts, USA.

NICHOLAS KENNY, Departments of Physiology and Chemistry, Colorado State University, Fort Collins, Colorado, USA.

P.L. KEYES, Departments of Physiology, Internal Medicine, and Pathology, The University of Michigan, Ann Arbor, Michigan, USA.

I. KHAN, Department of Physiology and Biophysics, College of Medicine, University of Illinois, Chicago, Illinois, USA.

FIRYAL S. KHAN-DAWOOD, Department of Obstetrics, Gynecology, and Reproductive Sciences, University of Texas Medical School, Houston, Texas, USA.

A. KRISHNA, Department of Physiology, Morehouse School of Medicine, Atlanta, Georgia, USA.

S.L. KUNKEL, Departments of Physiology, Internal Medicine, and Pathology, The University of Michigan, Ann Arbor, Michigan, USA.

CLAUDE LABRIE, Medical Research Council Group in Molecular Endocrinology, CHUL Research Center and Laval University, Quebec, Canada.

FERNAND LABRIE, Medical Research Council Group in Molecular Endocrinology, CHUL Research Center and Laval University, Quebec, Canada.

M. LAHAV, Faculty of Medicine, Technion–Israel Institute of Technology, Haifa, Israel.

LASSE LARSON, Department of Physiology, University of Göteborg, Göteborg, Sweden.

MARKUS LAUBER, Cecil H. and Ida Green Center for Reproductive Biology Sciences, and Departments of Biochemistry and Obstetrics and Gynecology, University of Texas Southwestern Medical Center, Dallas, Texas, USA.

F. LEDWITZ-RIGBY, Department of Biological Sciences, Northern Illinois University, DeKalb, Illinois, USA.

PETER C.K. LEUNG, Department of Obstetrics and Gynaecology, University of British Columbia, Vancouver, British Columbia, Canada.

JILL A. LOUKIDES, Department of Obstetrics and Gynecology, University of Maryland, Baltimore, Maryland, USA.

VAN LUU-THE, Medical Research Council Group in Molecular Endocrinology, CHUL Research Center and Laval University, Quebec, Canada.

R. LYLES, The Reproductive Resource Center of Greater Kansas City, Overland Park, Kansas, USA.

JOHN LYNCH, Department of Anatomy, University of Connecticut Health Center, Farmington, Connecticut, USA.

LAIRD D. MADISON, Thyroid Unit, Massachusetts General Hospital, Boston, Massachusetts, USA.

DENIS A. MAGOFFIN, Department of Obstetrics and Gynecology, Cedars-Sinai Medical Center/UCLA School of Medicine, Los Angeles, California, USA.

EVELYN T. MAIZELS, Department of Cell, Molecular, and Structural Biology, Northwestern University Medical School, Chicago, Illinois, USA.

B. MARCOTTE, Department of Molecular Endocrinology, CHUL Research Center and Laval University, Quebec, Canada.

CÉLINE MARTEL, Medical Research Council Group in Molecular Endocrinology, CHUL Research Center and Laval University, Quebec, Canada.

R.R. MAURER, U.S. Department of Agriculture, Agricultural Research Service, Roman L. Hruska U.S. Meat Animal Research Center, Clay Center, Nebraska, USA.

KELLY E. MAYO, Department of Biochemistry, Molecular Biology, and Cell Biology, Northwestern University, Evanston, Illinois, USA.

R.J. MCCORMICK, Department of Animal Science, University of Wyoming, Laramie, Wyoming, USA.

M.P. MCLEAN, Department of Physiology and Biophysics, College of Medicine, University of Illinois, Chicago, Illinois, USA.

JOSEPHINE B. MILLER, Department of Obstetrics and Gynecology, University of Illinois, Chicago, Illinois, USA.

EISHICHI MIYAMOTO, Department of Pharmacology, Kumamoto University Medical School, Kumamoto, Japan.

KOHJI MIYAZAKI, Department of Obstetrics and Gynecology, Kumamoto University Medical School, Kumamoto, Japan.

W.J. MURDOCH, Department of Animal Science, University of Wyoming, Laramie, Wyoming, USA.

BRUCE D. MURPHY, Reproductive Biology Research Unit, University of Saskatchewan, Saskatoon, Canada.

S. NELSON, Department of Physiology and Biophysics, College of Medicine, University of Illinois, Chicago, Illinois, USA.

PAMELA NELSON, Department of Obstetrics and Gynecology, Section of Reproductive Endocrinology, Yale University School of Medicine, New Haven, Connecticut, USA.

HIROAKI NITTA, Department of Animal Sciences, University of Illinois, Urbana, Illinois, USA.

ENSIO NORJAVAARA, Department of Physiology, University of Umeå, Umeå, Sweden.

TAKASHI OHBA, Department of Obstetrics and Gynecology, Kumamoto University Medical School, Kumamoto, Japan.

YASUTAKA OHTA, Department of Pharmacology, Kumamoto University Medical School, Kumamoto, Japan.

HITOSHI OKAMURA, Department of Obstetrics and Gynecology, Kumamoto University Medical School, Kumamoto, Japan.

JAN OLOFSSON, Department of Physiology, University of Umeå, Umeå, Sweden.

L.M. OLSON, Department of Pathology, The University of Chicago, Chicago, Illinois, USA.

YOSHIO OSAWA, Endocrine Biochemistry Department, Medical Foundation of Buffalo, Buffalo, New York, USA.

A.C. OTTOBRE, Department of Dairy Science, Ohio State University, Columbus, Ohio, USA.

J.S. OTTOBRE, Department of Dairy Science, Ohio State University, Columbus, Ohio, USA.

JEFFREY N. PACKMAN, Department of Obstetrics and Gynecology, University of Maryland School of Medicine, Baltimore, Maryland, USA.

J. PARINAUD, Inserm CJF 89-08, CHR La Grave, Toulouse Cedex, France.

T.G. PARMER, Department of Physiology and Biophysics, College of Medicine, University of Illinois, Chicago, Illinois, USA.

DONNA W. PAYNE, Department of Obstetrics and Gynecology, University of Maryland School of Medicine, Baltimore, Maryland, USA.

GEORGES PELLETIER, Medical Research Council Group in Molecular Endocrinology, CHUL Research Center and Laval University, Quebec, Canada.

JOHN J. PELUSO, Department of Obstetrics and Gynecology, University of Connecticut Health Center, Farmington, Connecticut, USA.

MARY LAKE POLAN, Department of Gynecology and Obstetrics, Stanford University School of Medicine, Stanford, California, USA.

JASON O. RAHAL, Department of Biochemistry, Molecular Biology, and Cell Biology, Northwestern University, Evanston, Illinois, USA.

D.G. REMICK, Departments of Physiology, Internal Medicine, and Pathology, The University of Michigan, Ann Arbor, Michigan, USA.

HANNAH RENNERT, Department of Obstetrics and Gynecology, University of Pennsylvania, Philadelphia, Pennsylvania, USA.

CAROL E. RESNICK, Department of Obstetrics and Gynecology, University of Maryland School of Medicine, Baltimore, Maryland, USA.

C.E. REXROAD, JR., U.S. Department of Agriculture, Agricultural Research Service, Beltsville Agricultural Research Center, Reproduction Laboratory, Beltsville, Maryland, USA.

ERIC RHÉAUME, Medical Research Council Group in Molecular Endocrinology, CHUL Research Center and Laval University, Quebec, Canada.

KATHERINE F. ROBY, Department of Physiology, University of Kansas Medical Center, Kansas City, Kansas, USA.

H.F. RODGERS, Department of Tissue Pathology, Prince Henry's Hospital, Melbourne, Victoria, Australia.

RAYMOND RODGERS, Cecil H. and Ida Green Center for Reproductive Biology Sciences, and Departments of Biochemistry and Obstetrics and Gynecology, University of Texas Southwestern Medical Center, Dallas, Texas, USA.

R.J. RODGERS, Prince Henry's Institute of Medical Research, Prince Henry's Hospital, Melbourne, Victoria, Australia.

MARIE R. RODWAY, Department of Obstetrics and Gynaecology, University of British Columbia, Vancouver, British Columbia, Canada.

DEBORAH A. ROESS, Departments of Physiology and Chemistry, Colorado State University, Fort Collins, Colorado, USA.

R.M. ROHAN, U.S. Department of Agriculture, Agricultural Research Service, Beltsville Agricultural Research Center, Reproduction Laboratory, Beltsville, Maryland, USA.

M. ROMANI, Department of Biological Sciences, Northern Illinois University, DeKalb, Illinois, USA.

MARIA SANCHO-TELLO, Department of Physiology, University of Kansas Medical Center, Kansas City, Kansas, USA.

P.G. SCHEID, Department of Biological Sciences, Northern Illinois University, DeKalb, Illinois, USA.

V.M. SCHMIT, Department of Obstetrics and Gynecology, The University of Chicago, Chicago, Illinois, USA.

DANIEL SCHOTT, Reproductive Biology Research Unit, University of Saskatchewan, Saskatoon, Canada.

J.R. SCHREIBER, Department of Obstetrics and Gynecology, The University of Chicago, Chicago, Illinois, USA.

NICHOLAS SCHULZ, ABL-Basic Research Program, NCI-Frederick Cancer Research and Development Center, Frederick, Maryland, USA.

DEBORAH L. SEGALOFF, Department of Physiology and Biophysics, The University of Iowa, Iowa City, Iowa, USA.

GUNNAR SELSTAM, Department of Physiology, University of Umeå, Umeå, Sweden.

JACQUES SIMARD, Medical Research Council Group in Molecular Endocrinology, CHUL Research Center and Laval University, Quebec, Canada.

EVAN R. SIMPSON, Cecil H. and Ida Green Center for Reproductive Biology Sciences, and Departments of Biochemistry and Obstetrics and Gynecology, University of Texas Southwestern Medical Center, Dallas, Texas, USA.

M.-A. SIRARD, Medical Research Council Group in Molecular Endocrinology, CHUL Research Center and Laval University, Quebec, Canada.

R. SRIDARAN, Department of Physiology, Morehouse School of Medicine, Atlanta, Georgia, USA.

R.K. SRIVASTAVA, Department of Physiology, Morehouse School of Medicine, Atlanta, Georgia, USA.

DAVID STIRLING, Cecil H. and Ida Green Center for Reproductive Biology Sciences, and Departments of Biochemistry and Obstetrics and Gynecology, University of Texas Southwestern Medical Center, Dallas, Texas, USA.

RICHARD L. STOUFFER, Division of Reproductive Biology and Behavior, Oregon Regional Primate Research Center, Beaverton, and Department of Physiology, Oregon Health Sciences University, Portland, Oregon, USA.

JEROME F. STRAUSS, III, Department of Obstetrics and Gynecology, University of Pennsylvania, Philadelphia, Pennsylvania, USA.

PAUL F. TERRANOVA, Department of Physiology, University of Kansas Medical Center, Kansas City, Kansas, USA.

O. TOPAZ, Faculty of Medicine, Technion–Israel Institute of Technology, Haifa, Israel.

Y. TREMBLAY, Department of Molecular Endocrinology, CHUL Research Center and Laval University, Quebec, Canada.

CLAUDE TRUDEL, Medical Research Council Group in Molecular Endocrinology, CHUL Research Center and Laval University, Quebec, Canada.

I.M. TURNER, Reproductive Endocrinology Laboratory, University of Edinburgh Centre for Reproductive Biology, Edinburgh, Scotland.

C.A. VANDEVOORT, Division of Reproductive Biology and Behavior, Oregon Regional Primate Research Center, Beaverton, Oregon, USA.

GEORGE F. VANDE WOUDE, ABL-Basic Research Program, NCI-Frederick Cancer Research and Development Center, Frederick, Maryland, USA.

A.K. VOSS, Department and Section of Physiology, Cornell University, Ithaca, New York, USA.

SERGE-ALAIN WANDJI, Départment de Zootechnie, CHUL Research Centre and Université Laval, Quebec, Canada.

SHU-YIN WANG, Department of Poultry and Avian Sciences, Cornell University, Ithaca, New York, USA.

MICHAEL R. WATERMAN, Cecil H. and Ida Green Center for Reproductive Biology Sciences, and Departments of Biochemistry and Obstetrics and Gynecology, University of Texas Southwestern Medical Center, Dallas, Texas, USA.

J. WEED, Department of Gynecology and Obstetrics, University of Kansas Medical Center, Kansas City, Kansas, USA.

J.A. WEGNER, Department of Physiology, University of Arizona, Tucson, Arizona, USA.

BRUCE A. WHITE, Department of Anatomy, University of Connecticut Health Center, Farmington, Connecticut, USA.

R.C. WIGGINS, Departments of Physiology, Internal Medicine, and Pathology, The University of Michigan, Ann Arbor, Michigan, USA.

T. WISE, U.S. Department of Agriculture, Agricultural Research Service, Roman L. Hruska U.S. Meat Animal Research Center, Clay Center, Nebraska, USA.

K.L. WYNE, Department of Pathology, The University of Chicago, Chicago, Illinois, USA.

RITSU YAMAMOTO, Department of Obstetrics and Gynecology, University of Pennsylvania, Philadelphia, Pennsylvania, USA.

DAVID ZHANG, Reproductive Biology Research Unit, University of Saskatchewan, Saskatoon, Canada.

HUI FEN ZHAO, Medical Research Council Group in Molecular Endocrinology, CHUL Research Center and Laval University, Quebec, Canada.

M. ZILBERSTEIN, Department of Physiology and Biophysics, College of Medicine, University of Illinois, Chicago, Illinois, and HGB NICHD, Bethesda, Maryland, USA.

Part I

Gonadotropin Receptors
and Transfactors

1

The Gonadotropin Receptors: Structural Insights Learned from the Cloning of Their cDNAs

DEBORAH L. SEGALOFF

Luteinizing hormone (LH) is a member of a family of glycoprotein hormones that also includes the pituitary hormones, follicle stimulating hormone (FSH) and thyroid stimulating hormone (TSH), as well as the placental hormone, human choriogonadotropin (hCG). All are composed of two dissimilar subunits, termed α and β, which are joined by noncovalent associations (1, 2). Within a given species, the α-subunits are identical, whereas the β-subunits are similar but distinct. Although both subunits are necessary for binding to the receptor, it is the β-subunit that confers binding specificity (3–5). Since the β-subunits of LH and hCG are nearly identical, the same receptor can bind either hormone, and hence it is formally referred to as the LH/CG receptor.

The LH/CG, FSH, and TSH receptors are all cell surface receptors that, upon binding hormone, activate adenylyl cyclase activity (6–10), presumably through coupling to a G_s protein. In studying the function and regulation of the LH/CG receptor, it became clear that a further understanding of these phenomenon necessitated learning the structure of this receptor.

The Structure of the LH/CG Receptor

From studies done in collaboration with M. Ascoli (11, 12, for reviews), the LH/CG receptor was determined to be a single glycoprotein with a molecular mass (on SDS polyacrylamide gels) of 93 kDa. In the course of these studies, a purification scheme for the rat luteal LH/CG receptor was developed (13). In collaboration with K. Nikolics and K.C. McFarland at Genentech, Inc., amino acid sequences were determined from both the intact purified receptor and from peptides derived from the purified receptor. With the collaboration of P. Seeburg and R. Sprengel at The University of Heidelberg (14), a full-length cDNA encoding the rat luteal LH/CG receptor was subsequently cloned. It should be pointed out that in France, Loosfelt et al. (15) independently reported the cloning of the porcine testicular LH/CG receptor cDNA. Although this discussion is centered on the rat luteal LH/CG receptor, it is important to note that the LH/CG receptors from these two sources have the same overall structure and share an 89% identity of amino acids.

The rat luteal LH/CG receptor cDNA encodes for a protein of 700 amino acids, the first 26 of which appear to be a signal peptide. The mature protein, therefore, is estimated to be 75 kDa. The difference between this and the 93 kDa that we observed for the native LH/CG receptor is presumably due to the glycoprotein nature of the receptor (16). Indeed, there are 6 potential sites for N-linked glycosylation within the N-terminal half of the receptor.

Hydrophathy analyses of the amino acid sequence showed that the C-terminal half of the LH/CG receptor contains 7 regions of hydrophobic amino acids, each of which is sufficiently long to span the plasma membrane. This is a notable feature common to other G-protein-coupled receptors (17). Indeed, a comparison of the amino acid sequence of the C-terminal half of the LH/CG receptor with other G-protein-coupled receptors shows that it is related to this family of proteins. Therefore, we postulate that this region of the LH/CG receptor similarly spans the plasma membrane 7 times, ending with a cytoplasmic C-terminal tail. Within the intracellular loops and the cytoplasmic tail, there are numerous serines, threonines, and tyrosines, which represent potential phosphorylation sites. In addition, within the cytoplasmic tail, there are two clusters of basic amino acids, which represent potential sites for tryptic cleavage.

Unlike other G-protein-coupled receptors that had been cloned at the time, however, the LH/CG receptor also contains a large relatively hydrophilic N-terminal domain postulated to be extracellular. Although the N-terminal half of the receptor does not share homology with other known receptors, it does contain a leucine-rich repeat motif that is observed in a number of other widely diverse proteins, collectively termed leucine-rich glycoproteins (14).

Functional Expression of the LH/CG Receptor cDNA

That the cDNA we cloned did encode for the LH/CG receptor was verified by expression studies in which the cDNA was placed into an expression vector under the transcriptional control of the cytomegalovirus promoter, and this was used to transiently transfect human kidney 293-cells.

When [^{125}I]hCG was allowed to bind to transfected 293-cells and then was crosslinked to the cells, a single radiolabeled hormone-receptor complex was

observed on SDS polyacrylamide gels. These data confirmed that the transfected 293-cells expressed a cell surface receptor that could specifically bind
hCG. When MA-10 Leydig tumor cells, which normally express functional
LH/CG receptors (18, for review), were similarly incubated with [^{125}I]hCG
and then crosslinked, a hormone-receptor complex of the same size was
observed. As we know the LH/CG receptor on MA-10 cells to be 93 kDa
(11, 16, 19), the LH/CG receptor expressed in the transfected 293-cells must
also be processed to the same molecular mass.

Two hormones, hCG and oLH, were determined to bind to transfected
293-cells with high affinity, 100 pM and 7.4 nM, respectively. The absolute
affinities and the relative difference in affinities between the two hormones is
comparable to that observed for the rat LH/CG receptor. Whether the binding
of hormone to the transfected 293-cells leads to the activation of adenylyl
cyclase activity was tested by measuring intracellular cAMP levels in cells
incubated with the different glycoprotein hormones. Mock transfected cells
did not show an elevation of cAMP in response to any glycoprotein hormone.
Cells transfected with the LH/CG receptor cDNA responded to hCG or oLH
with a dose-dependent and saturable increase in cAMP. The EC_{50} for both
hormones was calculated to be 36 pM.

These data confirmed that the cDNA that was cloned does indeed code for
the LH/CG receptor. These data also confirm our previous biochemical data
that had suggested that the LH/CG receptor is composed of a single polypeptide that both binds hormone and activates adenylyl cyclase (12). As summarized in a recent review, other reports purporting multiple subunits of the LH/
CG receptor can readily be explained by receptor proteolysis (11).

In addition to binding hormone and activating adenylyl cyclase activity,
the LH/CG receptor expressed in transfected 293-cells also displays a LH/
CG-dependent desensitization of LH/CG-stimulated adenylyl cyclase activity, an internalization of receptor-bound hCG, and a LH/CG-dependent
downregulation of receptors. Therefore, this cDNA encodes for a LH/CG
receptor with full biological activity. As such, site-directed mutagenesis can
now be utilized to determine which structural features of this receptor are
involved in these different biological functions.

The Orientation of the LH/CG Receptor as Revealed by Site-Specific Antibodies

From the deduced amino acid sequence of the LH/CG receptor cDNA, it
was postulated that the N-terminal half of the receptor was situated extracellularly and that the C-terminal tail was located intracellularly. In order
to test this hypothesis experimentally, site-specific polyclonal antibodies
were raised against synthetic peptides corresponding to discrete regions

of the receptor. These antibodies were then used in indirect immuno-fluorescence studies in primary cultures of rat luteal cells to detect the LH/CG receptor (20).

Anti-LHR02 was raised against a peptide corresponding to aa 194-207, which are located approximately midway in the N-terminal putative extra-cellular domain. By Western blotting, this antiserum was determined to be specific for the LH/CG receptor. When intact rat luteal cells were incubated with anti-LHR02, an intense immunofluorescence was observed, confirming that the N-terminal domain of the LH/CG receptor is indeed located extracellularly.

To examine the cellular disposition of the C-terminal tail of the receptor, anti-LHR06 was raised against a peptide corresponding to the extreme C-terminal 14 amino acids of the LH/CG receptor, as defined by the open reading frame of the cDNA. This antibody was also shown by Western blotting to be specific for the LH/CG receptor. When intact rat luteal cells were incubated with anti-LHR06, no immunofluorescence was observed. However, when the cells were permeabilized first with detergent and then incubated with antibody, an intense immunofluoresence was seen. These results demonstrate that the C-terminal tail of the LH/CG receptor is located intracellularly. Furthermore, this region of the receptor is accessible to antibody binding.

There is another important conclusion that can be made from the results with anti-LHR06. This has to do with the two potential sites for tryptic cleavage that are present within the cytoplasmic tail of the receptor (14). The presence of these sites raises the possibility that the mature receptor might be post-translationally modified to terminate at one of these positions. Since Western blots of a crude preparation of receptor (a detergent extract of rat luteal membranes in which the receptor has been purified only 10-fold by wheat germ agglutinin chromatography) that are probed with anti-LHR06 display only one 93-kDa band, and since the LH/CG receptor is visualized by anti-LHR06 in permeabilized rat luteal cells, we conclude that at least some of the mature receptor is not cleaved at one of these potential tryptic sites. It is possible, though, that cleavage at one of these sites might be involved in receptor regulation. This possibility is being examined.

Although we have not yet addressed the multiple membrane-spanning regions of the receptor, our immunofluorescence data demonstrate that the N-terminal domain of the LH/CG receptor is indeed located extracellularly and that the C-terminal tail is situated intracellularly.

The Role of the Extracellular Domain in Hormone Binding

The large N-terminal domain of the LH/CG rececptor has been shown to be located extracellularly, thus providing more reason to predict that this region would be involved in binding the large glycoprotein hormones. Although it is not unlikely that it is involved in binding hormone, it is not known whether it alone is sufficient for high-affinity binding. To test this directly, we constructed a cDNA encoding for a truncated LH/CG receptor, representing the extracellular domain. Expression of this cDNA in 293-cells resulted in a truncated receptor that bound hCG with a high affinity comparable to that of the full-length receptor (21).

These results demonstrate that not only is the extracellular domain involved in binding hormone, but that it is entirely sufficient for conferring high-affinity binding. This does not, however, preclude the possibility that once the hormone has bound to the extracellular domain, a region, or regions, of the extracellular domain and/or hormone interacts with the transmembrane regions of the receptor. Along these lines, it should be noted that the ligands for rhodopsin and for the adrenergic receptors have been shown to intercalcate within the plasma membrane and interact directly with amino acids within the transmembrane helices (22–25). By mechanisms not yet understood, the binding of agonists enables regions in the intracellular loops and N-terminal portion of the C-terminal tail to couple to the G-protein (26). Since the overall mechanism of receptor/G-protein coupling is not likely to be different among the different G-protein-coupled receptors, it does not seem unreasonable to predict that a direct interaction of the LH/CG receptor extracellular domain and/or hormone with the transmembrane region of the receptor might be necessary to invoke receptor-G_s coupling. Clearly, much more work needs to be done to elucidate the means by which LH or hCG binding to the LH/CG receptor leads to G_s coupling and activation.

A Comparison of the LH/CG, FSH, and TSH Receptors

Given that LH, hCG, FSH, and TSH are homologous proteins and given that they all bind to cell surface receptors that activate adenylyl cyclase, it was reasonable to predict that the FSH and TSH receptors would share both amino acid and structural homology with the LH/CG receptor.

Therefore, utilizing the rat luteal LH/CG receptor cDNA, it was possible to clone the FSH receptor from a rat Sertoli cell library (27). Similarly, the TSH receptor cDNA was cloned from a human thyroid library (28). Independently, two other laboratories have also reported the cloning of the TSH receptor cDNA (29–31). Importantly, the expression of the cDNAs for the FSH and TSH receptors confirmed that these receptors, too, are each composed of a single polypeptide that both binds hormone and activates adenylyl cyclase. Furthermore, as predicted, there is a significant homology between the 3 glycoprotein hormone receptors. Thus, each is composed of a large N-terminal extracellular domain that is attached to a region bearing homology with other receptors that couple to G-proteins and, thus, probably spans the plasma membrane 7 times, ending in a relatively short cytoplasmic C-terminal tail.

In comparing the two gonadotropin receptors, there is a 50% homology between the extracellular domains and a 80% homology between the C-terminal halves of the receptors. The homology between the LH/CG and FSH receptors is greater than that of either gonadotropin receptor with the TSH receptor for two reasons. First there is the trivial reason of the species being compared. Thus, the LH/CG and FSH receptors have both been cloned from the rat, whereas the TSH receptor has been cloned from the human and dog. Secondly, and more importantly, there is an insert of approximately 50 amino acids in the extracellular domain of the TSH receptor, which is not present in either of the two gonadotropin receptors.

The alignment of amino acids between the LH/CG and FSH receptors (27) does not, unfortunately, reveal any major insights into which amino acids might be involved in the binding of gonadotropins to these receptors. It is hoped that the construction and characterization of mutant and chimeric forms of the LH/CG and FSH receptors will yield valuable clues as to the structural requirements for hormone binding, especially as pertaining to the specificity of binding and the ability of glycosylated hormones (as opposed to deglycosylated derivatives) to elicit receptor/G-protein coupling.

Summary

In summary, the glycoprotein hormone receptors comprise a unique subclass of G-protein-coupled receptors. Although we have already learned much about these receptors from the cloning of their cDNAs, many questions remain. It should be pointed out, however, that it has been 15 years since hCG was first described to bind to the LH/CG receptor and only one year since the cloning of the LH/CG receptor cDNA was described. It is anticipated that the next few years should yield a wealth of new information about the structure, function, and regulation of these receptors.

References

1. Pierce JG. Gonadotropins: Chemistry and biosynthesis. In: Knobil E, Neill JD, Ewing LL, Greenwald GS, Markert CL, Pfaff DW, eds. The physiology of reproduction. New York: Raven Press, 1988:1335-48.
2. Strickland TW, Parsons TF, Pierce JG. Structure of LH and hCG. In: Ascoli M, ed. Luteinizing hormone action and receptors. Boca Raton, FL: CRC Press, 1985:1-16.
3. Pierce JG, Bahl OP, Cornell JS, Swaminathan N. Biologically active hormones

prepared by recombination of the α chain of human chorionic gonadotropin and the hormone specific chain of bovine thyrotropin or of bovine luteinizing hormone. J Biol Chem 1971;246:2321-4.

4. Reichert LE. Biological studies on the relatedness of the subunits of human follicle stimulating hormone and chorionic gonadotropin. Endocrinology 1972;90:1119-22.

5. Williams JF, Davies TF, Catt KJ, Pierce JG. Receptor-binding activity of highly purified bovine luteinizing hormone and thyrotropin, and their subunits. Endocrinology 1980;106:1353-9.

6. Hunzicker-Dunn M, Birnbaumer L. The stimulation of adenylyl cyclase and cAMP-dependent protein kinases in luteinizing hormone actions. In: Ascoli M, ed. Luteinizing hormone action and receptors. Boca Raton, FL: CRC Press, 1985:57-134.

7. Pereira ME, Segaloff DL, Ascoli M, Eckstein F. Inhibition of choriogonadotropin-activated steroidogenesis in cultured Leydig tumor cells by the Rp diastereoisomer of adenosine 3',5'-cyclic phosphorothioate. J Biol Chem 1987; 262:6093-100.

8. Ascoli M, Pignataro OP, Segaloff DL. The inositol phosphate/diacylglycerol pathway in MA-10 Leydig tumor cells. Activation by arginine vasopressin and lack of effect of epidermal growth factor and human choriogonadotropin. J Biol Chem 1989;264:6674-81.

9. Reichert LE, Jr, Dattatreyamurty B. The follicle-stimulating hormone (FSH) receptor in testis: Interaction with FSH, mechanism of signal transduction, and properties of the purified receptor. Biol Reprod 1989;40:13-26.

10. Filetti S, Takai N, Rapoport B. Influence of cell density on desensitization of the thyroid cell cyclic adenosine 3',5'-monophosphate response to thyrotropin stimulation. Endocrinology 1981;109:1156-63.

11. Ascoli M, Segaloff DL. On the structure of the luteinizing hormone/chorionic gonadotropin receptor. Endocr Rev 1989;10:27-44.

12. Segaloff DL, Sprengel R, Nikolics K, Ascoli M. The structure of the lutropin/choriogonadotropin receptor. Recent Prog Horm Res 1990;46:261-303.

13. Rosemblit N, Ascoli M, Segaloff DL. Characterization of an antiserum to the rat luteal luteinizing hormone/chorionic gonadotropin receptor. Endocrinology 1988;123:2284-90.

14. McFarland KC, Sprengel R, Phillips HS, et al. Lutropin-choriogonadotropin receptor: An unusual member of the G protein-coupled receptor family. Science 1989;245:494-9.

15. Loosfelt H, Misrahi M, Atger M, et al. Cloning and sequencing of porcine LH-hCG receptor cDNA: Variants lacking transmembrane domain. Science 1989; 245:525-8.

16. Kim I-C, Ascoli M, Segaloff DL. Immunoprecipitation of the lutropin/choriogonadotropin receptor from biosynthetically labeled Leydig tumor cells: A 92-kDa glycoprotein. J Biol Chem 1987;262:470-7.

17. Caron MG. The guanine nucleotide regulatory protein-coupled receptors for nucleosides, nucleotides, amino acids and amine neurotransmitters. Curr Opin in Cell Biol 1989;1:159-66.

18. Ascoli M. Functions and regulation of cell surface receptors in cultured Leydig

tumor cells. In: Conn PM, ed. The receptors. Boca Raton, FL: Academic Press, 1985:368-400.

19. Ascoli M, Segaloff DL. Effects of collagenase on the structure of the lutropin/ choriogonadotropin receptor. J Biol Chem 1986;261:3807-15.

20. Rodriguez MC, Segaloff DL. The orientation of the LH/CG receptor as revealed by site-specific antibodies. Endocrinology 1990;127:674-81.

21. Xie YB, Wang H, Segaloff DL. The extracellular domain of the lutropin/ choriogonadotropin receptor expressed in transfected cells binds choriogonadotropin with high affinity. Submitted.

22. Strader CD, Sigal IS, Dixon RAF. Structural basis of β-adrenergic receptor function. FASEB J 1989;3:1825-32.

23. Wong SK-F, Slaughter C, Ruoho AE, Ross EM. The catecholamine binding site of the β-adrenergic receptor is formed by juxtaposed membrane-spanning domains. J Biol Chem 1988;263:7925-8.

24. Dohlman HG, Caron MG, Strader CD, Amlaiky N, Lefkowitz RJ. Identification and sequence of a binding site peptide of the β2-adrenergic receptor. Biochemistry 1988;27:1813-7.

25. Frielle T, Daniel KW, Caron MG, Lefkowitz RJ. Structural basis of β-adrenergic receptor subtype specificity studies with chimeric β1/β2-adrenergic receptors. Proc Natl Acad Sci USA 1988;85:9494-8.

26. O'Dowd BF, Hnatowich M, Regan FW, Leader WM, Caron MG, Lefkowitz RJ. Site-directed mutagenesis of the cytoplasmic domains of the human β2-adrenergic receptor: Localization of regions involved in G protein-receptor coupling. J Biol Chem 1988;263:15985-92.

27. Sprengel R, Braun T, Nikolics K, Segaloff DL, Seeburg PH. The testicular receptor for follicle stimulating hormone: Structure and functional expression of cloned cDNA. Mol Endocrinol 1990;4:525-30.

28. Frazier AL, Robbins LS, Stork PJ, Sprengel R, Segaloff DL, Cone RD. Isolation of TSH and LH/CG receptor cDNA's from human thyroid: Regulation by tissue specific splicing. Mol Endocrinol (in press).

29. Nagayami Y, Kaufman KD, Seto P, Rapoport B. Molecular cloning, sequence and functional expression of the cDNA for the human thyrotropin receptor. Biochem Biophys Res Commun 1989;165:1184-90.

30. Libert F, Lefort A, Gerard C, et al. Cloning, sequencing and expression of the human thyrotropin (TSH) receptor: Evidence for binding of autoantibodies. Biochem Biophys Res Commun 1989;165:1250-5.

31. Parmentier M, Libert F, Maenhaut C, et al. Molecular cloning of the thyrotropin receptor. Science 1989;246:1620-2.

2

Hormonal Regulation of Gonadotropin Gene Expression

J. LARRY JAMESON, THOMAS W.H. KAY, DEBRA S. DRUST,
LAIRD D. MADISON, AND CHRIS ALBANESE

The glycoprotein hormones include TSH, LH, FSH, and CG (1, 2). TSH is produced by the thyrotrope cells of the pituitary gland and stimulates the biosynthesis and secretion of thyroid hormone from the thyroid gland. LH and FSH are produced in the gonadotrope cells and stimulate gametogenesis and sex steroid production from the gonads. Chorionic gonadotropin (CG) is a placental hormone that is important for maintenance of the corpus luteum of pregnancy. The physiology of the pituitary glycoprotein hormones has been summarized in Figure 1.

TSH secretion is tightly regulated by the hypothalamic/pituitary/thyroid axis. Thyrotropin releasing hormone (TRH) stimulates TSH secretion, which, in turn, stimulates production of thyroid hormones from the thyroid gland. Thyroid hormones feedback at the level of the hypothalamus and the pituitary gland to suppress TSH secretion. Similarly, the gonadotropins are regulated as part of a hypothalamic/pituitary/gonadal axis. GnRH stimulates secretion of both LH and FSH. The gonadotropins are secreted in a pulsatile manner that reflects the pattern of GnRH secretion by the hypothalamus. Indeed, a number of elegant studies have demonstrated that pulsatile GnRH stimulation is necessary for gonadotropin secretion as continuous exposure to GnRH desensitizes the gonadotrope and results in suppressed gonadotropin levels (3). In the female, the gonadotropins stimulate follicular development and regulate ovulation and sex steroid production. In the male, the gonadotropins stimulate spermatogenesis and testosterone production. The recent discovery of the inhibins, activins, and follistatin provide an additional level of feedback control of FSH secretion.

Each of the glycoprotein hormones are heterodimers that are comprised of a common α-subunit and distinct β-subunits that confer biological specificity

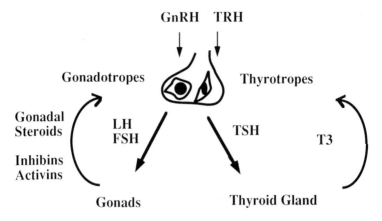

FIGURE 1. Hormonal regulation of the pituitary glycoprotein hormones.

(1). The α-subunit is encoded by a single gene located on chromosome 6. The β-subunit genes, although structurally similar, are located on separate chromosomes. The TSH β and FSH β genes are single copy genes located on chromosomes 3 and 11, respectively. In contrast, the LH β and CG β genes comprise a cluster located on chromosome 19. The LH β/CG β cluster consists of a single LH β and 6 copies of duplicated CG β genes or pseudo-genes.

The regulation of glycoprotein hormone gene expression has now been studied extensively (2). This family of hormone genes provides a useful model system for addressing a variety of aspects that are common to many other genes (Table 1). For example, because the glycoprotein hormones require heterodimers for biological activity, the α- and β-subunit genes must be coordinately expressed in response to both positive and negative hormonal stimuli. This feature of their physiology has led to the hypothesis that the α- and β-genes share common regulatory pathways that modulate tran-

TABLE 1. Features of glycoprotein hormone (GPH) gene expression.

α-Gene	β-Genes
Expressed in several pituitary and placental cell types	Expression is restricted to specific pituitary and placental cells
Coordinant expression with multiple β-genes	Coordinant expression with the α-gene
Responds to a wide array of physiological stimuli that encompasses all of the GPHs	Respond to physiological stimuli that are specific for a given GPH
Expressed ectopically in malignancy	Only CG β is expressed ectopically

scription and/or mRNA stability. Secondly, although the β-subunit genes are structurally similar, they exhibit cell-specific expression and distinct patterns of responses to hormonal stimulation, consistent with their different physiological functions. The α-gene, being common to each of the glycoprotein hormones, is of particular interest for analyses of hormonal regulation in that it must respond to a variety of different hormonal signals. This chapter reviews our studies of transcriptional regulation of the α-gene and characterization of some of the transcription factors that interact with the α-gene promoter. We also describe our preliminary characterization of positive regulatory elements in the α-gene that respond to GnRH and TRH, as well as negative regulatory elements in the α-gene that mediate repression by thyroid hormone.

Delineation of a cAMP Response Element in the α-Gene Promoter

The α-gene is expressed in the placenta in conjunction with the CG β-subunit to produce chorionic gonadotropin. Several trophoblastic placental cell lines that allow detailed analyses of CG biosynthesis and secretion are available. Early studies demonstrated that CG secretion was markedly stimulated in placental cell lines by treatment with derivatives of cAMP. Subsequently, several groups demonstrated that the effects of cAMP were mediated largely at the level of biosynthesis, including transcriptional stimulation of the α- and CG β-genes and subsequent elevation of mRNA levels (4, 5). The cloning of the α-gene and the development of transient expression assays using heterologous reporter genes, such as CAT, provided an opportunity to map the DNA sequences involved in cAMP stimulation (4, 6). Deletion mutants of the α-gene promoter localized the cAMP-responsive region to an area approximately 150 base pairs upstream from the start of transcription (6–9). Inspection of this area revealed an 18-bp repeated sequence that contained the palindrome, TGACGTCA.

The functional properties of this palindromic cAMP response element (CRE) sequence have now been characterized in detail. Insertion of the CRE upstream of heterologous sequences, such as the TK promoter or the SV40 promoter, demonstrated that it functions as an enhancer element that is orientation and relatively distance independent (7–10). Similar DNA sequences have been defined in other cAMP-responsive genes, and it is now apparent that the TGACGTCA palindrome represents a consensus sequence for cAMP responsiveness (11). To investigate the DNA sequence determinants for cAMP responsiveness, we used oligonucleotide cassettes to perform detailed mutagenesis of the CRE (10, 12). These studies demonstrated that essentially all mutations within the palindromic sequence greatly reduced basal activity and most mutations substantially decreased the degree of cAMP responsiveness as well. A somewhat surprising finding in these studies was the observation that a variety of mutations adjacent to the palindrome also had profound effects on the function of the CRE. These effects of DNA context are likely to be physiologically relevant by restricting or activating CREs or CRE-like elements in specific genes. As described below, it is now apparent that the transcription factors that interact with the CRE comprise a large family, and it is possible that adjacent DNA sequences provide an additional measure of specificity for protein binding.

In addition to its function as a cAMP-stimulated element, the CRE functions as an important basal regulatory element and also exerts some degree of cell-specific expression. For example, the CRE functions optimally when linked to the native α-promoter and when expressed in placental cells, as opposed to other cell types such as fibroblasts (7, 9, 13). It is also noteworthy that the CRE in the human gene differs by a single nucleotide from the homologous sequence in the rat, mouse, and bovine genes. This single base mutation has been suggested as a possible basis for the fact that the α-gene is expressed in the placenta in humans, but not in these other species. In support of this model, Bokar et al. (14) have demonstrated that the palindromic CRE sequence that is found in the human gene confers placental specific expression in transgenic mice, whereas the sequence observed in other mammals restricts expression to the pituitary gland. Thus, the CRE functions as a regulatory element that confers cell-specific expression, basal expression, and cAMP stimulation.

Characterization of CRE Binding Proteins

DNA regulatory sequences in general correspond to target sequences for transcription factors. Using DNase I footprinting studies, the CRE of the α-gene has been demonstrated to interact with nuclear proteins extracted from a variety of different cell lines (Fig. 2) (9, 13).

The DNA binding properties of the CRE binding protein (CREB) have been analyzed in greater detail using gel mobility shift assays. Mutations that alter CREB binding to the CRE correlate well with mutations that alter CRE function in transient expression assays (10, 12, 15). The CREB is relatively abundant and is remarkably resilient to denaturation. For example, extracts that have been heated retain CREB binding (15). Furthermore, the CREB is readily detected in so-called Southwestern blots, in which nuclear proteins are transferred from SDS gels to nitrocellulose filters and subsequently hybridized with radiolabeled CRE probes (16). This latter feature made the CREB an ideal candidate for expression cloning in which placental λgt 11 libraries were screened with the radiolabeled CRE sequence (16). The previ-

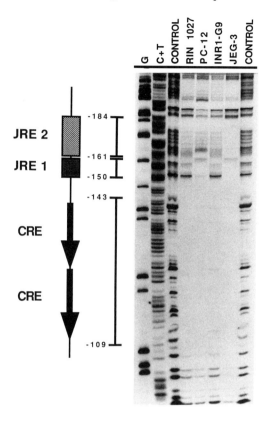

FIGURE 2. DNase I protection of the α-gene promoter by proteins extracted from different cell types. Cell lines from which nuclear extracts were obtained are shown at the top of the figure and include islet cell lines (RIN 1027, INR1-G9), an adrenal medullary cell line (PC-12), and a choriocarcinoma cell line (JEG-3). (From Jameson JL, Powers AC, Gallagher GD, Habener JF, Enhancer and promoter element interactions dictate cyclic AMP-mediated and cell-specific expression of the glycoprotein hormone α-gene, Mol Endocrinol 1989;3:763–72.)

ous mutagenesis studies were particularly valuable in this endeavor since the isolated clone was demonstrated to bind to functional CRE sequences, but not to a variety of sequences that included mutations either within the palindrome or in the adjacent bases that altered the CRE context. The cloning of CREB revealed it to be a 43-kDa protein that contains a carboxyterminal leucine zipper structure that is adjacent to a basic region involved in DNA binding (Fig. 3).

The leucine zipper motif in CREB resembles that found in a variety of other transcription factors including ATF, jun, fos, and C/EBP. As initially postulated by McKnight and colleagues (17), the leucine zipper is thought to

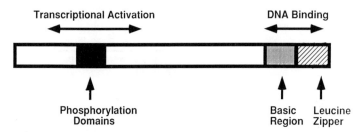

FIGURE 3. Schematic illustration of the structure of CREB.

be involved in the formation of homodimers and heterodimers of various transcription factors. The N-terminal portion of CREB contains a relatively acidic region that contains a number of potential phosphoacceptor sites. Recent studies by the laboratories of Habener (unpublished data) and Montminy (18) have demonstrated the presence of a protein kinase A site in CREB that modulates the transcriptional response to cAMP. It is now recognized that CREB is a member of a large family of related transcription factors that includes the ATF factors that interact with the adenovirus promoter among many others. Some of the features of this rapidly evolving family have been summarized in Table 2, but detailed analyses remain to be performed.

Upstream Regulatory Elements

Although the CREs are critical for α-gene transcription, deletion studies have demonstrated the importance of upstream DNA sequences for maximal expression (9, 19, 20). DNase I footprinting studies initially demonstrated a footprinted region adjacent to the CRE between −183 and −150 bp in the α-promoter (Fig. 2). Delegeane and colleagues (9) demonstrated that this upstream regulatory element (URE) footprint was relatively restricted to placental cells. The URE has somewhat unusual properties in that it is nonfunctional when studied in isolation, but when coupled to the CRE, it enhances expression approximately 10-fold (9, 13). Using a combination of gel mobility shift assays and methylation interference studies to delineate the protein contact regions within the URE, this area has been shown to interact with distinct proteins that bind in a mutually exclusive manner, suggesting that it is comprised of at least two overlapping protein-binding domains (20). Nevertheless, each of the URE binding proteins can activate CRE-mediated expression, providing an additional level of diversity for α-gene expression. The URE proteins have not been further characterized or cloned. Moreover,

TABLE 2. Family of CRE binding proteins.

Name	DNA Binding Site	M_r (kDa)	Signal Response	Dimer Properties	References
CREB 1 (327 aa)	TGACGTCA	38	+cAMP	Homodimer	Hoeffler et al., Science 1988;242:1430
CREB 1 (341 aa)	TGACGTCA	43	+cAMP	Homodimer	Gonzales et al., Nature 1989;337:749
CREB 2 (351 aa)	TGACGTCA		−cAMP	Homodimer	Leiden et al., Clin Res 1990;465A
				CREB 1:CREB 2	
CREBP 1 (HB16) (ATF 2)	TGACGTCA	55–63	?cAMP	Homodimer	Maekawa et al., EMBO J 1989;8:2023
				Jun-CREBP 1	Kara et al., MCB 1990;10:1347
CREBP 2 (mXBP)	TGACGTCA	45	?cAMP	Homodimer	Ivashkiv et al., MCB 1990;10:1609
				Jun-CREBP 2	
ATF 1,2,3,4,7	TGACGTCA			Homodimers	Hai et al., Genes Dev 1989;3:2083
				ATF 2-ATF 3	
ATF 5 (c-fos), 6	CRE Trimer				Hai et al., Genes Dev 1989;3:2083
ATF 8	TGA-GTCA				Hai et al., Genes Dev 1989;3:2083
120 kDa	TGACGTCA	120	?cAMP		Andrisani et al., JBC 1990;265:3212
Jun	TGA-GTCA	39	+TPA	Jun-Jun	Bohmann et al., Science 1988;238:1386
				Jun-Fos	
Jun B	TGA-GTCA		−TPA		Ryder et al., PNAS 1988:85:1487
Jun D	TGA-GTCA				Nakabeppu et al., Cell 1988;55:907
					Hirai et al., EMBO J 1989;8:1433
Fos	TGA-GTCA	55	+TPA	Jun-Fos	Chiu et al., Cell 1988;54:541
Fos B	TGA-GTCA				Zerial et al., EMBO J 1989;8:805
Fra 1	TGA-GTCA				Cohen et al., Genes Dev 1989;3:173

there are additional regulatory elements upstream of –183 bp that have yet to be characterized in the α-promoter.

Downstream Promoter Elements and Combinatorial Regulation

As mentioned above, the enhancer elements in the upstream region of the α-promoter function optimally when coupled to the α-promoter as opposed to heterologous promoters, such as TK or SV40. These experiments have led to the concept that the upstream and downstream region of the α-promoter interact to provide cell-specific expression (7, 13). The transcription factors that interact with the proximal region of the α-promoter have not been characterized in detail. However, a CAAT box binding region has been identified by DNase I footprinting (9) and gel mobility shift studies (19). Recently, Kennedy et al. (21) provided evidence that the protein that interacts with this CAAT binding region may be relatively specific for the α-promoter. Future studies of the proximal promoter region will be important to further delineate interactions with upstream enhancer elements.

Transcriptional Regulation by GnRH and TRH

The absence of cell lines that produce TSH or gonadotropins has greatly limited studies of pituitary glycoprotein hormone gene expression. However, we have recently adapted transfection procedures to allow transient expression assays in primary cultures of pituitary cells (22). Using the sensitive reporter enzyme luciferase, we demonstrated that the α-promoter directs specific expression in gonadotropes and thyrotropes as assessed by double labeled immunofluorescence. When transfected into rat pituitary cells, α-LUC expression was stimulated by treatment with either GnRH or TRH (22). These results suggest that the hypothalamic releasing hormones exert their effects, in part, at the transcriptional level. Although this system is limited by transfection efficiency, it has allowed preliminary mapping of GnRH response elements in the α-promoter upstream of the UREs and CREs.

For studies of TRH regulation of α-promoter activity, we have employed GH3 cells that contain TRH receptors and express the α-promoter at levels that can be readily measured. Similar to the studies with GnRH, TRH responsiveness appears to reside in multiple areas of the α-promoter upstream of the CREs. These experiments suggest that the signal transduction pathways by GnRH and TRH in the pituitary gland may converge on transcription factors that are distinct from CREB and involve a novel class of transcription factors that interact with the upstream portion of the α-gene.

Negative Regulation of the α-Gene by the T3 and Glucocorticoid Receptors

In addition to its positive regulation by GnRH, TRH, and cAMP, the α-gene is also subject to negative regulation by hormones that are produced by the thyroid gland and gonads. Thyroid hormone has been demonstrated to suppress TSH α- and β-gene expression at the transcriptional level (23), and these effects are direct in that they do not require on-going protein synthesis. The model has been put forth that T3 interacts with its nuclear thyroid hormone receptor that subsequently binds to the promoter to directly repress gene transcription. The recent cloning of the thyroid hormone receptor has allowed this model to be tested. We used a receptor deficient cell line (JEG-3) to demonstrate that thyroid hormone suppressed transcription of the α-gene and that the repression required both hormone and co-expression of thyroid hormone receptors (24). Mutations in the DNA binding domain of the T3 receptor prevented negative regulation consistent with the model that the T3 receptor must bind to DNA sequences in the α-gene to repress transcription. Deletion studies of the α-promoter localized the putative negative thyroid hormone response element (nTRE) to a proximal region of the promoter between −100 and +1. Because the levels of expression were relatively low with additional deletion mutants, the nTRE was localized further using binding studies of the T3 receptor to α-promoter DNA sequences. The receptor was shown to bind to a specific DNA sequence between −22 and −7 bp (Fig. 4). This receptor binding region is located between the TATA box and the transcriptional initiation site. These studies suggest a model for negative regulation in which the activated thyroid hormone receptor interacts with the α-promoter near the site of transcription initiation and thereby interferes with transcription. Studies are currently on-going to examine this hypothesis further.

Unlike the CRE consensus sequence, which is highly conserved in different genes and exhibits stringent DNA sequence determinants for CREB

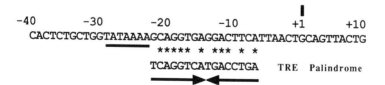

FIGURE 4. Schematic illustration of the nTRE sequence in the α-promoter. (From Chatterjee VKK, Lee JK, Rentoumis A, Jameson JL, Negative regulation of the thyroid-stimulating hormone α gene by thyroid hormone: Receptor interaction adjacent to the TATA box, Proc Natl Acad Sci USA 1989;86:9114–8.)

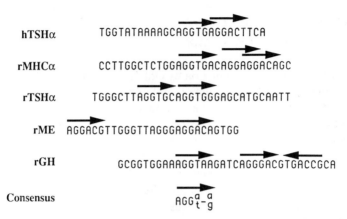

FIGURE 5. T3 response elements (TREs) from different genes. (Key: hTSH α = human glycoprotein hormone [TSH] α-gene; rMHC α = rat α-myosin heavy-chain gene; rTSH α = rat glycoprotein hormone [TSH] α-gene; rME = rat malic enzyme gene; and rGH = rat growth hormone gene.)

binding, the target DNA sequences for thyroid receptor action are surprisingly variable. TRE elements from a variety of T3 responsive genes are compared in Figure 5. It is apparent that each TRE is slightly different, and attempts to derive a consensus sequence are difficult. This variability in naturally occurring TREs is also reflected in relatively promiscuous binding of the T3 receptor to DNA elements that are not thought to mediate T3 regulation. One of the challenges for future studies is to better understand the mechanisms that confer specific T3 receptor action.

Akerblom et al. (25) have described glucocorticoid mediated repression of α-promoter activity. In this instance, glucocorticoid-mediated repression maps to the CRE region of the α-promoter, leading to the suggestion that the glucocorticoid receptor represses transcription by blocking the access of CREB to the CRE. Thus, feedback regulation by steroid and thyroid hormones may involve interference with positive transcription factors. Although appealing in concept, this mechanism for transcriptional repression remains to be examined in detail.

At this stage, the α-promoter represents a well-characterized model system for studies of cell-specific expression and hormonal regulation by a variety of signals including GnRH, TRH, and cAMP, as well as transcriptional repression by steroid and thyroid hormone receptors (Fig. 6). From these studies, it is apparent that transcriptional regulation represents complex pathways that involve multiple interacting transcription factors that can be activated by distinct cellular signaling pathways. These studies of the α-promoter provide an invaluable road map for more detailed analyses of specific DNA regulatory

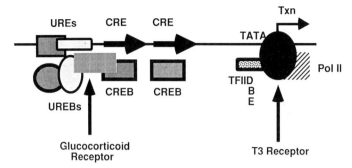

FIGURE 6. Summary of the regulatory elements and transcription factors that interact with the human glycoprotein hormone α-gene.

elements and transcription factors. It is likely that the transcription factors identified to date may in reality comprise families of proteins that will recognize specific promoters and will differ in various cell types.

References

1. Pierce JG, Parsons TF. Glycoprotein hormones: Structure and function. Annu Rev Biochem 1981;50:465-95.
2. Gharib SD, Wierman ME, Shupnik MA, Chin WW. Molecular biology of the pituitary gonadotropins. Endocr Rev 1990;11:177-99.
3. Belchetz P, Plant T, Hakai Y, Keough E, Knobil E. Hypophysial responses to continuous and intermittent delivery of hypothalamic gonadotropin releasing hormone. Science 1978;202:631-3.
4. Jameson JL, Jaffe RC, Gleason SL, Habener JF. Transcriptional regulation of chorionic gonadotropin α- and β-subunit gene expression by 8-bromo-adenosine 3', 5'-monophosphate. Endocrinology 1986;119:2560-7.
5. Milsted A, Cox RP, Nilson JH. Cyclic AMP regulates transcription of the genes encoding human chorionic gonadotropin with different kinetics. DNA 1987; 6:213-9.
6. Darnell RB, Boime I. Differential expression of the human gonadotropin α gene in ectopic and eutopic cells. Mol Cell Biol 1985;5:3157-67.
7. Deutsch PJ, Jameson JL, Habener JF. Cyclic AMP responsiveness of human gonadotropin-α gene transcription is directed by a repeated 18 base pair enhancer: α-promoter receptivity to the enhancer confers cell-preferential expression. J Biol Chem 1987;262:12169-74.
8. Silver BJ, Bokar JA, Virgin JB, Vallen EA, Milsted A, Nilson JH. Cyclic AMP regulation of the human glycoprotein hormone alpha-subunit gene is mediated by an 18-base-pair element. Proc Natl Acad Sci USA 1987;84:2198-202.
9. Delegeane AM, Ferland LH, Mellon PL. Tissue-specific enhancer of the human glycoprotein hormone alpha-subunit gene: Dependence on cyclic AMP-inducible elements. Mol Cell Biol 1987;7:3994-4002.

10. Deutsch PJ, Hoeffler JP, Jameson JL, Lin JC, Habener JF. Structural determinants for transcriptional activation by cAMP-responsive DNA elements. J Biol Chem 1988;263:18466-72.
11. Roesler WJ, Vandenbark GR, Hanson RW. Cyclic AMP and the induction of eukaryotic gene transcription. J Biol Chem 1988;263:9063-6.
12. Deutsch PJ, Hoeffler JP, Jameson JL, Habener JF. Cyclic AMP and phorbol ester-stimulated transcription mediated by similar DNA elements that bind distinct proteins. Proc Natl Acad Sci USA 1988;85:7922-6.
13. Jameson JL, Powers AC, Gallagher GD, Habener JF. Enhancer and promoter element interactions dictate cyclic AMP-mediated and cell-specific expression of the glycoprotein hormone α-gene. Mol Endocrinol 1989;3:763-72.
14. Bokar JA, Keri RA, Farmerie TA, et al. Expression of the glycoprotein hormone alpha-subunit gene in the placenta requires a functional cyclic AMP response element, whereas a different cis-acting element mediates pituitary-specific expression. Mol Cell Biol 1989;9:5113-22.
15. Bokar JA, Roesler WJ, Vandenbark GR, Kaetzel DM, Hanson RW, Nilson JH. Characterization of the cAMP responsive elements from the genes from the α subunit of glycoprotein hormones and phosphoenolpyruvate carboxykinase (GTP): Conserved features of nuclear protein binding between tissues and species. J Biol Chem 1988;263:19740-47.
16. Hoeffler JP, Meyer TE, Yun Y, Jameson JL, Habener JF. Cyclic AMP-responsive DNA-binding protein: Structure based on a cloned placental cDNA. Science 1988;242:1430-3.
17. Landschultz WH, Johnson PF, McKnight SL. The leucine zipper: A hypothetical structure common to a new class of DNA binding proteins. Science 1988;240:1759-64.
18. Gonzales GA, Montminy MR. Cyclic AMP stimulates somatostatin gene transcription by phosphorylation of CREB at serine 133. Cell 1989;59:675-80.
19. Jameson JL, Jaffe RC, Deutsch PJ, Albanese C, Habener JF. The gonadotropin α-gene contains multiple protein binding domains that interact to modulate basal and cAMP-responsive transcription. J Biol Chem 1988;263:9879-86.
20. Jameson JL, Albanese C, Habener JF. Adjacent but distinct protein binding domains in the glycoprotein hormone α gene interact independently with a cAMP-responsive enhancer. J Biol Chem 1989;264:16190-6.
21. Kennedy GC, Andersen B, Nilson JH. The human alpha subunit glycoprotein hormone gene utilizes a unique CCAAT binding factor. J Biol Chem 1990; 265:6279-85.
22. Burrin JM, Jameson JL. Regulation of transfected glycoprotein hormone α gene expression in primary pituitary cell cultures. Mol Endocrinol 1989;3:1643-51.
23. Shupnik MA, Ridgway EC. Thyroid hormone control of thyrotropin gene expression in rat anterior pituitary cells. Endocrinology 1987;121:619-24.
24. Chatterjee VKK, Lee JK, Rentoumis A, Jameson JL. Negative regulation of the thyroid-stimulating hormone α gene by thyroid hormone: Receptor interaction adjacent to the TATA box. Proc Natl Acad Sci USA 1989;86:9114-8.
25. Akerblom IE, Slater EP, Beato M, Baxter JD, Mellon PL. Negative regulation by glucocorticoids through interference with a cAMP responsive enhancer. Science 1988;241:350-3.

3

Inositol Lipid Metabolism and Calcium Signaling in Rat Ovarian Cells

MARIE R. RODWAY AND PETER C.K. LEUNG

Steroidogenesis in the ovary is controlled by multiple endocrine, paracrine, and autocrine regulatory factors. Endocrine stimulation by the gonadotropins, luteinizing hormone (LH), and follicle stimulating hormone (FSH) is transduced through activation of adenylate cyclase and generation of cyclic adenosine monophosphate (cAMP) (1, for review). Cyclic AMP may bind to A-kinase, cause cleavage of the catalytic and regulatory subunits, and together with the regulatory subunit, interact with DNA at transcription enhancer sequences; or activated A-kinase may phosphorylate transacting factors that subsequently interact with transcription enhancer sequences; or cAMP may have direct actions at the post-translational level (2).

The recent discovery that hormones effective in the ovary also use products of polyphosphoinositide breakdown as second messengers (3–16) makes mechanistic studies of effects of one hormone on the action of another possible. Gonadotropin releasing hormone (GnRH) and prostaglandin $F_{2\alpha}$ ($PGF_{2\alpha}$) are believed to act principally as modulators of gonadotropin action in the ovary, although they also have direct effects on steroid hormone production.

This chapter includes a brief discussion of components of the phosphoinositide second messenger system and a discussion of agents that are believed to exert their effects through activation of this pathway in rat ovarian cells.

Transduction of Information Through PIP_2 Breakdown

Agonist binding to the G-protein-linked receptor induces activation of phosphoinositide/phospholipase C (PLC), which hydrolyses phosphatidyl inositol 4,5-bisphosphate (PIP_2) into diacylglycerol (DG) and inositol phosphates, including inositol 1,4,5-trisphosphate (IP_3) (17). At least 7 PLC isoenzymes with different tissue distribution and calcium sensitivity have been purified and characterized. Multiple PLC isoenzymes have been found in each tissue studied (18).

DG activates protein kinase C (PKC). Subspecies of PKC that have been found are different in mode of activation, sensitivity to calcium, catalytic activity towards endogenous substrates, cell type distribution, and intracellular location (19). PKC has been found in rat ovarian tissues (20). After activation, PKC phosphorylates and activates proteins (19). One of the proteins found to be phosphorylated by PKC may be SCP_2, which is a sterol carrier responsible for transportation of cholesterol to the inner mitochondrial membrane (21).

DG can be phosphorylated to phosphatidic acid (PA) with subsequent production of arachidonic acid (AA), or it can be hydrolysed to monoacylglycerol, which is subsequently hydrolysed to release AA. AA may also be produced from the direct action of phospholipase A_2 (PLA_2) on phospholipids (22). AA is the precursor for synthesis of eicosanoids such as leukotrienes, through the lipoxygenase pathway, and the thromboxanes and prostaglandins, through the cyclooxygenase pathway. Eicosanoids can in turn act as paracrine or autocrine agents (23).

At least 20 IP have been found; however, at present there is clear evidence of a second messenger role only for IP_3 and inositol 1,3,4,5-tetraphosphate (IP_4). IP_3 and IP_4 can increase $[Ca^{++}]_i$, either by releasing calcium from intracellular stores or by increasing uptake of calcium from the extracellular space. The primary site of action of IP_3 has been identified as intracellular calcium stores. The endoplasmic reticulum is more likely than the mitochondria to be the site of IP_3 releasable calcium stores. However, recent evidence suggests distinct organelles (calciosomes) may be the site of IP_3 releasable calcium (17, for review). IP_3 may also cause calcium entry into the cell at the plasma membrane. IP_4 may have a role in the movement of calcium at the plasma membrane and at internal calcium stores (17).

Hormones that Induce PIP_2 Breakdown in the Ovary

GnRH

The classic role of GnRH is as a regulator of LH/FSH release at the pituitary. However, it has been known for some time that GnRH also has direct actions at the gonadal level (24, for review). FSH promotes steroidogenesis and maturation of the granulosa cell. Prolactin, insulin, testosterone, and estrogen modulate this process. GnRH inhibits this maturation by inhibiting FSH-stimulated estrogen and progestin production, apparently through an effect on steroidogenic enzymes (aromatase, side-chain cleavage, 3β-HSD, and

20α-HSD) as well as by suppression of cAMP formation and stimulation of cAMP breakdown (25).

Although the major effect of GnRH in primary cultures of granulosa cells is suppression of FSH-stimulated steroidogenesis and, therefore, maturation of the granulosa cell, GnRH alone has multiple effects on cells in culture. GnRH stimulates progesterone, pregnenolone, 20α-OH-progesterone, estradiol, and prostaglandin production; lactate formation and plasminogen activator activity is also enhanced by GnRH (24).

GnRH action in the ovary is believed to be mediated by increased inositol lipid metabolism (3, 4, 10, 15). GnRH has been shown to enhance PA/phosphatidyl inositol turnover in cultured rat granulosa (3, 4, 13, 14) and luteal (10) cells. The ED_{50} in luteal cells corresponds with the potency of GnRH to inhibit LH/hCG induced cAMP and progesterone accumulation (12).

Increased production of inositol 4-phosphate (IP), inositol 1,4-bisphosphate (IP_2), and IP_3 in concert with increased PIP_2 breakdown has been demonstrated in response to GnRH in rat ovarian cells (9, 14). The accumulation of InsP was concentration dependent and could be prevented by a GnRH antagonist. PIP_2 breakdown also produces DG, which is the physiological activator of PKC. GnRH stimulates production of DG in GnRH treated granulosa cells (9). Activation of PKC is believed to be at least partially responsible for the actions of GnRH in ovarian cells (12). Inhibitors of PKC, such as H-7, have been used to investigate the role of PKC in GnRH action. The stimulatory effect of GnRH on progesterone production after 5 h of treatment was reduced by 60% (26) when H-7 was present.

The activation of PKC induced by GnRH in the ovary has been investigated by using phorbol esters such as 12-O-tetradecanoylphorbol-13-acetate (TPA) and permeant diacylglycerols, such as dioctanylglycerol, 1-oleoyl-2-acetoyl-sn-3-glycerol, and 1-oleoyl-2-acetylglycerol, which activate PKC directly (19, 27). TPA, similar to GnRH, increased progesterone accumulation by approximately 2.5-fold; there was no synergistic or additive effect of TPA on GnRH-stimulated progesterone accumulation (26, 28–30). During short-term incubations (30 min), no effect of phorbol esters or permeant diacylglycerols was seen on progesterone synthesis stimulated by gonadotropins (31). In longer cultures of rat granulosa cells (up to 24 h), GnRH inhibited FSH-stimulated progesterone production (32). TPA inhibited progesterone production stimulated by LH, FSH, cholera toxin, 8-bromo-cAMP, and dibutyrl cAMP (28, 32, 33) with or without 1-methyl-3-isobutyl-xanthine, which blocked phosphodiesterase (34). The ability of TPA to attenuate FSH-stimulated progesterone production at shorter time points (5 h) may have been due to the concentration of TPA used (34). Although TPA is believed to mimic the DG activation of PKC, a recent report has shown that TPA and DG have distinctly different effects on progestin formation (27). If this is the case, then inhibition of progestin formation by GnRH may

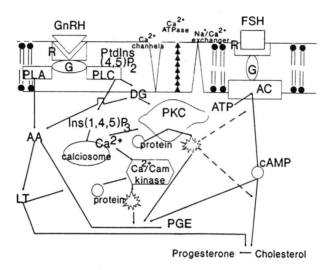

FIGURE 1. Generation of some of the second messengers in rat ovarian cells. GnRH and FSH bind to cell surface receptors (R), which cause production of second messengers. FSH activates adenylate cyclase (AC), which produces cAMP from ATP. GnRH induces formation of diacylglycerol (DG) and IP_3 by the activation of G-protein (G) bound phosphoinositide/phospholipase C (PLC). GnRH may also activate phospholipase A_2 (PLA) and produce phosphatidic acid, from which AA may be generated. DG activates protein kinase C (PKC), which phosphorylates and activates proteins. DG can also be metabolized to AA. AA is the precursor of leukotrienes (LT), prostaglandins, and other metabolites. IP_3 binds to receptors and releases calcium from intracellular stores such as calciosomes on the endoplasmic reticulum. Increased $[Ca^{++}]_i$ activates calcium/calmodulin (Ca^{++}/Cam)-dependent protein kinase, which also phosphorylates and activates proteins. Calcium movement at the plasma membrane may occur via calcium ATPase, the sodium/calcium exchanger or calcium channels (voltage or receptor activated). Activated PKC inhibits the formation of cAMP and the production of progesterone from cAMP. Activated PKC, increased $[Ca^{++}]_i$, AA, and cAMP all stimulate the production of prostaglandin E (PGE). (Solid lines indicate stimulation of production; broken lines indicate inhibition of production.)

be the result of the action of another second messenger, such as calcium, which is known to attenuate gonadotropin-stimulated progesterone production (see Fig. 1).

TPA did not affect basal or LH-stimulated cAMP accumulation for up to 5 h, which was identical to the results obtained using a GnRH agonist in the same experiments (28). However, after day 2 of culture, TPA inhibited a FSH-induced increase in cAMP (35, 36) as did GnRH (37–39). TPA may directly affect steroidogenic enzyme activity. Stimulation (33) or inhibition of 3β-HSD activity has been seen (40, 41). TPA stimulated (33), inhibited

(42), or had no effect on 20α-HSD activity (41). GnRH and TPA both inhibited maturation responses, such as cellular aggregation and expression of LH receptors. GnRH and TPA both blocked FSH inhibition of the synthesis of adherens junction proteins, vinculin, α-actinin, and actin (43). TPA and GnRH increased PGE accumulation but were not additive (29, 30, 32). Both increased PG synthase activity (TPA by half as much as GnRH agonist) (29). The effect of TPA on PGE_2 production was additive with LH or FSH (28, 30, 32). Based on the similarity between the effects of TPA and GnRH on granulosa cell function, we conclude that some of the actions of GnRH result from the production of DG and its activation of PKC.

Calcium is also believed to be important in GnRH activity. Intracellular calcium has been measured by Quin-2 fluorescence in suspensions of rat granulosa cells (9). GnRH caused a 2-fold increase in $[Ca^{++}]_i$ as compared with resting concentrations. Fura-2, a calcium sensitive fluorescent indicator has also been used to show a GnRH alteration in intracellular free calcium levels in individual rat granulosa cells (44). Five-fold changes in intracellular free calcium were measured within 20 sec of administration of GnRH using Fura-2 microspectrofluorimetry. This alteration in intracellular free calcium was transient (hormone was washed away from the cells within about 15 sec) and returned to baseline levels after about 80 sec. The specificity of this increase in $[Ca^{++}]_i$ has been verified by using a specific GnRH blocker (44). Experiments with a low calcium perifusion buffer suggested that the immediate source of the $[Ca^{++}]_i$ was intracellular stores. High concentrations (up to 10^{-5}M) of blockers of L-type calcium channels, verapamil, nifedipine, and diltiazem failed to affect the $[Ca^{++}]_i$ response to GnRH (45). Extracellular calcium may be required for the inhibitory effect of GnRH on LH-stimulated cAMP, progesterone, and PGE_2 production. However, reduced extracellular calcium also decreased isoproterenol-induced cAMP production, suggesting that the decreased production of progesterone occurs even in the absence of agents believed to use calcium as a second messenger (39).

The effect of increased concentration of $[Ca^{++}]_i$ was investigated using the calcium ionophore, A23187. Calcium ionophores increased basal progesterone production, as did phorbol esters and GnRH (26, 28, 34). Calcium ionophores did not have additive effects with GnRH- or TPA-stimulated progesterone production (29, 32). FSH-, 8-bromo-cAMP-, or cholera toxin-stimulated progesterone production was attenuated by A23187, with and without 1-methyl-3-isobutylxanthine in rat granulosa cells (26, 32, 34). This effect was similar to the effect of GnRH on gonadotropin-stimulated progesterone production (24). However, A23187 had no further effect on TPA inhibition of progesterone production stimulated by LH, cholera toxin, or dibutyrl cAMP (33, 34). A23187 apparently has the same effects as TPA on progesterone production. The mechanism by which A23187 has its effects on inhibition of gonadotropin-stimulated progesterone production is not clear.

However, high amounts of calcium can activate PKC in the absence of DG (22). Calcium may have distinct effectors for the enhancement of progesterone and PGE production because A23187 synergises with TPA or GnRHa in the production of PGE, but not progesterone (29).

The stimulatory effect of GnRH on progesterone production may be mediated by AA in the rat ovary (46–50). Administration of exogenous AA increased progesterone production (48, 51, 52), and GnRH, TPA, or A23187 increased AA release from rat granulosa cells (29, 48). The concentration of TPA required was high (over 10^{-6}M) but A23187 was effective at much lower concentrations (10^{-8}M) (47), suggesting that increased $[Ca^{++}]_i$ leads to increased AA production. TPA or A23187 had additive effects with GnRH on AA production (29, 48). Progesterone production in the presence of AA with TPA was greater than either agent alone (48). The PLA_2 activator, melittin, which increases AA production, stimulated progesterone production by rat granulosa cells (30, 32). Additional support for the involvement of AA production in the stimulatory effect of GnRH on progesterone production came from the inhibition of GnRH stimulation of progesterone production with nordihydroguaiaretic acid, which blocked formation of lipoxygenase metabolites of AA (48, 50). The GnRH stimulation of progesterone production was not blocked by indomethacin, a blocker of the cyclooxygenase pathway. Treatment of rat granulosa cells with lipoxygenase metabolites of AA resulted in stimulation of progesterone production (50). AA partially reversed the inhibition of FSH-stimulated progesterone caused by GnRH or TPA, in short- but not in long-term incubations (49). GnRH-stimulated PGE_2 production may also be dependent on production of AA and its metabolites (50). Lipoxygenase metabolites of AA stimulated production of progesterone and PGE_2 in cultured rat granulosa cells; TPA-stimulated production of PGE_2 was stimulated further by AA metabolites (49).

Thus, the actions of GnRH in rat ovarian cells are complex. The inhibition of gonadotropin-stimulated cAMP and progesterone production may involve PIP_2 breakdown and subsequent increases in $[Ca^{++}]_i$ and PKC activation. Stimulation of progesterone and PGE_2 production by GnRH appears to be mediated in part by AA and its metabolites.

$PGF_{2\alpha}$

Prostaglandins are produced in theca, interstitial, and granulosa cells of rat ovaries (53), and $PGF_{2\alpha}$ receptors are found in rat corpus luteum (54, 55). $PGF_{2\alpha}$ may play a role in regression of luteal cells and atresia in granulosa cells (56). Prostaglandins can regulate the secretory capability of granulosa cells (25, 56).

$PGF_{2\alpha}$ may cause luteolysis by inhibiting LH-induced cAMP and progesterone production (57). Rather than stimulating the degradation of cAMP,

$PGF_{2\alpha}$ inhibited production (58). The effect of $PGF_{2\alpha}$ was presumably not at the level of the LH receptor, because similar effects of $PGF_{2\alpha}$ have been seen on cAMP generation stimulated by treatment with isoproterenol and sodium fluoride (59, 60). Inhibition of cAMP production by $PGF_{2\alpha}$ is also not a result of direct inhibition of adenylate cyclase activity in membranes or homogenates prepared from corpus luteum of rats (61, 62). Therefore, this inhibition is probably mediated by production of second messengers that inhibit adenylate cyclase. Progesterone content of the corpus luteum is decreased by a reduction in the supply of precursors and stimulation of metabolism of progesterone. A decreased supply of precursors, caused by decreased cholesterol ester synthesis and decreased tissue content of cholesterol ester, occurs in ovaries of gonadotropin-stimulated immature rats that have been treated with $PGF_{2\alpha}$ (63). The sensitivity of the corpus luteum to the luteolytic effects of $PGF_{2\alpha}$ increased as the corpus luteum aged (59).

The question of how $PGF_{2\alpha}$ exerts its luteolytic effect has not been answered conclusively. However, there is evidence that $PGF_{2\alpha}$ uses $PtdIns(4,5)P_2$ breakdown as a transducing mechanism in rat luteal and granulosa cells (12, 64).

In rat granulosa cells, $PGF_{2\alpha}$ rapidly stimulated ^{32}P incorporation into phosphatidic acid and phosphatidylinositol (11, 13). Concentrations that inhibit LH-induced progesterone secretion in luteal cells markedly increased labeling of phosphatidylinositol and phosphatidic acid with ^{32}P as early as 2 min after $PGF_{2\alpha}$ addition (11). The ED_{50} of 60 nM for PA labeling was in close agreement with the potency of $PGF_{2\alpha}$ in inhibition of LH-induced progesterone secretion measured at an ED_{50} value of 40 nM (12). Increased formation of IP, IP_2, and IP_3 was seen in response to $PGF_{2\alpha}$ in rat luteal cells (65).

The luteolytic effect of $PGF_{2\alpha}$ in rat luteal cells can be duplicated using a phorbol ester, TPA, and the calcium ionophore A23187. TPA mimicked the effect of $PGF_{2\alpha}$ on LH-stimulated cAMP and progesterone secretion from luteal cells (66). Calcium ionophores also have effects similar to $PGF_{2\alpha}$ on LH-stimulated cAMP and progesterone accumulation (66–68). Progesterone production in response to 8-bromo-cAMP or dibutyrl cAMP was almost inhibited by treatment of cells with A23187 or TPA (66).

Calcium may be important in the effect of $PGF_{2\alpha}$ on ovarian cells. Fura-2-labeled rat luteal cells in suspension increased $[Ca^{++}]_i$ in response to $PGF_{2\alpha}$ (10^{-6}M). The response to $PGF_{2\alpha}$ was not eliminated by EGTA in the extracellular medium, but was decreased by dimethyl bis-(O-aminophenoxy) ethane-N,N,N',N'-tetraacetic acid (BAPTA), which chelated intracellular calcium. Depletion of intracellular calcium, by using a calcium ionophore and including EGTA in the medium, eliminated the increase in $[Ca^{++}]_i$ in response to $PGF_{2\alpha}$. The pattern of $[Ca^{++}]_i$ was biphasic in suspensions of rat luteal cells; the initial increase occurred in 20 sec and was followed by a decrease to an elevated basal level in about 1 min (69). Studies on individual rat granulosa and luteal cells have been done using Fura-2 micro-spectrofluorimetry. Cells responded rapidly (30 sec average) to $PGF_{2\alpha}$, with a 3-fold increase in $[Ca^{++}]_i$, and recovered in about 90 sec. The increased $[Ca^{++}]_i$ was not larger with increased $PGF_{2\alpha}$ concentrations. The source of the increased calcium may be intracellular stores. However, because the response to $PGF_{2\alpha}$ can be eliminated with prolonged perifusion with a low calcium buffer, extracellular calcium must be important at least in refilling the intracellular calcium stores (70). Attempts have been made to identify the immediate source of the calcium. A blocker of L-type calcium channels, verapamil, had no effect on the inhibition of LH-stimulated cAMP formation by $PGF_{2\alpha}$ (67, 71). Radioactive calcium uptake studies showed no effect of $PGF_{2\alpha}$ on calcium uptake (71). TMB-8 (8-(N,N-diethylamino)-octyl-3,4,5-trimethoxybenzoate), which inhibited intracellular calcium release and the action of intracellular calcium, did not prevent $PGF_{2\alpha}$ inhibition of LH-induced cAMP accumulation (72). Calmodulin inhibitors trifluoroperzaine, pimozide (diphenylbutylpiperidine), and N-(6-aminohexyl)-5-chloro-1-naphthalenesulphonamide (W-7) had no effect on $PGF_{2\alpha}$ inhibition of cAMP formation (72).

$PGF_{2\alpha}$ stimulated a calcium-dependent phosphorylation of a specific protein in luteal membranes of rat ovary (73), suggesting that an endogenous protein kinase is involved in $PGF_{2\alpha}$ action. Phosphorylation occurred within 5 min of hormone administration, concurrent with $PGF_{2\alpha}$-induced PIP_2 breakdown, and may be another aspect of the mechanism of action of $PGF_{2\alpha}$.

The role of PIP_2 breakdown and calcium in $PGF_{2\alpha}$-induced inhibition of LH-stimulated cAMP production is not clear. The increase in $[Ca^{++}]_i$ can be eliminated without affecting the decrease in LH-stimulated cAMP production caused by $PGF_{2\alpha}$ (69). Other studies also question the involvement of PIP_2 breakdown in the action of $PGF_{2\alpha}$. Maximum sensitivity of luteal cells to $PGF_{2\alpha}$-induced PIP_2 turnover does not correspond to maximum sensitivity of LH-stimulated cAMP production to $PGF_{2\alpha}$ inhibition (see 64). Results from studies involving cAMP accumulation, ATP levels, and subcellular distribution of PKC activity following treatment of rat luteal cells in culture with TPA and $PGF_{2\alpha}$ suggest that the luteolytic effect of $PGF_{2\alpha}$ was not transduced by activation of PKC (74). In these studies, staurosparine, a PKC inhibitor, reversed TPA inhibition of LH-stimulated cAMP accumulation but had no effect on $PGF_{2\alpha}$ inhibition of LH-stimulated cAMP accumulation. Prolonged treatment with TPA caused a loss of response to TPA without changing the effect of $PGF_{2\alpha}$; however, the authors acknowledged that TPA may not activate all PKC fractions. Interestingly, cells that increased cAMP production in response to LH may not be the cells that have $PGF_{2\alpha}$ receptors (75, 76).

These data question the involvement of PIP_2 breakdown at least in the in-hibition of LH-stimulated cAMP caused by $PGF_{2\alpha}$. However, $PGF_{2\alpha}$ does affect PIP_2 metabolism in rat ovarian cells. The possibility that PKC and $[Ca^{++}]_i$ may transduce other effects of $PGF_{2\alpha}$ cannot be ruled out.

Other Hormones

LH. Although LH is well known to activate adenylate cyclase (1), it may also activate PLC. Davis et al. find that LH increased synthesis (5, 7) and degradation (7) of phosphoinositides in rat granulosa cells isolated from mature graafian follicles. Increases in formation of IP_3 occur in response to LH (8). Others, however, have not seen increased $[Ca^{++}]_i$ in response to LH in rat granulosa and luteal cells (44).

Angiotensin II. Angiotensin II may affect ovarian steroid hormone production via specific receptors on subpopulations of granulosa cells. Four-fold increases in $[Ca^{++}]_i$ in response to angiotensin II but not angiotensin I have been seen in rat granulosa cells. $[Ca^{++}]_i$ returned to baseline levels after about 75 sec. Specificity of this increase in $[Ca^{++}]_i$ was verified using an angiotensin II antagonist (77).

Summary

Specific receptors for numerous endocrine, paracrine, and autocrine regulators have been found on rat ovarian cells. Physiological effects of the gonadotropins (LH and FSH), GnRH, and $PGF_{2\alpha}$ have been well documented. GnRH and $PGF_{2\alpha}$ have been reported to cause enhanced metabolism of PIP_2 and increases in $[Ca^{++}]_i$. Agents that activate PKC or increase $[Ca^{++}]_i$ may have the same effects as these physiologically active agonists. We conclude that GnRH and $PGF_{2\alpha}$ use PIP_2 breakdown as a transducing mechanism in the rat ovary. In the case of LH, it is possible that the PLC system is involved in addition to the well-established second messenger role of the adenylate cyclase system. Other agents may also make use of one or both signal transduction pathways to regulate ovarian functions.

References

1. Gore-Langton RE, Armstrong DT. Follicular steroidogenesis and its control. In: Knobil E, Neill J, eds. The physiology of reproduction. New York: Raven Press, 1988:331-85.
2. Strauss JF, III, Golos TG, Silavin SL, Soto EA, Takagi K. Involvement of cyclic AMP in the functions of granulosa and luteal cells: Regulation of steroidogenesis. Prog Clin Biol Res 1988;267:177-200.
3. Naor Z, Yavin E. Gonadotropin releasing hormone stimulates phospholipid labeling in cultured granulosa cells. Endocrinology 1982;11:1615-19.

4. Davis JS, Farese RV, Clark MR. Gonadotropin-releasing hormone (GnRH) stimulates phosphatidylinositol metabolism in rat granulosa cells, mechanism of action of GnRH. Proc Natl Acad Sci USA 1983;80:2049-53.

5. Davis JS, Farese RV, Clark MR. Stimulation of phospholipid synthesis by luteinizing hormone in isolated rat granulosa cells. Endocrinology 1983;112: 2212-14.

6. Davis JS, West LA, Farese RV. Gonadotropin-releasing hormone rapidly alters polyphosphoinositide metabolism in rat granulosa cells. Biochem Biophys Res Commun 1984;122:1289-95.

7. Davis JS, West LA, Farese RV. Effects of luteinizing hormone on phospho-inositol metabolism in rat granulosa cells. J Biol Chem 1984;259:15028-34.

8. Davis JS, Weakland LL, West LA, Farese RV. Luteinizing hormone stimulates the formation of inositol trisphosphate and cyclic AMP in rat granulosa cells. Biochem J 1986;238:597-604.

9. Davis JS, West LA, Farese RV. Gonadotropin-releasing hormone (GnRH) rapidly stimulates the formation of inositol phosphates and diacylglycerol in rat granulosa cells: Further evidence for the involvement of Ca^{2+} and protein kinase. Endocrinology 1986;118:2561-71.

10. Leung PCK, Raymond V, Labrie F. Stimulation of phosphatidic acid and phosphatidylinositol labeling in luteal cells by luteinizing hormone releasing hormone. Endocrinology 1983;112:1138-40.

11. Raymond V, Leung PCK, Labrie F. Stimulation by prostaglandin $F_{2\alpha}$ of phosphatidic acid-phosphatidylinositol turnover in rat luteal cells. Biochem Biophys Res Commun 1983;116:39-46.

12. Leung, PCK. Mechanism of gonadotropin-releasing hormone and prostaglandin action on luteal cells. Can J Physiol Pharmacol 1985;63:249-56.

13. Minegishi T, Leung PCK. Effects of prostaglandins and luteinizing hormone-releasing hormone on phosphatidic acid-phosphatidylinositol labeling in rat granulosa cells. Can J Physiol Pharmacol 1985a;63:320-4.

14. Ma F, Leung PCK. Luteinizing hormone-releasing hormone enhances polyphosphoinositide breakdown in rat granulosa cells. Biochem Biophys Res Commun 1985;130:1201-8.

15. Leung PCK, Wang J. Inositol lipids and LHRH action in the rat ovary. J Reprod Fertil [Suppl] 1989;37:287-93.

16. Leung PCK, Wang J. The role of inositol lipid metabolism in the ovary. Biol Reprod 1989;40:703-8.

17. Berridge MJ, Irvine RF. Inositol phosphates and cell signalling. Nature 1989;341:197-205.

18. Crooke ST, Bennett CB. Mammalian phosphoinositide-specific phospholipase C isoenzymes. Cell Calcium 1989;10:309-23.

19. Nishizuka Y. The molecular heterogeneity of protein kinase C and its implications for cellular regulation. Nature 1988;334:661-5.

20. Shinohara O, Knecht M, Catt KJ. Calcium and phospholipid-dependent protein kinase activity and substrate phosphorylation in the rat ovary. In: Toft DO, Ryan RJ, eds. 5th Ovarian Workshop. Champaign, IL: Ovarian Workshops,1984: 433-48.

21. Steinschneider A, McLean MP, Billheimer JT, Azhar S, Gibori G. Protein kinase

C catalyzed phosphorylation of sterol carrier protein 2. Endocrinology 1989; 125:569-71.

22. Nishizuka Y, Takai Y, Kishimoto A, Kikkawa U, Kaibuchi K. Phospholipid turnover in hormone action. Recent Prog Horm Res 1984;40:301-45.

23. Berridge MJ. Inositol trisphosphate and diacylglycerol: Two interacting second messengers. Annu Rev Biochem 1987;56:159-93.

24. Hsueh AJW, Jones PCW. Extrapituitary actions of gonadotropin-releasing hormone. Endocr Rev 1981;2:437-61.

25. Hsueh AJW, Adashi EY, Jones PBC, Welsh TH. Hormonal regulation of the differentiation of cultured ovarian granulosa cells. Endocr Rev 1984;5:76-127.

26. Wang J, Leung PCK. Role of protein kinase C in luteinizing hormone-releasing hormone (LHRH)-stimulated progesterone production in rat granulosa cells. Biochem Biophys Res Commun 1987;146:939-44.

27. Komorowski JI, Tsang BK. Divergent effects of 1-Oleoyl-2-Acetylglycerol and tumor-promoting phorbol ester on rat granulosa cell steroidogenesis in vitro. Biol Reprod 1990;43:73-9.

28. Kawai Y, Clark MR. Phorbol ester regulation of rat granulosa cell prostaglandin and progesterone accumulation. Endocrinology 1985;116:2320-6.

29. Kawai Y, Clark MR. Mechanisms of action of gonadotropin releasing hormone on rat granulosa cells. Endocr Res 1986a;12:195-209.

30. Wang J, Lee V, Leung PCK. Differential role of protein kinase C in the action of luteinizing hormone-releasing hormone on hormone production in rat ovarian cells. Am J Obstet Gynecol 1989a;160:984-9.

31. Shinohara O, Knecht M, Feng P, Catt KJ. Activation of protein kinase C potentiates cyclic AMP production and stimulates steroidogenesis in differentiated ovarian granulosa cells. J Steroid Biochem 1986;24:161-8.

32. Wang J, Leung PCK. Synergistic stimulation of prostaglandin E_2 production by calcium ionophore and protein kinase C activator in rat granulosa cells. Biol Reprod 1989a;40:1000-6.

33. Kawai Y, Clark MR. The mechanisms by which phorbol ester inhibits LH stimulation of progesterone production in rat granulosa cells. Endocr Res 1986b;12:211-28.

34. Leung PCK, Minegishi T, Wang J. Inhibition of follicle-stimulating hormone and adenosine-3',5'-cyclic monophosphate-induced progesterone production by calcium and protein kinase C in the rat ovary. Am J Obstet Gynecol 1988;158: 350-6.

35. Shinohara O, Knecht M, Catt KJ. Inhibition of gonadotropin-induced granulosa cell differentiation by activation of protein kinase C. Proc Natl Acad Sci USA 1985;82:8518-22.

36. Knecht M, Katz MS, Catt KJ. Gonadotropin-releasing hormone inhibits cyclic nucleotide accumulation in cultured rat granulosa cells. J Biol Chem 1981; 256:34-6.

37. Knecht M, Catt KJ. Gonadotropin-releasing hormone: Regulation of adenosine-3',5'-monophosphate in ovarian granulosa cells. Science 1981;214:1346-8.

38. Gore-Langton RE, Lacroix M, Dorrinton JH. Differential effects of luteinizing hormone-releasing hormone on follicle-stimulating hormone-dependent responses in rat granulosa cells and Sertoli cells in vitro. Endocrinology 1981;108:812-5.

39. Ranta T, Knecht M, Darvon J-M, Baukal AJ, Catt KJ. Calcium dependence of the inhibitory effect of gonadotropin-releasing hormone on luteinizing hormone-induced cyclic AMP production in rat granulosa cells. Endocrinology 1983; 113:427-9.

40. Jones PBC, Hsueh AJW. Pregnenolone biosynthesis by cultured rat granulosa cells: Modulation by follicle-stimulating hormone and gonadotropin-releasing hormone. Endocrinology 1982;111:713-21.

41. Welsh TH, Jr, Jones PBC, Hsueh AJW. Phorbol ester inhibition of ovarian and testicular steroidogenesis in vitro. Cancer Res 1984;44:885-92.

42. Jones PBC, Hsueh AJW. Direct stimulation of ovarian progesterone-metabolizing enzyme by gonadotropin-releasing hormone in cultured granulosa cells. J Biol Chem 1981;256:1248-54.

43. Ben-Ze'ev A, Amsterdam A. In vitro regulation of granulosa cell differentiation. Involvement of cytoskeletal protein expression. J Biol Chem 1987;262:5366-76.

44. Wang J, Baimbridge KG, Leung PCK. Changes in cytosolic free calcium ion concentrations in individual rat granulosa cells: Effect of luteinizing hormone-releasing hormone. Endocrinology 1989b;124:1912-7.

45. Wang J, Rodway MR, Baimbridge KG, Leung PCK. The sources of LHRH-induced changes of cytosolic free calcium ion concentrations in rat granulosa cells. Submitted.

46. Minegishi T, Leung PCK. Luteinizing hormone-releasing hormone stimulates arachidonic acid release in rat granulosa cells. Endocrinology 1985b;117:2001-7.

47. Minegishi T, Wang J, Leung PCK. Luteinizing hormone-releasing hormone (LHRH)-induced arachidonic acid release in rat granulosa cells. Role of calcium and protein kinase C. FEBS Lett 1987;214:139-42.

48. Wang J, Leung PCK. Role of arachidonic acid in luteinizing hormone-releasing hormone action: Stimulation of progesterone production in rat granulosa cells. Endocrinology 1988;122:906-11.

49. Wang J, Leung PCK. Arachidonic acid as a stimulatory mediator of luteinizing hormone-releasing hormone action in the rat ovary. Endocrinology 1989b;124: 1973-9.

50. Wang J, Ho Yuen B, Leung PCK. Stimulation of progesterone and prostaglandin E_2 production by lipoxygenase metabolites of arachidonic acid. FEBS Lett 1989c;244:154-8.

51. McPhail LC, Clayton CC, Snyderman R. A potential second messenger role for unsaturated fatty acids: Actions of Ca^{2+}-dependent protein kinase. Science 1984;224:622-5.

52. Murakami K, Routtenberg A. Direct activation of purified protein kinase C by unsaturated fatty acids (oleate and arachidonate) in the absence of phospholipids and Ca^{2+}. FEBS Lett 1985;192:189-93.

53. Curry TE, Jr, Malik A, Clark MR. Ovarian prostaglandin synthase: Immunohistochemical localization in the rat. Am J Obstet Gynecol 1987;157:537-43.

54. Wright K, Luborsky-Moore JL, Behrman HR. Specific binding of prostaglandin $F_{2\alpha}$ to membranes of rat corpora lutea. Mol Cell Endocrinol 1979;13:25-34.

55. Bussmann LE. Prostaglandin $F_{2\alpha}$ receptors in corpora lutea of pregnant rats and relationship with induction of 20α-hydroxysteroid dehydrogenase. J Reprod Fertil 1989;85:331-41.

56. Armstrong DT. Prostaglandins and follicular functions. J Reprod Fertil 1981;62:283-91.
57. Niswender GD, Nett TM. The corpus luteum and its control. In: Knobil E, Neill J, eds. The physiology of reproduction. New York: Raven Press, 1988:489-525.
58. Behrman HR. Prostaglandins in hypothalamo-pituitary and ovarian function. Annu Rev Physiol 1979;41:685-700.
59. Lindner HR, Zor U, Kohen F, Bauminger S, Amsterdam A, Lahav M, Salomon Y. Significance of prostaglandins in the regulation of cyclic events in the ovary and uterus. Adv Prostaglandin Thromboxane Leukotriene Res 1980;8:1371-90.
60. Khan I, Rosberg S. Acute suppression by $PGF_{2\alpha}$ on LH, epinephrine and fluoride stimulation of adenylate cyclase in rat luteal tissue. J Cycl Nucl Res 1979; 5:55-61.
61. Aakvaag A, Torjesen PA. Prostaglandin-induced luteolysis in the superluteinized rat ovary. In: McKerns KW, ed. Reproductive processes and contraception. New York: Plenum Press, 1981:677-90.
62. Behrman HR, Luborsky JL, Aten RF, et al. Luteolytic hormones are calcium-mediated, guanine nucleotide antagonists of gonadotropin-sensitive adenylate cyclase. Adv Prostaglandin Thromboxane Leukotriene Res 1985;15:601-4.
63. Behrman HR, Yoshinaga K, Greep RO. Extraluteal effects of prostaglandins. Ann NY Acad Sci 1971;180:426-35.
64. Lahav M, West LA, Davis JS. Effects of prostaglandin $F_{2\alpha}$ and a gonadotropin-releasing hormone agonist on inositol phospholipid metabolism in isolated rat corpora lutea of various ages. Endocrinology 1988;123:1044-52.
65. Leung PCK, Minegishi T, Ma F, Zhou FZ, Ho-Yuen B. Induction of polyphosphoinositide breakdown in rat corpus luteum by prostaglandin $F_{2\alpha}$. Endocrinology 1986;119:12-8.
66. Sender Baum M, Rosberg S. A phorbol ester, phorbol 12-myristate 13-acetate, and a calcium ionophore, A23187, can mimic the luteolytic effect of prostaglandin $F_{2\alpha}$ in isolated rat luteal cells. Endocrinology 1987;120:1019-26.
67. Dorflinger LJ, Albert PJ, Williams AT, Behrman HR. Calcium is an inhibitor of luteinizing hormone-sensitive adenylate cyclase in the luteal cell. Endocrinology 1984;114:1208-15.
68. Soodak LK, Musicki B, Behrman HR. Selective amplification of luteinizing hormone by adenosine in rat luteal cells. Endocrinology 1988;122:847-54.
69. Pepperell JR, Preston SL, Behrman HR. The antigonadotropic action of prostaglandin $F_{2\alpha}$ is not mediated by elevated cytosolic calcium levels in rat luteal cells. Endocrinology 1989;125:144-51.
70. Rodway MR, Baimbridge KG, Leung PCK. Alterations in cytosolic free calcium ion concentrations in response to prostaglandin $F^{2\alpha}$ ($PGF_{2\alpha}$) in rat ovarian cells [Abstract]. 35th Annual Meeting. Canadian Fertility and Andrology Society, 1989.
71. Lahav M, Weiss E, Rafaeloff R, Barzilai D. The role of calcium ion in luteal function in the rat. J Steroid Biochem 1983;19:805-10.
72. Lahav M, Rennert H, Sabag K, Barzilai D. Calmodulin inhibitors and 8-(N,N-diethylamine)-octyl-3,4,5-trimethoxybenzoate do not prevent the inhibitory effect of prostaglandin $F_{2\alpha}$ on cyclic AMP production in isolated rat corpora lutea. J Endocrinol 1987;113:205-12.

73. Sender Baum M. Prostaglandin $F_{2\alpha}$ administered in vivo induced Ca2+-dependent protein phosphorylation in rat luteal tissue. Endocrinology 1989;124:555-7.

74. Musicki B, Aten RF, Behrman HR. The antigonadotropic actions of $PGF_{2\alpha}$ and phorbol ester are mediated by separate processes in rat luteal cells. Endocrinology 1990;126:1388-95.

75. Smith CJ, Greer TB, Banks TW, Sridaran R. The response of large and small luteal cells from the pregnant rat to substrates and secretagogues. Biol Reprod 1989;41:1123-32.

76. Wiltbank MC, Guthrie PB, Mattson MP, Kater SB, Niswender GD. Hormonal regulation of free intracellular calcium concentrations in small and large ovine luteal cells. Biol Reprod 1989;41:771-8.

77. Wang J, Baimbridge KG, Leung PCK. Perturbation of intracellular calcium ion concentrations in single rat granulosa cells by angiotensin II. Endocrinology 1989d;124:1094-6.

4

Interactions Among the cAMP and IP$_3$/DAG Intracellular Signaling Systems in Bovine Luteal Cells

JOHN S. DAVIS

The mammalian corpus luteum is a transient gland. During the estrous or menstrual cycle, it develops, secretes progesterone for a period of time characteristic of the species, and then declines. This decline or luteolysis is prevented when pregnancy ensues and the extended life of the corpus luteum allows it to provide the steroids needed for ovum implantation and the maintenance of pregnancy. The corpus luteum is also recognized as a gland responsible for secreting a number of important biologically active peptides (oxytocin and relaxin). The survival and regression of the corpus luteum depend on a delicate balance between trophic and luteolytic factors. In the cow and the human, the trophic factors that control luteal function (1–3) have been demonstrated to be predominately luteinizing hormone (LH) and human chorionic gonadotropin (hCG). Prostaglandin $F_{2\alpha}$ (PGF$_{2\alpha}$) is recognized as the primary luteolytic factor in many species (1–3), although multiple mechanisms or factors appear to be involved.

Research studying the effects of gonadotropins and prostaglandins on luteal function in vivo and in vitro with primary cultures of luteal cells and highly purified preparations of large and small luteal cells has received a great deal of attention. Understanding the biochemical mechanisms responsible for the actions of gonadotropins and prostaglandins is necessary in order to fully understand the regulation of steroid and peptide hormone secretion in the corpus luteum. Specific gonadotropin and prostaglandin receptors have been characterized in luteal cells but their post-receptor transmembrane signaling events are just beginning to be identified.

The initial biochemical events associated with gonadotropin action in luteal cells are universally held to be the result of the activation of adenylate cyclase and the formation of cAMP (Fig. 1). This is not, however, the only signaling

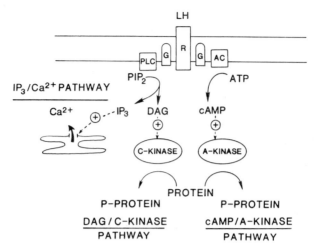

FIGURE 1. Transmembrane signaling systems mediating the actions of gonadotropins in bovine luteal cells.

system that is activated in response to gonadotropins. We (4–6) and others (7) have shown that LH and hCG also activate the inositol phospholipid/phospholipase C pathway, giving rise to increases in inositol 1,4,5-trisphosphate (IP_3) and intracellular calcium (5, 8). $PGF_{2\alpha}$ stimulates the latter signaling pathway without activating adenylate cyclase in luteal cells (6). This chapter reviews our current knowledge of the recently described inositol phospholipid signaling pathway in the bovine corpus luteum and explores some of the interactions among the signaling pathways in gonadotropin-stimulated luteal cells.

Overview of the Inositol Phospholipid Signaling Pathway

In animal cells, inositol lipids play an important role in the regulation of cellular function (9–22). Three myoinositol-containing lipids are phosphatidyl inositol (PI), phosphatidyl inositol 4-phosphate (PIP), and phosphatidyl inositol 4,5-bisphosphate (PIP_2). Although these lipids usually account for less than 10% of total cellular phospholipids (with PI representing 90% of inositol lipids), they are highly metabolically active. In 1953, Hokin and Hokin (13) discovered that acetylcholine stimulated the incorporation of radioactive phosphorus into PI in the pancreas. In 1970, Holub discovered that PI was unique in terms of its characteristic enrichment with arachidonate at the sn-2 position of the glycero (3) phosphoinositol backbone (14). The PI response was subsequently observed in many tissues in response to various stimuli, but its function remained an enigma until 15 years ago when Michell (15) suggested that agonist-induced PI hydrolysis may play an important role in calcium gating. A few years later, Low (16) discovered that PI could serve as a hydrophobic anchor for membrane protein. In 1979, Farese (17) observed that hormone-stimulated synthesis of PI, PIP, and PIP$_2$ played an integral role in cellular response to a number of hormones (ACTH, AII, and insulin). About the same time, Nishizuka (18) discovered that a product of phosphoinositide hydrolysis, 1,2-diacylglycerol (DAG), could activate protein kinase C (PKC). A few years later, this group demonstrated that tumor-promoting phorbol esters could substitute for DAG at very low concentrations and activate PKC in vitro and in vivo. In 1983, Berridge observed that another product of PIP$_2$ hydrolysis, IP$_3$, stimulated intracellular calcium mobilization (9). Three years later, a number of laboratories reported the presence of multiple distinct forms of PKC (18–20), suggesting an even greater diversity in cellular signaling pathways. Subsequent to these independent observations have been a flood of information on the regulation of inositol phospholipids, cations, and PKC and their importance in cellular regulation. The relationships between the actions of hormones and cell events are (9–22) *(a)* increased synthesis/degradation of inositol phospholipids; *(b)* altered cationic flux (Ca^{++}, Na$^+$, and H$^+$); *(c)* increased protein kinase activity; *(d)* increased transport of nutrients; *(e)* control of cell growth and differentiation; and *(f)* control of cellular processes (i.e., ligand-receptor coupling, secretion, and metabolism).

Prostaglandins

The important role that prostaglandins of the F series play in corpus luteum regression in vivo is well documented. The mechanism of action PGF$_{2\alpha}$ in the bovine corpus luteum in vitro appears to involve the activation of a guanine nucleotide-sensitive phospholipase C, which causes the hydrolysis of PIP$_2$ and increases IP$_3$. This response has been observed in bovine (23, 24), rat (25, 26), ovine (27), and human (28) luteal cells. In the cow, both large and small luteal cells respond to PGF$_{2\alpha}$ with increases in IP$_3$ and intracellular calcium (8, 23, 24 and Table 1). Experiments in bovine luteal cells (manuscript in preparation) have provided evidence suggesting that the hormone-responsive phospholipase C in ovarian tissues is coupled to a

TABLE 1. Effects of LH and PGF$_{2\alpha}$ in bovine luteal cells.

Cellular Responses	Small Luteal Cells		Large Luteal Cells	
	LH	PGF$_{2\alpha}$	LH	PGF$_{2\alpha}$
cAMP	+++	None	Slight	None
IP$_3$	++	+++	Slight	+++
Progesterone	+++	+	+	None

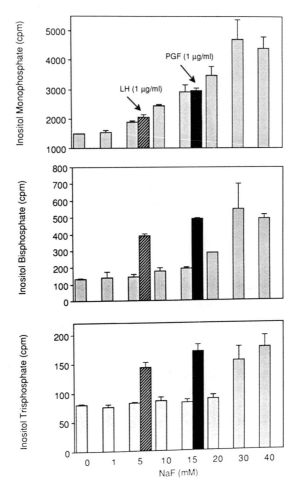

FIGURE 2. Stimulatory effects of NaF, LH, and PGF$_{2\alpha}$ on inositol phosphate accumulation in bovine luteal cells. Luteal cells were treated with 10-mM LiCl and incubated with increasing concentrations of NaF (1–40 mM) for 30 min. The effects of LH (1 µg/mL) and PGF$_{2\alpha}$ (1 µM) are shown for comparative purposes.

guanine nucleotide regulatory G-protein (29): *(a)* NaF stimulates concentration-dependent increases in the formation of IP, IP$_2$, and IP$_3$ in bovine luteal cells (Fig. 2); *(b)* the effects of NaF and other hormones (LH and PGF$_{2\alpha}$) are not additive; *(c)* GTPγS stimulates IP$_3$ formation in saponin-permeabilized cells but not in intact cells; and *(d)* GTPγS is required for hormone-induced PLC activity in permeabilized cells. Hormone-induced PLC activation was relatively insensitive to cholera or pertussis toxins, suggesting the involvement of a G-protein distinct from those associated with the AC system.

The rapid nature of the response and the presence of multiple forms of

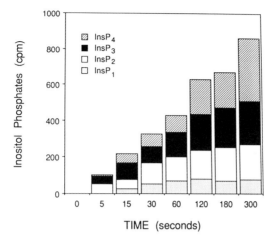

FIGURE 3. Acute increases in inositol phosphate accumulation in PGF$_{2\alpha}$-stimulated bovine luteal cells. Luteal cells were prelabeled with [^{3}H]inositol for 3 h prior to the addition of PGF$_{2\alpha}$ (1 μM). Incubations were performed in the absence of LiCl. The chart demonstrates the relative contribution of inositol mono-, bis-, tris-, and tetrakis-phosphates to the total amount of inositol phosphates.

inositol phosphates are indicative of the intricate nature of inositol phosphate metabolism. The time-course of PGF$_{2\alpha}$ action on this signaling system is shown in Figure 3. The increases in IP$_3$ observed in PGF$_{2\alpha}$-treated bovine luteal cells are due to the presence of two IP$_3$ isomers, I(1,4,5)P$_3$ and I(1,3,4)P$_3$ (30). The earliest increases occur in the I(1,4,5)P$_3$ isomer, which is consistent with observations that one of the initial effects of PGF$_{2\alpha}$ in luteal cells is the hydrolysis of PIP$_2$ (23–25). The rapid increases in I(1,4,5)P$_3$ are also coincident with the rapid increases observed in intracellular calcium (8, 23). I(1,4,5)P$_3$ is metabolized by two pathways in bovine luteal cells (30): *(a)* dephosphorylation via inositol polyphosphate-5-phosphatase to I(1,4)P$_2$ and *(b)* phosphorylation via I(1,4,5)P$_3$-3-kinase to I(1,3,4,5)P$_4$ (Fig. 4). These conclusions are supported by the observations that *(a)* the addition of [^{3}H]I(1,4,5)P$_3$ to permeabilized luteal cells results in the formation of both I(1,4)P$_2$ and I(1,3,4,5)P$_4$ as well as I(1,3,4)P$_3$; *(b)* bovine luteal cytosol contains an enzyme that phosphorylates I(1,4,5)P$_3$ to form I(1,3,4,5)P$_4$; and *(c)* the formation of I(1,4,5)P$_3$ temporally precedes the formation of either I(1,4)P$_2$ or I(1,3,4,5)P$_4$ in PGF$_{2\alpha}$-treated cells. Thus, I(1,4,5)P$_3$ accumulation in PGF$_{2\alpha}$-treated luteal cells is rapidly attenuated by metabolism via a phosphomonoesterase specific for the 5 position of inositol and a kinase that is specific for the 3 position. The activity of bovine luteal I(1,4,5)P$_3$-3-kinase is greatest in the presence of calcium and calmodulin raising the possibility that PGF$_{2\alpha}$-induced increases in intracellular calcium are sufficient to activate the enzyme. A flow chart of the possible metabolic pathways involved in luteal inositol lipid metabolism is shown in Figure 4. This pathway was

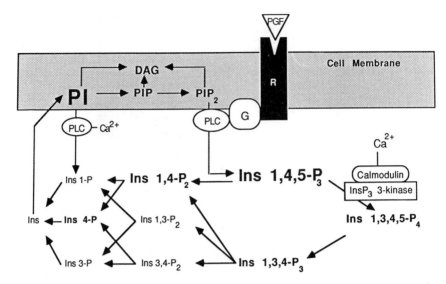

FIGURE 4. Proposed pathways of inositol phospholipid and inositol phosphate metabolism in PGF$_{2\alpha}$-stimulated bovine luteal cells.

developed based on the detection of radioactive inositol metabolites after labeling cells for up to 3 h with [^{3}H]inositol. This pathway, however, may be more complex and include higher polyphosphorylated inositol phosphates (i.e., IP$_5$ and IP$_6$) that may be detected only following the labeling of luteal cells to constant specific radioactivity (31).

The existence of multiple pathways for I(1,4,5)P$_3$ metabolism in bovine luteal cells offers a rapid and sensitive means to regulate the accumulation of I(1,4,5)P$_3$. This may be physiologically relevant since the activation of inositol phospholipid hydrolysis and inositol phosphate formation in bovine luteal cells is continuous in the presence of PGF$_{2\alpha}$. Continuous increases in I(1,4,5)P$_3$, and thus intracellular calcium, could damage the luteal cells. However, following an initial rapid rise, I(1,4,5)P$_3$ accumulation is reduced (30), consistent with the submaximal elevations in intracellular calcium still apparent many minutes after treatment with PGF$_{2\alpha}$ (23). Unregulated levels of IP$_3$ and intracellular calcium could explain part of the luteolytic actions of PGF$_{2\alpha}$.

Other prostaglandins play an important role in luteal function. In contrast to the luteolytic role of PGF$_{2\alpha}$, PGE$_2$, and PGI$_2$ exert luteotropic effects on luteal function (3). PGE$_2$ and PGI$_2$ provoke increases in cAMP, IP$_3$ and intracellular Ca^{++} in bovine luteal cells (32). When used at maximally effective concentrations, PGE$_2$ and PGI$_2$ produce cAMP levels that reach only one twentieth (5%) of that observed with LH, but produce equivalent increases in IP$_3$ and calcium mobilization. Since activation of protein kinase C stimulates progesterone secretion alone and augments the steroidogenic response to suboptimal concentrations of LH (33–37), activation of this signaling system may augment steroidogenesis in the presence of modest cAMP levels.

Gonadotropins

The gonadotropins, LH and hCG, stimulate the formation of intracellular second messengers derived from both adenylate cyclase and inositol phospholipid/phospholipase C (Fig. 1). The activation of adenylate cyclase and the resultant increases in cAMP accumulation are well documented and appear to be consistent responses across species (38). In comparison, the stimulation of inositol phospholipid hydrolysis and resultant increases in IP$_3$ and DAG have only recently been described and appear to be species specific. Stimulatory effects of gonadotropins on inositol phospholipid metabolism have been reported in bovine (4–6) and porcine (7) corpora lutea, but are absent in rat corpora lutea (26, 39) and cultured human granulosa/luteal cells (28).

The occupancy of gonadotropin receptors in isolated bovine luteal cells results in prompt increases in intracellular cAMP, IP$_3$, and Ca^{++}. The concentration-response relationships among these intracellular messengers are identical in response to LH. The concentrations of LH required for half-maximal (EC$_{50}$) increases in IP$_3$ and cAMP are 5.5 nM and 4.9 nM, respectively. The EC$_{50}$ value for the progesterone response to LH is 40 pM, indicating that the steroidogenic response to LH is a very sensitive index of gonadotropin action. hCG (40) and chemically deglycosylated hCG analogues (41), which act as partial agonists in other gonadotropin responsive tissues, elicit similar cAMP and IP$_3$ responses in bovine luteal cell preparations. Deglycosylated hCG analogues were also equally effective in antagonizing the stimulatory effects of hCG and LH on both cAMP and IP$_3$ accumulation (41). These studies indicate that gonadotropin receptor occupancy is closely coupled to the activation of cellular signaling systems. The results also suggest (but do not prove) that a single gonadotropin receptor may mediate the formation of both cAMP and IP$_3$. In accordance with the data presented above, similar concentration-dependent increases in cAMP, IP$_3$, and progesterone were observed in purified preparations of gonadotropin-responsive bovine small luteal cells (6), suggesting that these responses occur in a single population of luteal cells (Table 1).

The ability of LH to increase inositol phospholipid hydrolysis and IP$_3$ formation could not be reproduced by exogenously applied cAMP analogues or agents that increase adenylate cyclase activity (i.e., cholera toxin and forskolin) (5, 6). Despite the inability of cAMP analogues and forskolin to increase intracellular IP_3, bovine luteal cells respond to these agents with demonstrable increases in intracellular calcium (5, 8). The magnitudes of these increases, however, are less than those observed with LH. Mechanisms, in addition to IP_3, appear to be operating in the regulation of intracellular calcium in gonadotropin-stimulated luteal cells.

Interactions Among Signaling Systems

Pretreatment of luteal cells with LH for 1–3 h resulted in a significant reduction (50–60%) in LH-sensitive adenylate cyclase activity (Fig. 5). In contrast, LH pretreatment did not alter IP_3 levels in subsequent incubations with LH (Fig. 5), indicating that the rapid homologous desensitization of LH-sensitive adenylate cyclase was not associated with concomitant desensitization of LH-sensitive phospholipase C. Previous reports suggest that the desensitization of LH-sensitive adenylate cyclase does not appear to be the result of selective alterations in hormone-receptor coupling. However, desensitization of transmembrane signaling systems may result from the actions of the intracellular second messengers formed after ligand binding.

To evaluate this hypothesis, we have compared the effects of agonist-induced activation of adenylate cyclase and phospholipase C to the effects of

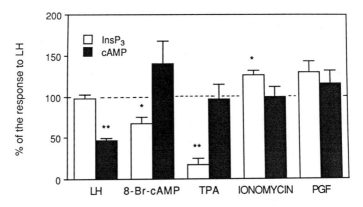

FIGURE 5. Modulation of LH-sensitive transmembrane signaling systems in bovine luteal cells. Luteal cells were pretreated with control media or the agents shown. The pretreatments were 60 min with LH (1 µg/mL) or 8-bromo-cAMP (5 mM), 15 min with TPA (50 nM), 15 min with ionomycin (0.1 µM), or 3 h with $PGF_{2\alpha}$ (1 µM). After pretreatment, the cells were washed 3 times and incubated for 15 min at 37°C. The media was changed, and aliquots of cells from each pretreatment group were incubated for 30 min in the presence or absence of LH (1 µg/mL). The results are expressed as a percentage of the LH-induced IP_3 and cAMP responses observed in the control pretreatment group. (*$P < 0.05$; **$P < 0.01$ vs. control.)

exogenous second messengers on LH-stimulated signaling systems. Pretreatment with exogenous cAMP, 8-bromo-cAMP (5 mM), for 60 min had no inhibitory effect on LH-sensitive adenylate cyclase activity (Fig. 5). Other studies have shown that direct activation of adenylate cyclase with forskolin had no inhibitory effect on LH-sensitive adenylate cyclase (42) in bovine luteal cells. The results demonstrate that cAMP is not a mediator of the acute homologous desensitization of adenylate cyclase. However, pretreatment with high concentrations of 8-bromo-cAMP (5 mM) reduced (33%) LH-sensitive phospholipase C activity (Fig. 5). While these results indicate a possible feedback regulation of LH-sensitive phospholipase C by cAMP in luteal cells, it is important to note that physiological accumulation of endogenous cAMP in response to LH had no subsequent inhibitory effects on LH-sensitive phospholipase C.

PGF$_{2\alpha}$, a physiological agonist that stimulates phospholipase C, mobilizes intracellular calcium (23) and activates PKC (43) but does not alter levels of cAMP (6) in bovine luteal cells, had no effect on LH-sensitive adenylate cyclase or phospholipase C (Fig. 5). These observations are important in light of the antigonadotropic effects exerted by PGF$_{2\alpha}$ in vivo (1–3). Similar results were observed in other studies using ionomycin (0.1 μM) to specifically induce calcium mobilization. Ionomycin had no effect on cAMP levels, but it enhanced IP$_3$ accumulation in LH-treated cells (Fig. 5). Pretreatment with the PKC activator, 12-0-tetradecanoylphorbol 13-acetate (TPA) (50 nM), for up to 3 h did not change gonadotropin receptor affinity (42) or reduce the stimulatory effect of LH on adenylate cyclase (Fig. 5). TPA, however, almost completely (90%) inhibited inositol phospholipid hydrolysis in LH-treated cells (44). Surprisingly, TPA has little effect on PGF$_{2\alpha}$-stimulated IP$_3$ accumulation, indicating that TPA does not exert a nonspecific inhibitory effect on luteal phospholipase C and that the stimulatory effects of LH and PGF$_{2\alpha}$ on inositol phospholipid hydrolysis are controlled by separate mechanisms (unpublished results). The effects of TPA, therefore, appear to be pharmacologic and possibly involve changes in cell membrane lipid turnover or the activation of a distinct PKC isoform (18–20) that is not available for activation by treatment with LH or PGF$_{2\alpha}$. In summary, our results demonstrate that physiological or pharmacological increases in cAMP, calcium mobilization, and PKC activation were insufficient to desensitize LH-stimulated adenylate cyclase in bovine luteal cells.

Gonadotropin-responsive bovine luteal cells provide a unique model for examining the regulation of the adenylate cyclase and phospholipase C transmembrane signaling systems. The coupling mechanisms of adenylate cyclase and phospholipase C in bovine luteal cells possess some similarities and interactions among the systems are apparent (Fig. 6). LH induces a rapid homologous desensitization of the LH-sensitive adenylate cyclase system without inhibiting the LH-sensitive phospholipase C system. This response

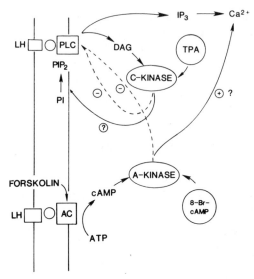

FIGURE 6. Interactions among the cAMP and IP$_3$/DAG second messenger systems in bovine luteal cells.

presumably involves a functional modification of the hormone-receptor complex (i.e., phosphorylation of the gonadotropin receptor or the G-protein(s) that regulate adenylate cyclase activity).

Protein Kinase C

PKC is an ubiquitous serine/threonine protein kinase in animal tissues requiring Ca^{++} and phospholipid for activity (18–20). DAG and phorbol ester compete for the same binding site and increase the affinity of PKC for Ca^{++}, thereby permitting activation of the enzyme at physiologic Ca^{++} levels. Although PKC was originally purified as a monomeric protein with an apparent molecular weight of 80 kDa, recent reports demonstrate that PKC is encoded by a family of closely related, but distinct genes (18–20). Additionally, three types of PKC isozymes (I–III) have been isolated from a variety of tissues using immunological approaches and chromatography on hydroxylapatite. Thus, previous studies using apparently homogeneous PKC were, in fact, conducted with a mixture of different molecular species of PKC. Based on product/precursor relationships of the PKC isozymes and cloned cDNAs, it is now certain that the types I–III PKC isozymes are products of γ-, β-, and α-type genes, respectively. Alternative splicing of the β-type gene has been shown to result in βI and βII PKCs, which differ only in their C-terminal 52 amino acids. The sequences of the four PKC molecules are closely related and show 70–95% sequence homology. In the past few years, at least three other genes (δ, ϵ, and ζ), which also share homology to PKC, have been isolated (18, 19).

The calcium and phospholipid requirements for PKC activity have been studied in crude and partially purified preparations of ovarian PKC from the rat, pig, sheep, cow, and human (45–50). These studies have also demonstrated that endogenous proteins serve as substrates in cell free assays, suggesting involvement of specific phosphoproteins in the action of PKC. PKC has been partially purified from porcine (46, 49) and bovine corpus luteum (Table 2). A recent report by Dowd et al. (51) suggested that the primary phorbol binding site in bovine luteal cells is PKC. Furthermore, small luteal cells possess a single high-affinity binding site comparable to the high-affinity binding of phorbol esters in partially purified luteal PKC preparations. PKC activity and phorbol binding sites in bovine large luteal cells remain to be demonstrated but are present in ovine large luteal cells (50). Wheeler and Veldhuis (49) have suggested the presence of multiple PKC species in porcine luteal tissue, but the identities of the PKC subspecies were unknown. We have identified two prominent forms of PKC (α and β or types III and II, respectively) in the bovine corpus luteum (Table 2). The characterization, cellular distribution, and regulation of the PKC isozymes in luteal cells remain to be examined.

The effects of PKC activators (usually phorbol esters) on steroid secretion appear to be species specific as well as dependent on the state of cellular differentiation. With regard to bovine corpora lutea, phorbol esters exert stimulatory effects on bovine small luteal cells (3, 33–37) but have no effect on basal progesterone synthesis in large luteal cells (3, 35, 36). Diacylglycerols and exogenous phospholipase C also stimulate progesterone secretion in small cells (3, 37) but have no effect in large cells (3). These observations, using pharmacological probes for PKC, are intriguing because they are not consistent with the effects of PGF$_{2\alpha}$. PGF$_{2\alpha}$ stimulates phosphoinositide hydrolysis in both large and small luteal cells (24), increases progesterone secretion in small luteal cells, but inhibits progesterone secretion in large cells (3, 36). The diverse actions of PGF$_{2\alpha}$ and activators of PKC on steroid production could be explained, in part, by

TABLE 2. Bovine luteal protein kinase C isozymes.

Purification Procedure	Specific Activity (nM/min/mg)	Total Activity (nM/min)	Fold Purification
Crude Extract	0.1	0.8	1
Mono Q	3.1	6.3	31
Hydroxylapatite			
Type II PKC	95	0.9	950
Type III PKC	83	0.3	830

PKC isozymes that are variably expressed in large and small luteal cells and/or PKC isozymes with differential sensitivity to phorbol esters and endogenously produced DAGs. Caution must be exercised when comparing the response (or a lack thereof) to hormones with the response to probes such as phorbol esters. Hormones may exert their effects through multiple physiologic mechanisms (i.e., $PGF_{2\alpha}$ stimulates Ca^{++} and PKC; LH stimulates cAMP, Ca^{++}, and PKC), whereas the pharmacologic agent exerts its effects at one intracellular target, PKC (hopefully, with few nonspecific actions). The response to hormones may also be compartmentalized, whereas the response to the lipophilic phorbol esters may activate PKC in multiple cellular compartments.

Acknowledgments. The secretarial assistance of Sheryl Johnson is gratefully acknowledged. This work was supported by the Research Service of the Department of Veterans Affairs, NIH HD-22248, the Wesley Medical Research Institutes, and the Wesley Foundation.

References

1. Rothchild I. The regulation of the mammalian corpus luteum. Recent Prog Horm Res 1981; 37:183-298.
2. Niswender GD, Nett TM. The corpus luteum and its control. In: Knobil E, Neil J, eds. The physiology of reproduction. New York: Raven Press, 1988:489-525.
3. Hansel W, Dowd JP. New concepts of the control of corpus luteum function. J Reprod Fertil 1986;78:755-68.
4. Davis JS, Farese RV, Marsh, JM. Stimulation of phospholipid labeling and steroidogenesis by luteinizing hormone in isolated bovine luteal cells. Endocrinology 1981;109:469-75.
5. Davis JS, Weakland LL, Farese RV, West LA. Luteinizing Hormone (LH) increases inositol trisphosphate (IP3) and cytosolic free Ca^{2+} in isolated bovine luteal cells. J Biol Chem 1987;262:8515-21.
6. Davis JS, Alila HW, West LA, Corradino RA, Weakland LL, Hansel W. Second messenger systems and progesterone secretion in the small cells of the bovine corpus luteum: Effects of LH and $PGF_{2\alpha}$. J Steroid Biochem 1989;32:643-9.
7. Allen RB, Su HC, Snitzer J, Dimino MJ. Rapid decreases in phosphatidylinositol in isolated luteal plasma membranes after stimulation by luteinizing hormone. Biol Reprod 1988;38:79-83.
8. Alila HW, Corradino RA, Hansel W. Differential effects of luteinizing hormone on intracellular free Ca^{2+} in small and large bovine luteal cells. Endocrinology 1989;124:2314-20.
9. Berridge MJ, Irvine RF. Inositol phosphates and cell signalling. Nature (London) 1989;341:197-205.
10. Bleasdale JE, Eichberf J, Hauser G, eds. Inositol and phosphoinositides, metabolism and regulation. New Jersey: Humana Press, 1985.

11. Kuo JF. Phosphoinositides and cellular regulation; vol 1. Boca Raton, FL: CRC Press, 1985.

12. Rana RS, Hokin LE. Role of phosphoinositides in transmembrane signalling. Physiol Rev 1990;70:115-64.

13. Hokin MR, Hokin LE. Enzyme secretion and the incorporation of ^{32}P into the phospholipids of pancreas slices. J Biol Chem 1953;203:967-77.

14. Holub BJ. Nutritional regulation of the composition, metabolism, and the function of cellular phosphatidylinositol. In: Bleasdale JE, Eichberf I, Hauser G, eds. Inositol and phosphoinositides, metabolism and regulation. New Jersey: Humana Press, 1985:31-47.

15. Michell RH. Inositol phospholipids and cell surface receptor function. Biochim Biophys Acta 1975;415:81-147.

16. Low MG. The glycosyl-phosphatidylinositol anchor of membrane proteins. Biochim Biophys Acta 1989;988:427-54.

17. Farese RV. De novo phospholipid synthesis as an intracellular mediator system. In: Kuo JF, ed. Phospholipids and cellular regulation; vol. 1. Boca Raton, FL: CRC Press, 1985;207-28.

18. Nishizuka Y. The family of protein kinase C for signal transduction. JAMA 1989;262:1826-33.

19. Parker PJ, Kour G, Marais RM, et al. Protein kinase C—a family affair. Mol Cell Endocrinol 1989;65:1-11.

20. Coussens L, Parker PJ, Rhee L, et al. Multiple, distinct forms of bovine and human protein kinase C suggest diversity in cellular signalling pathways. Science 1986;233:859-66.

21. Berridge MJ. Growth factors, oncogenes and inositol lipids. Cancer Surv 1986;5:413-30.

22. Putney JW, ed. Receptor biochemistry and methodology. Phosphoinositides and receptor mechanism. New York: Liss, 1986.

23. Davis JS, Weakland LL, Weiland DA, Farese RV, West LA. Prostaglandin F$_{2\alpha}$ stimulates phosphatidylinositol 4,5-bisphosphate hydrolysis and mobilizes intracellular Ca^{2+} in bovine luteal cells. Proc Natl Acad Sci USA 1987;84:3728-32.

24. Davis JS, Alila HW, West LA, Corridino RV, Hansel W. Acute effects of prostaglandin F$_{2\alpha}$ on inositol phospholipid hydrolysis in large and small cells of bovine corpus luteum. Mol Cell Endocrinol 1988;58:43-50.

25. Leung PCK, Minegishi T, Ma F, Zhou F, Ho-Yen B. Induction of polyphosphoinositide breakdown in rat corpus luteum by prostaglandin F$_{2\alpha}$. Endocrinology 1986;119:12-8.

26. Lahav M, West LA, Davis JS. Effect of prostaglandin F$_{2\alpha}$ and a gonadotropin-releasing hormone agonist on inositol phospholipid metabolism in isolated rat corpora lutea of various ages. Endocrinology 1988;123:1044-52.

27. McCann TJ, Flint APF. Prostaglandin F$_{2\alpha}$, cyclic adenosine monophosphate and inositol trisphosphate in sheep corpus luteum [Abstract]. Biol Reprod 1987; 36(suppl 1):163.

28. Davis JS, Tedesco TA, West LA, Maroulis GB, Weakland LL. Effects of human chorionic gonadotropin, prostaglandin F$_{2\alpha}$ and protein kinase C activators on the cyclic AMP and inositol phosphate second messenger systems in cultured human granulosa-luteal cells. Mol Cell Endocrinol 1989;65:187-93.

29. Davis JS, Weakland LL, West LA. GTP-binding protein coupled hydrolysis of PI and PIP$_2$ in bovine luteal cells: Effects of NaF and GTPγS [Abstract]. 70th Annual Meeting of the Endocrine Society. New Orleans, 1988.

30. Duncan RH and Davis JS. Prostaglandin F$_{2\alpha}$ stimulates inositol 1,4,5-triphosphate and inositol 1,3,4,5-tetratrisphosphate formation in bovine luteal cells. Submitted.

31. Stephens LR, Downes CP. Product-precursor relationships amongst inositol polyphosphates. Biochem J 1990;265:435-52.

32. West LA, Weakland LL, Duncan RA, Davis JS. Dual activation of adenylate cyclase and phospholipase C by prostaglandins of E and I series in bovine luteal cells. In: Hirshfield A, ed. VII Ovarian Workshop: Paracrine communication in the ovary oncogenesis and growth factors. New York: Plenum Press, 1989: 369-74.

33. Benhaim A, Herrou M, Mittre H, Leymaire P. Effect of phorbol esters on steroidogenesis in small bovine luteal cells. FEBS Lett 1987;223:321-6.

34. Brunswig B, Mukhopadhyay AK, Budnik HG, Leidenberger FA. Phorbol ester stimulates progesterone production by isolated bovine luteal cells. Endocrinology 1986;118:743-9.

35. Hansel W, Alila HW, Dowd JP, Yang X. Control of steroidogenesis in small and large bovine luteal cells. Austr J Biol Sci 1987;40:331-47.

36. Alila HW, Dowd J, Corradino RA, Harris WV, Hansel W. Control of progesterone production in small and large bovine luteal cells separated by flow cytometry. J Reprod Fertil 1988;82:645-55.

37. Benhaim A, Bonnamy PJ, Mittre H, Leymaire P. Involvement of the phospholipase C second messenger system in the regulation of steroidogenesis in small bovine luteal cells. Mol Cell Endocrinol 1990;68:105-11.

38. Marsh, JM. The role of cyclic AMP in gondal function. Adv Cyclic Nucleotide Res 1975;6:137-99.

39. Schuler LA, Flickinger GL, Straus JF, III. Effect of luteinizing hormone on the lipid composition of rat ovaries. J Endocrinol 1978;78:233-40.

40. Davis JS, West LA, Weakland LL, Farese RV. Human chronic gonadotropin activates the inositol 1,4,5-trisphosphate-Ca^{2+} intracellular signalling system in bovine luteal cells. FEBS Lett 1986;208:287-91.

41. Davis JS, Ryan RJ. Deglycosylated forms of hCG act as partial agonists and competitive antagonists of LH- and hCG-stimulated second messenger systems in bovine luteal cells [Abstract]. Biol Reprod 1990;42(suppl 1):137.

42. Budnik LT, Mukhopadhyay AK. Desensitization of LH-stimulated cyclic AMP accumulation in isolated bovine luteal cells—effect of phorbol ester. Mol Cell Endocrinol 1987;54:51-61.

43. Veldhuis JD. Prostaglandin F$_{2\alpha}$ initiates polyphosphatidylinositol hydrolysis and membrane translocation of protein kinase C in swine ovarian cells. Biochem Biophys Res Commun 1987;149:112-7.

44. Davis JS, Conway WA, West LA. Protein kinase C activators uncouple gonadotropin-stimulated inositol phospholipid hydrolysis in isolated bovine luteal cells. 18th Miami Winter Symposium. ISCU Short Reports, 1986;4:220-1.

45. Clark MR, Kawai Y, Davis JS, Le Maire WJ. Ovarian protein kinases. In: Toft,

DO, Ryan, RJ, eds. 5th Ovarian Workshop. Champaign, IL: Ovarian Workshops, 1984:383-401.
46. Wheeler MB, Veldhuis JD. Catalytic and receptor-binding properties of the calcium-sensitive phospholipid-dependent protein kinase (protein kinase C) in swine luteal cytosol. Mol Cell Endocrinol 1987;50:123-9.
47. Davis JS, Clark MR. Activation of protein kinase in the bovine corpus luteum by phospholipid and Ca^{2+}. Biochem J 1983;214:569-74.
48. Noland TA Jr, Dimino MJ. Characterization and distribution of protein kinase C in ovarian tissue. Biol Reprod 1986;35:863-72.
49. Wheeler MB, Veldhuis JD. Purification of three forms of chromatographically distinct protein kinase C from the swine ovary. Mol Cell Endocrinol 1989;61:117-22.
50. Wiltbank FF, Knicherbocker N, Niswender GD. Regulation of the corpus luteum by protein kinase C, I. Phosphorylation activity and steroidogenic action in large and small ovine luteal cells. Biol Reprod 1989;40:1194-1200.
51. Dowd JP, Alila HW, Hansel W. Phorbol ester receptors in bovine luteal cells: Relationship to protein kinase C. Mol Cell Endocrinol 1990;69:199-206.

5

Variant Diacylglycerol-Dependent Protein Phosphotransferase Activity in Ovarian Tissues

EVELYN T. MAIZELS, VICTORIA JACKIW,
JOSEPHINE B. MILLER, RICHARD E. CUTLER, JR.,
ELLEN M. CARNEY, AND MARY HUNZICKER-DUNN

Protein phosphorylation has been implicated as a key response to gonadotropic stimulation of ovarian cells. The second messenger systems, which would act by control of protein phosphorylation, include the adenylate cyclase/cAMP/A-kinase system (1) and the phosphoinositide hydrolysis system (2). Hydrolysis of phospatidylinositol 4,5-bisphosphate leads to the generation of 1,2-diacylglycerol, activation of diacylglycerol-dependent protein kinases (the C-kinases) (2, 3), and the generation of inositol 1,4,5-triphosphate, promoting release of Ca^{++} (2) and activation of Ca^{++}/calmodulin-dependent kinases (1). Ovarian tissues have been shown to contain protein kinases in each of the above classes. The functional significance of each class of protein kinases is not yet fully defined, but the existence of hormone-regulated parameters for each class of kinase in the ovary suggests that the kinases participate in the mediation of or modulation of hormone-regulated cellular responses. Ovarian A-kinases are regulated acutely (4) and chronically (5) by gonadotropic stimulation. Estrogen is also required for stimulated levels of mRNA for A-kinase regulatory subunit (RIIβ) in the rat granulosa cell (6). Ca^{++}/calmodulin kinase III, which phosphorylates the protein synthesis elongation factor EF_2, is regulated by estrogen in the rat corpus luteum of pregnancy (7). Levels of lipid-derived second messengers, 1,2-diacylglycerol (DAG) and inositol 1,4,5-triphosphate, are regulated by gonadotropin, prostaglandin, and GnRH exposure in ovarian cells (8–11).

Lipid-dependent protein kinases have been documented in ovarian tissues (12–17). C-kinase is the recognized receptor for DAG (3). C-kinase, or protein kinase C, was first described as a proenzyme for a proteolytically activated kinase, protein kinase M, now recognized to be a proteolytically generated fragment containing the catalytic region of the intact enzyme. Recognition that the intact C-kinase could be catalytically active in the presence of Ca^{++} and phospholipid led C-kinase to be referred to as Ca^{++}-activated phospholipid-dependent protein kinase. Kinetic studies revealed a role for DAG in the activation of C-kinase. The recognition of structural similarity of active tumor-promoting phorbol esters to DAG and the demonstration that C-kinase was subject to activation by phorbol ester led to recognition of C-kinase as the major cellular phorbol ester receptor (3).

The early description of the C-kinase activation mechanism implicated DAG as a factor that increases the sensitivity of C-kinase to Ca^{++} such that lower Ca^{++} concentrations are sufficient to activate the enzyme (in the presence of phospholipid) (3). Further kinetic studies refined the classical model of C-kinase activation. In the more recent classical C-kinase activation models, the binding of DAG, or its analog phorbol ester, is considered to comprise activation of C-kinase, and the role of Ca^{++} is to promote binding of C-kinase to phospholipid, in phospholipid-containing micelles, vesicles, or membranes. The binding step allows access of the lipid-soluble activating species, DAG or phorbol ester, to the appropriate site on the enzyme (18). In both the older classical Ca^{++}-activation model and the more recent classical diacylglycerol/phorbol ester-activation model, Ca^{++} is a positive effector, required directly or indirectly for the activation of C-kinase.

A variety of studies have suggested that the classical description of C-kinase activation does not completely describe the set of activities attributable to C-kinase or C-kinase-like enzymes. Ca^{++}-independent as well as Ca^{++}-dependent C-kinase activities have been described. Alternate C-kinase activators in addition to the DAG/phorbol esters have been documented, including free fatty acids (19), polyphosphorylated phosphatidylinositol derivatives (20, 21), and lysophospholipids (22). According to Murakami et al. (19), activation of C-kinase by free fatty acid was not dependent on Ca^{++}. A purified phorbol ester receptor was shown to possess Ca^{++}-independent kinase activity (23). Two classes of substrates were subject to phosphorylation by purified C-kinase in the absence of Ca^{++} (24). Phosphorylation of a peptide substrate by partially purified C-kinase was shown to be maximal in the presence of EGTA and phorbol esters (25).

Additional kinase activities regulated by phospholipid and phospholipid/ (DAG or phorbol ester) have been described. These include a Mn^{++}-dependent phospholipid-dependent protein kinase (26), the protease-activated S6 kinase PAK II (27) and a phorbol ester-sensitive kinase activity resolvable from C-kinase (28).

The recognition that C-kinase exists as a multienzyme family rather than a single entity was based on both biochemical and genetic observations (29 and 30, for reviews). There are mechanistic as well as physiological implications to the multiplicity of C-kinase forms. Mechanistically, the existence of

Ca^{++}-independent as well as Ca^{++}-dependent forms of C-kinase could reconcile the findings of both Ca^{++}-independent and Ca^{++}-dependent activities attributable to C-kinase (29, 30). The physiological roles for the different forms of C-kinase are not defined, but different patterns of distribution during development, as well as different tissue and cellular distribution patterns suggest the isotypes may have different functions. Three forms of C-kinase, called types I, II and III, were resolved biochemically by hydroxylapatite chromatography (31). Four closely-related members of the C-kinase family were originally delineated by genetic means, comprising α, $\beta 1$, $\beta 2$, and γ isotypes of C-kinase. α, β, and γ are products of independent genes. $\beta 1$ and $\beta 2$ forms arise from a common gene by alternate splicing. Hydroxylapatite-resolved type I C-kinase activity has been attributed to the γ isotype, type II activity to the $\beta 1/\beta 2$ isotypes, and type III activity has been attributed to the α isotype. The four original members of the C-kinase family demonstrate some minor biochemical differences, but, as reviewed by Parker et al. (30), the majority of studies indicate these isotypes to be Ca^{++}-dependent. Additional members of the C-kinase family, comprising δ, ϵ, and ζ isotypes, have lower degrees of structural homology and biochemical similarity to the originally described members of the C-kinase family (32). The ϵ C-kinase is a Ca^{++}-independent kinase form (33, 34). The other additional members show some similar missing gene sequences (C2 region), relative to the classical isotypes. The missing sequences are located in the regulatory region of the molecule, so these distant C-kinase isotypes may be Ca^{++}-independent as well (29). Several groups have reported hydroxylapatite-resolved lipid-dependent kinase activities in addition to the recognized C-kinase isotypes (35–37).

We initiated studies to identify endogenous substrates for lipid-dependent protein kinases in ovarian soluble extracts. We observed a rat ovarian phosphorylation activity with certain characteristics in common with the C-kinases as classically described, but demonstrating variant responsiveness to Ca^{++} (38). We have found the variant phospholipid/diacylglycerol-dependent phosphorylation activity in soluble extracts prepared from a variety of ovarian tissues. The phosphorylation of an endogenous substrate ($M_r = 80,000$ in rat extracts; $M_r = 76,000$ in rabbit extracts) was observed in the presence of EGTA, phosphatidylserine and DAG. Inclusion of Ca^{++} blocked rather than enhanced phosphate incorporation into the endogenous substrate. This variant lipid-dependent phosphorylation system was found to be regulated by in vivo estrogen exposure in the rabbit corpus luteum of pseudopregnancy (manuscript in preparation). The estrogen regulatory response as well as the prominence of the variant lipid-dependent phosphorylation reaction in rabbit luteal soluble extracts has led us to pursue definition of the variant lipid-dependent protein phosphotransferase activity of the rabbit corpus luteum.

Materials and Methods

Biochemical reagents were purchased from Sigma Chemical Company (St. Louis, MO) unless otherwise indicated. [γ^{32}P]ATP (ammonium salt, specific activity 1000–4000 Ci/mM) and [^{125}I]protein A were purchased from ICN Chemical and Radioisotope Division (Irvine, CA). SDS polyacrylamide gel electrophoresis reagents and hydroxylapatite were purchased from Bio-Rad (Richmond, CA). Female New Zealand white rabbits (7 kg) were obtained from American-Scientific (retired breeders) and used on day 7 of pseudo-pregnancy. Pseudopregnancy was induced by injection of 100 IU human chorionic gonadotropin from Ayerest Laboratories, Inc. (NY) in 0.9% (w/v) NaCl.

Soluble Extract Preparation. Rabbit luteal cytosol was prepared by homogenization of corpora lutea from 4 day-7 pseudopregnant rabbits in 36 volumes of homogenization buffer (10-mM Tris (pH 7.0), 3-mM $MgCl_2$, 0.32-M sucrose, and 25-mM benzamidine), followed by centrifugation at $105,000 \times g$ for 60 min at 4°C. Supernatant was collected for use as soluble extract. Protein concentrations in soluble extracts, measured by the method of Lowry et al. (39), ranged from 1.2 to 1.6 mg/mL, using crystalline bovine serum albumin as a standard.

DEAE Cellulose Chromatography. Rabbit luteal soluble extracts (total protein of 13.7 to 21 mg) were applied to columns (2 cm × 6 cm) of Whatman DE 52 DEAE cellulose equilibrated in 10-mM potassium phosphate, pH 7.0. Columns were washed, then eluted with 60-mL gradients (10-mM–300-mM $KHPO_4$, with 1.0-mM EGTA and 25-mM benzamidine), collecting 0.75-mL fractions. Column fraction aliquots were assayed for protamine phosphotransferase activity and histone III-S phosphotransferase activity as indicated. Conductivities of eluted fractions were determined using a radiometer conductivity meter calibrated against the phosphate elution buffers.

Protamine Phosphotransferase Assay. 50-μL column fraction aliquots were assayed in a final volume of 260μL in the presence of 26.7-mM α-glycerol phosphate (pH 7.0), 0.8-mM dithiothreitol, 8.0-mM MgAc, 2.6-mM theophylline, 7.8-mM NaF, 0.3-μM cAMP, 50-μM [γ^{32}P]ATP (40 cpm/pM), and 100-μg/sample protamine, by incubation at 37°C for 10 min. Reactions were stopped by the addition of 3 mL cold 10% trichloroacetic acid and 1% sodium docedyl sulfate. The precipitated [^{32}P]phosphoproteins were collected by vacuum filtration on Millipore HAWP 025, 0.45-μm pore-size filters and quantitated by liquid scintillation spectrometry.

Histone III-S Phosphotransferase Assay. 100-μL column fraction aliquots were assayed in a final volume of 230 μL in the presence of 43.4-mM αglycerolphosphate (pH 7.0), 8.7-mM $MgCl_2$, 70-μM [γ^{32}P]ATP (70 cpm/ pM), 50-μg/sample histone III-S, with or without 43-μg/mL phosphatidylserine and 1.1-μg/mL 1,2-diolein, and with or without 0.434-mM $CaCl_2$. +Ca^{++} samples contained 1.3×10^{-5}M free Ca^{++}, calculated using Kd = 2.1×10^{-7}M for Ca^{++}/EGTA complex and Kd = 9.0×10^{-3}M for Mg^{++}/EGTA complex at pH 7.0 (40). −Ca^{++} samples contained 0.47-mM EGTA and no calcium additions. Samples were incubated for 10 min at 37°C, then stopped by the addition of cold 25% trichloroacetic acid. The precipitated [^{32}P]phosphoproteins were collected by vacuum filtration on Millipore HAWP 025, 0.45-μm pore-size filters and quantitated by liquid scintillation spectrometry.

Phosphorylation Incubation (In Vitro Phosphorylation of Endogenous Substrate). Phosphorylation of column fraction aliquots was carried out in an incubation volume of 220 μL, containing 100 μL of reaction buffer (10-μM α-glycerol phosphate buffer (pH 7.0), 100-nM dithiothreitol, 2-μM $MgCl_2$, 1-nM ATP), 100-μL eluant aliquot, and additions as indicated below. Preincubation was performed for 3 min at 37°C, then experimental incubation was initiated by the addition of [γ^{32}P]ATP (5.0 μCi per 0.22-mL sample) in the presence or absence of various test additions. Additions included phospholipid (phosphatidylserine, 45 μg/mL), 1,2-diolein (1,2-*sn*- or *rac*-dioleoylglycerol, 1.1 μg/mL) and either $CaCl_2$ (0.45 mM) or EGTA (0.45 mM). +Ca^{++} samples contained 1.4×10^{-5}M free Ca^{++}, calculated using Kd = 2.1×10^{-7}M for Ca^{++}/EGTA complex and Kd = 9.0×10^{-3}M for Mg^{++}/EGTA complex at pH 7.0 (40). −Ca^{++} samples contained 0.9-mM EGTA (final) and no calcium additions. Incubation was performed at 37°C for 1 min, then terminated by addition of 100 μL of SDS stop solution (3% SDS, 150-mM Tris-HCl (pH 6.8), 2.4-mM EDTA, 3% β-mercaptoethanol, 30% glycerol, and 0.5% bromphenol blue) and heat denaturation (100°C, 5 min).

Electrophoresis, Autoradiography and Quantitation of ^{32}P Incorporation. [^{32}P]phosphoproteins were separated by SDS polyacrylamide gel electrophoresis as described by Rudolph and Krueger (41), using 4 or 5% stacking gels and 8.5% separating gels. Molecular weight standards were myosin heavy-chain, β-galactosidase, phosphorylase b, bovine serum albumin, ovalbumin, carbonic anhydrase, and soybean trypsin inhibitor. Autoradiography was performed by exposure of dried gels to Kodak XRP-5 or XAR-5 film for 2 to 14 days. Quantitation of ^{32}P incorporation was performed by densitometric scanning of autoradiograms, using Zeineh laser densitometer with a Hewlett Packard 3390A integrator.

Western Immunoblot. Following SDS-PAGE in the presence of prestained electrophoresis standards (Diversified Biotech), proteins were electrophoretically transferred from the gel slabs to Nytran sheets (0.2 μm,

Schleicher and Schuell) in 25-mM Tris base, 192-mM glycine, 20% (v/v) methanol, pH 8.3, at room temperature overnight at 0.1 A in Hoeffer transfer apparatus. Nytran sheets were blocked in buffer containing 10-mM potassium phospate (pH 7.4), 0.15-M NaCl (PBS), and 5% (w/v) Carnation nonfat dry milk, at 4°C for 30 min. Primary antibody (sheep anti-protein kinase C, obtained from Dr. K. Leach, Upjohn Co., Kalamazoo, MI, used at 1:500 dilution) was added to fresh blocking buffer and incubated with blots overnight at 4°C on a Nutator (Adams). Blots were washed successively in PBS buffer, in PBS buffer containing 0.15% Triton X-100, and PBS buffer. Blots were then incubated with secondary antibody (goat anti-sheep antibody, used at 1:500 dilution) in fresh blocking buffer at room temperature for 30 min, subjected to the washing protocol described above, incubated with fresh blocking buffer containing [^{125}I]protein A (about 1-μCi per lane) for 30 min at room temperature, washed, dried, and exposed to Kodak XAR-5 film.

Results

In order to resolve and define the complement of soluble rabbit luteal protein kinase activities, soluble extracts were prepared from pseudopregnant rabbit corpora lutea and subjected to DEAE cellulose chromatography. Eluant fractions were evaluated for phosphotransferase activities by several different techniques. Protamine phosphotransferase assay detects both cAMP-dependent protein kinases (A-kinases) and C-kinases. Ca^{++}- and lipid-dependent histone III-S phosphotransferase assay detects C-kinases. C-kinase was also assessed immunologically by Western blot analysis. Endogenous substrate phosphorylation, performed in the presence of EGTA, phosphatidylserine and 1,2-diolein, was used as a measure of variant lipid-dependent phosphotransferase activity.

DEAE cellulose chromatographic separation of rabbit luteal cytosol resolved several peaks of protamine phosphotransferase activity (Fig. 1, panels A–C). The second shoulder of the first phosphotransferase peak revealed characteristics of C-kinase. That shoulder of protamine phosphotransferase activity was not regulated by cAMP, as shown in panel B. The second shoulder of the first protamine phosphotransferase peak corresponded to a peak of Ca^{++}- and lipid-dependent histone III-S phosphotransferase activity as shown in panel C. We have also shown that luteal Ca^{++}- and lipid-dependent histone III-S phosphotransferase activity co-eluted from DEAE cellulose with lower levels of lipid-dependent histone III-S phosphotransferase activity assayed in the presence of EGTA (not shown).

To confirm the presence of C-kinase in eluted fractions, the DEAE eluant fraction aliquots were subjected to SDS polyacrylamide gel electrophoresis, electrotransfer, and Western blot analysis, using a polyspecific polyclonal

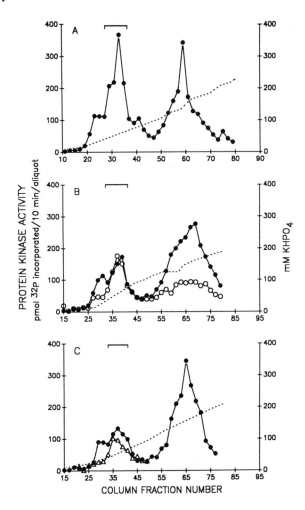

FIGURE 1. DEAE cellulose column profile of phosphotransferase activities. Each of the panels represents a separate DEAE cellulose column profile. (Closed circles indicate protamine phosphotransferase activity, assayed in the presence of 0.3-μM cAMP; open circles (panel B) indicate protamine phosphotransferase activity, assayed in the absence of cAMP; open triangles (panel C) indicate histone III-S phosphotransferase activity assayed in the presence of Ca^{++}, phosphatidylserine, and 1,2-diolein; and dashed lines indicate $KHPO_4$ concentration determined by conductivity measurement.) Eluant fractions of column shown in panel A were used for Western immunoblot analysis and endogenous substrate phosphorylation incubations.

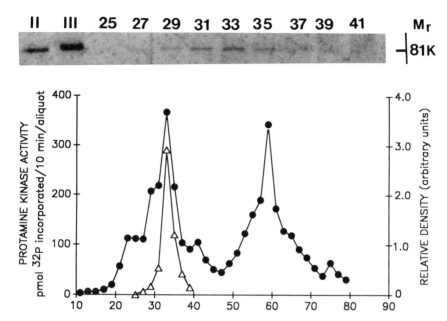

FIGURE 2. Western immunoblot showing the presence of immunoreactive C-kinase in the DEAE cellulose eluant fractions. Western immunoblot was performed according to methods given in text. In the autoradiogram shown in the upper panel, fraction numbers are indicated above lanes. Control lanes (indicated as II and III) contained rat spleen hydroxylapatite-resolved type II and type III C-kinase peaks, respectively. The lower panel shows densitometric quantitation of immunoblot autoradiogram at the $M_r = 81,000$ migration position (indicated as open triangles). Protamine kinase profile (closed circles), as shown in Figure 1, panel A, is included for comparison.

anti-C-kinase antiserum. Results are shown in Figure 2. Several immunoreactive bands were observed in eluant fractions. We noted the presence of an 80- to 82-kDa immunoreactive band, maximal in the fractions corresponding to the peak of C-kinase identified by protamine phosphotransferase assay.

DEAE cellulose eluant fractions from the column shown in panel A were evaluated for lipid-dependent endogenous 76-kDa phosphotransferase activity. Column fraction aliquots were subjected to phosphorylation incubations in the presence of EGTA, phosphatidylserine, and 1,2-diolein, followed by SDS-PAGE and autoradiography. The resulting autoradiogram is shown in Figure 3, panel a. Lipid-dependent 76-kDa phosphotransferase activity is maximal in fraction 33. This fraction corresponds to the peak of C-kinase, identified by protamine phosphotransferase assay (Fig. 1) and immunoreactivity (Fig. 2).

Effector dependence of the peak of 76-kDa phosphotransferase activity was evaluated. Aliquots of DEAE column fraction 32 were subjected to phosphory-

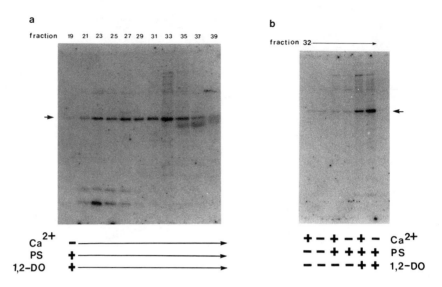

FIGURE 3. Endogenous substrate phosphorylation in DEAE cellulose eluant fractions. *(a)*: Phosphorylation incubations performed on column fractions aliquots (fraction numbers indicated above lanes). *(b)*: Phosphorylation incubations using phosphotransferase peak (fraction 32) in the presence or absence of various effectors. ($+Ca^{++}$ = 0.45-mM $CaCl_2$, 1.4×10^{-5}M free Ca^{++}; $-Ca^{++}$ = 0.9-mM EGTA; PS = phosphatidylserine, 45 µg/mL; 1,2-DO = 1,2-diolein, 1.1 µg/mL; arrow indicates the migration position of endogenous 76-kDa phosphorylation substrate.)

lation incubation in the presence or absence of Ca^{++}, in the presence or absence of phosphatidylserine, and in the presence or absence of 1,2-diolein. The resulting autoradiogram is shown in Figure 3, panel *b*. Maximal phosphorylation of the 76-kDa substrate was seen in the presence of EGTA, phosphatidylserine and 1,2-diolein. This pattern of responsiveness to effectors corresponds to the variant effector dependence, which we have previously observed in the evaluation of endogenous substrate phosphorylation by unresolved soluble extracts of ovarian tissues. We have thus confirmed that the DEAE-resolved lipid-dependent 76-kDa phosphotransferase activity demonstrated the variant effector dependence previously described in cytosol.

Discussion

We have previously observed that ovarian soluble extracts, which are subjected to phosphorylation conditions, catalyze the lipid-dependent phosphorylation of an endogenous substrate as demonstrated by SDS-PAGE and autoradiography. This lipid-dependent phosphotransferase activity resembled C-kinase as classically described in that it required phosphatidylserine and was active in the presence of the 1,2-diacylglycerol/1,2-diolein. However, in contrast to C-kinase activities as classically described, the ovarian lipid-dependent phosphotransferase activity was maximal in the presence of EGTA and was reduced by the inclusion of Ca^{++} over a wide range of Ca^{++} concentrations.

Luteal soluble extracts were subjected to DEAE cellulose chromatography to effect partial purification of C-kinase and the lipid-dependent endogenous substrate phosphotransferase activity. At the level of DEAE cellulose chromatography, the activities of interest co-eluted. At this level of purification we observed a single peak of C-kinase, assessed by protamine kinase assay and Western immunoblot analysis, corresponding to the peak of Ca^{++}- and lipid-dependent histone kinase activity in a parallel column. We have also measured lipid-dependent histone III-S kinase activity in the presence of EGTA in rabbit luteal DEAE-resolved eluant fractions (not shown). The EGTA and lipid-dependent histone activity was demonstrated to co-elute with the Ca^{++} and lipid-dependent histone kinase activity at this level of purification.

Lipid-dependent endogenous substrate phosphotransferase activity was assessed in the DEAE-resolved eluant fractions and found to co-elute with C-kinase. Effector dependence was evaluated, and it followed the variant pattern that we have previously described with maximal activity in the presence of EGTA, phosphatidylserine, and 1,2-diolein. The inclusion of added Ca^{++} inhibited rather than enhanced phosphorylation of the endogenous substrate. We have concluded that the variant response pattern, retained following DEAE chromotography, is not due to a DEAE-resolvable Ca^{++}-dependent inhibitor of C-kinase in unpurified extracts. These results confirm observations made on rat luteal DEAE-resolved lipid-dependent kinase (38).

The relation of the variant luteal lipid-dependent phosphotransferase activity to the C-kinase family is not yet defined. Further resolution of the complement of luteal lipid-dependent phosphotransferase activities can be obtained using hydroxylapatite gel chromatography. Phosphotransferase activity associated with C-kinase or the variant endogenous-substrate lipid-dependent phosphotransferase, which appeared as a single peak following DEAE cellulose chromatography, eluted from hydroxylapatite resin under a compound peak comprised of two or possibly more protamine phosphotransferase shoulders (manuscript in preparation).

Several arguments suggest that the observed ovarian variant lipid-dependent phosphotransferase is a member of the broader C-kinase family. The various members of the C-kinase family resolvable by hydroxylapatite are recognized to elute in a single peak from DEAE cellulose columns (42). Co-elution of the ovarian lipid-dependent phosphotransferase with C-kinase from DEAE cellulose is consistent with the membership of the ovarian variant lipid-dependent phosphotransferase in the broader C-kinase family. Likewise, sensitivity of the ovarian phosphotransferase to the 1,2-diacylglycerol/1,2-diolein in the presence of phosphatidylserine is consistent with membership in the broader C-kinase family. The ovarian lipid-dependent 76-kDa phosphotransferase activity would not likely comprise the type I (γ) form of C-kinase, which has been described to be restricted to the central nervous system (29). The ovarian phosphotransferase activity is not likely to correspond to either the type II (β1, β2) C-kinases or type III (α) C-kinase on the basis of sensitivity to effectors (30). In addition, the ^{32}P-labeled variant lipid-dependent phosphorylation substrate, detected in a comparable DEAE-resolved rat luteal phosphotransferase preparation, could be distinguished from autophosphorylated C-kinase types II and III on the basis of minor size differences (38). The ovarian lipid-dependent phosphotransferase activity does not comprise the ε form of C-kinase. The variant ovarian activity a shows lipid-dependent histone III-S phosphotransferase activity, while ε C-kinase is not a histone kinase (34). Furthermore, autophosphorylated ε C-kinase migrates on SDS-PAGE as a 90-kDa band, a higher migration position than our observed phosphoprotein band (33). Antiserum to nPKC (identical to ε C-kinase) is poorly reactive to not reactive with samples of resolved ovarian lipid-dependent 76-kDa phosphotransferase activity (manuscript in preparation). Other C-kinase forms include the δ and ζ forms (32), which have not been completely characterized, and a recently-described additional member (37). Other related described kinases include the S6-kinase protease activated kinase type II described by Traugh and coworkers (27); a heparin-agarose purified, Ca^{++}-independent, lipid-dependent histone kinase purified from membrane extracts of several tissues (43); and a hydroxylapatite-resolved, Ca^{++}-inhibited, lipid-dependent kinase described in brain extracts (35).

Acknowledgments. We thank Dr. Karen Leach (Upjohn Co., Kalamazoo, MI) for the gift of the anti-C-kinase antiserum used in the present study. The research reported in this chapter was supported by NIH grant HD-11356 (to MHD), by NSF grant DCB-415927 (to JBM), and by University of Illinois CRB grant 4031 (to JBM).

References

1. Edelman AM, Blumenthal DK, Krebs EG. Protein serine/threonine kinases. Annu Rev Biochem 1987;56:567-613.
2. Berridge MJ. Inositol trisphosphate and diacylglycerol: Two interacting second messengers. Annu Rev Biochem 1987;56:159-93.
3. Nishizuka Y. The role of protein kinase C in cell surface signal transduction and tumour promotion. Nature 1984;308:693-8.

4. Hunzicker-Dunn M. Selective activation of rabbit ovarian protein kinase iso-zymes in rabbit ovarian follicles and corpora lutea. J Biol Chem 1981;256: 12185-93.
5. Richards JS, Jahnsen T, Hedin L, et al. Ovarian follicular development: From physiology to molecular biology. Recent Prog Horm Res 1987;43:231-76.
6. Hedin L, McKnight GS, Lifka J, Durica JM, Richards JS. Tissue distribution and hormonal regulation of messenger ribonucleic acid for regulatory and catalytic subunits of adenosine 3', 5'-monophosphate-dependent protein kinases during ovarian follicular development and luteinization in the rat. Endocrinology 1987;120:1928-35.
7. Rao MC, Palfrey HC, Nash NT, Greisman A, Jayatilak, PG, Gibori G. Effects of estradiol on calcium-specific protein phosphorylation in the rat corpus luteum. Endocrinology 1987;120:1010-8.
8. Davis JS, Weakland LL, Farese RV, West LA. Luteinizing hormone increases inositol trisphosphate and cytosolic free Ca^{2+} in isolated bovine luteal cells. J Biol Chem 1987;262:8515-21.
9. Davis JS, Weakland LL, Weiland DA, Farese RV, West LA. Prostaglandin $F_{2\alpha}$ stimulates phosphatidylinositol-4, 5-biphosphate hydrolysis and mobilizes intra-cellular Ca^{2+} in bovine luteal cells. Proc Natl Acad Sci USA 1987;84:3728-32.
10. Leung PCK, Minegishi T, Ma F, Zhow F, Ho-Yuen B. Induction of polyphospho-inositide breakdown in rat corpus luteum by prostaglandin $F_{2\alpha}$. Endocrinology 1986;119:12-8.
11. Ma F, Leung PCK. Luteinizing hormone-releasing hormone enhances poly-phosphoinositide breakdown in rat granulosa cells. Biochem Biophys Res Commun 1985;130:1201-8.
12. Davis JS, Clark MR. Activation of protein kinase in the bovine corpus luteum by phospholipid and Ca^{2+}. Biochem J 1983;214:569-74.
13. Wheeler MB, Veldhuis JD. Catalytic and receptor-binding properties of the calcium-sensitive phospholipid-dependent protein kinase (protein kinase C) in swine luteal cytosol. Mol Cell Endocrinol 1987;50:123-9.
14. Noland TA, Jr, Dimino MJ. Characterization and distribution of protein kinase C in ovarian tissue. Biol Reprod 1986;35:863-72.
15. Hoyer PB, Kong W. Protein kinase A and C activities and endogenous substrates in ovine small and large luteal cells. Mol Cell Endocrinol 1989;62:203-15.
16. Su H-D, Mazzei GJ, Vogler WR, Kuo JF. Effect of tamoxifen, a nonsteroidal antiestrogen on phospholipid/calcium-dependent protein kinase and phosphory-lation of its endogenous substrate proteins from the rat brain and ovary. Biochem Pharmacol 1985;34:3649-53.
17. Dowd JP, Alila HW, Hansel W. Phorbol ester receptors in bovine luteal cells: Relationship to protein kinase C. Mol Cell Endocrinol 1990;69:199-206.
18. Bell RM. Protein kinase C activation by diacylglycerol second messengers. Cell 1986;45:631-2.
19. Murakami K, Chan SY, Routtenberg A. Protein kinase C activation by cis-fatty acid in the absence of Ca^{2+} and phospholipids. J Biol Chem 1986;261:15424-9.
20. O'Brian CA, Arthur WL, Weinstein IB. The activation of protein kinase C by the polyphosphoinositides phosphatidylinositol 4,5-diphosphate and phospha-tidylinositol 4-monophosphate. FEBS Lett 1987;214:339-42.

21. Chauhan A, Chauhan VPS, Deshmukh DS, Brockerhoff H. Phosphatidylinositol 4,5-bisphosphate competitively inhibits phorbol ester binding to protein kinase C. Biochemistry 1989;28:4952-6.
22. Oishi K, Raynor RL, Charp PA, Kuo JF. Regulation of protein kinase C by lysophospholipids: Potential role in signal transduction. J Biol Chem 1988; 263:6865-71.
23. Shoyab M, Boaze R. Isolation and characterization of a specific receptor for biologically active phorbol and ingenol esters. Arch Biochem Biophys 1984;234: 197-205.
24. Bazzi MD, Nelsestuen GL. Role of substrate in imparting calcium and phospholipid requirements to protein kinase C activation. Biochemistry 1987;26:1974-82.
25. O'Brian CA, Lawrence DS, Kaiser ET, Weinstein IB. Protein kinase C phosphorylates the synthetic peptide arg-arg-lys-ala-ser-gly-pro-pro-val in the presence of phospholipid plus either Ca^{2+} or a phorbol ester tumor promotor. Biochem Biophys Res Commun 1984;124:296-302.
26. Klemm DJ, Elias L. A distinctive phospholipid-stimulated protein kinase of normal and malignant murine hemopoietic cells. J Biol Chem 1987;262:7580-85.
27. Gonzatti-Haces MI, Traugh JA. Ca^{2+}-independent activation of protease-activated kinase II by phospholipids/diolein and comparison with the Ca^{2+}/phospholipid-dependent protein kinase. J Biol Chem 1986;261:15266-72.
28. Malviya AN, Louis J-C, Zwiller J. Separation from protein kinase C—a calcium-independent TPA-activated phosphorylating system. FEBS Lett 1986;199:213-6.
29. Nishizuka Y. The molecular heterogeneity of protein kinase C and its implications for cellular regulation. Nature 1988;334:661-5.
30. Parker PJ, Kour G, Marais RM, et al. Protein kinase C—a family affair. Mol Cell Endocrinol 1989;65:1-11.
31. Huang K-P, Nakabayashi H, Huang FL. Isozymic forms of rat brain Ca^{2+}-activated and phospholipid-dependent protein kinase. Proc Natl Acad Sci USA 1986;83:8535-9.
32. Ono Y, Fujii T, Ogita K, Kikkawa U, Igarashi K, Nishizuka Y. The structure, expression and properties of additional members of the protein kinase C family. J Biol Chem 1988;263:6927-32.
33. Ohno S, Akita Y, Konno Y, Imajoh S, Suzuki K. A novel phorbol ester receptor/protein kinase, nPKC, distantly related to the protein kinase C family. Cell 1988;53:731-41.
34. Schaap D, Parker PJ, Bristol A, Kriz R, Knopf J. Unique substrate specificity and regulatory properties of PKC-ε: A rationale for diversity. FEBS Lett 1989;243:351-7.
35. Farago A, Farkas G, Meszaros G, Buday L, Antoni F, Seprodi J. Isoenzyme patterns of protein kinase C and a phospholipid-dependent but Ca^{2+}-inhibited enzyme fraction in the crude extracts of different tissues. FEBS Lett 1989;243:328-32.
36. Ryves WJ, Garland LG, Evans AT, Evans FJ. A phorbol ester and a daphnane ester stimulate a calcium-independent kinase activity from human mononuclear cells. FEBS Lett 1989;245:159-63.
37. Hashimoto K, Kishimoto A, Aihara H, Yasuda I, Mikawa K, Nishizuka Y.

Protein kinase C during differentiation of human promyelocytic leukemia cell line, HL-60. FEBS Lett 1990;263:31-4.

38. Maizels ET, Miller JB, Cutler RE, Jr., et al. Calcium-independent phospholipid/diolein-dependent phosphorylation of a soluble ovarian M_r = 80,000 substrate protein: Biochemical characteristics. Biochim Biophys Acta 1990 (in press).

39. Lowry OH, Rosebrough NJ, Farr AL, Randall RJ. Protein measurement with the Folin phenol reagent. J Biol Chem 1951;193:265-75.

40. Grynkiewicz G, Poenie M, Tsien RY. A new generation of Ca^{2+} indicators with greatly improved fluorescence properties. J Biol Chem 1985;260:3440-50.

41. Rudolph SA, Krueger BK. Endogenous protein phosphorylation and dephosphorylation. Adv Cyclic Nucleotide Res 1979;10:107-33.

42. Marais RM, Parker PJ. Purification and characterization of bovine brain protein kinase C isotypes α, β and γ. Eur J Biochem 1989;182:129-37.

43. Gschwendt M, Leibersperger H, Marks F. Differentiative action of K252a on protein kinase C and a calcium-unresponsive, phorbol ester/phospholipid-activated protein kinase. Biochem Biophys Res Commun 1989;164:974-82.

6

Endocrine, Paracrine, and Autocrine Regulators of the Macaque Corpus Luteum

RICHARD L. STOUFFER

The 1980s witnessed important advances in our understanding of the function and regulation of the primate corpus luteum during the menstrual cycle and early pregnancy. The corpus luteum in women and nonhuman primates produces at least four substances that may have important endocrine actions during the luteal phase of the cycle or in early pregnancy: progesterone, estradiol, inhibin, and relaxin. Following the lead of research on the antecedent follicle, investigators are considering whether local factors combine with classical hormones to control the function or lifespan of the corpus luteum. Novel approaches are providing intriguing evidence that the primate corpus luteum consists of dynamic subpopulations of luteal cells that differ in function as well as responsiveness to endocrine and paracrine factors. This report will focus on the subcellular, cellular, and whole animal studies in the author's laboratory that employed the rhesus monkey as a model for understanding primate luteal function. Recent advances have not solved, indeed have generated, many controversies, and critical gaps in our knowledge will be illustrated.

Luteal Development and the LH Surge

It seems assured that the mid-cycle surge of luteinizing hormone (LH) from the anterior pituitary is the initiator of ovulation and luteinization of the periovulatory follicle. Yet few studies have been directed towards understanding the cascade of events underlying luteal development following the LH surge. Variability in the length of the follicular phase (8–16 days) and labor-intensive procedures required to time precisely the onset, magnitude, and duration of the LH surge in spontaneous cycles make such studies difficult. The development of treatment regimens that stimulate the growth of multiple preovulatory follicles (1) for oocyte collection and in vitro fertilization (IVF) offers a model for such research. Since spontaneous surges do not generally occur in these artificial cycles, one can precisely define the point at which follicles are first exposed to the ovulatory/luteinization stimulus as the time of hCG injection. Events that follow within minutes to days can be investigated in detail with tissue from a dozen or more luteinizing follicles.

Based on earlier studies examining the distribution of progesterone receptors (PR) in the macaque ovary (see later discussion; 2), we used the artificial IVF cycles to test the hypothesis that the mid-cycle LH surge induces the expression of PR in luteinizing granulosa cells in the developing corpus luteum (3). Exogenous human gonadotropins (FSH and LH, Serono Metrodin and Pergonal) were administered to monkeys for 9 days to stimulate development of large follicles (1). Granulosa cells were collected by follicle aspiration either before or 27 h after an hCG bolus of 1000 IU (Serono Profasi) designed to initiate ovulatory maturation. Cells collected before the hCG bolus failed to stain immunocytochemically for the presence of PR and produced little progesterone during 24-h incubation in vitro in the absence of gonadotropins. In contrast, the majority (up to 80%) of granulosa cells collected after the hCG bolus were intensely PR positive and produced large quantities of progesterone in vitro. The data suggest that the ovulatory stimulus (i.e., the LH surge in spontaneous cycles or the hCG bolus in artificial cycles) not only stimulates the developing luteal tissue to synthesize progesterone for endocrine actions outside the ovary, but also promotes PR expression for local effects of progesterone in luteal cells. Thus, one action of the LH surge may be to promote cellular recognition of paracrine or autocrine factors that become predominant in the developing corpus luteum.

The duration of the LH surge in normal ovarian cycles of women and rhesus monkeys (48–50 h; 4) is considerably longer than that in rats and rabbits (4–8 h; 5) or sheep and cows (10–16 h; 6). Whether the prolonged LH surge is required for ovulatory maturation of the follicle and its enclosed oocyte in primates is not known. Zelinski-Wooten (7) and Aladin Chandrasekher and colleagues (8) have provided studies titrating the periovulatory LH requirements for follicles in artificial IVF cycles of rhesus monkeys. Again, exogenous pituitary gonadotropins (hFSH and hLH) were given for 9 days to stimulate development of large follicles. On day 10, animals received (a) 1000-IU hCG im, (b) 1 or 3 sc injections of 100-μg GnRH (Serono Relisorm) at 3-h intervals, or (c) 2 sc injections of 50-μg GnRH agonist (GnRHa, TAP Lupron) at 8-h intervals. As summarized in Table 1, hCG treatment markedly elevated circulating gonadotropin levels for 3–4 days. GnRH injection increased circulating levels of bioactive LH

TABLE 1. Comparison of protocols that produce surge levels of gonadotropins with subsequent periovulatory events in follicles of rhesus monkeys during artificial IVF cycles.

Ovulatory Stimulus[1]	Interval of Gonadotropin Surge (hours)	Oocyte Maturation[2] (% M1 + M2)	Granulosa Cells[3]		Luteal Phase[4] (days)
			PR Expression (±)	Progesterone Production (ng/mL)	
None	0	13	–	19	0
GnRH, 100 µg × 1	6	0	–	35	0
GnRH, 100 µg × 3	10	43	2(–), 1(+)	61	2(0), 1(7)
GnRHa, 50 µg × 2	+14	12	–	105	0
hCG, 1000 IU	96	86	+	680	12

Source: Adapted from references 7 and 8.

[1] On day 10 of artificial IVF cycles, monkeys (n = 3–6 group) received various treatments to elevate circulating gonadotropin levels; see text for details.

[2] Percent oocytes that reached metaphase I or II (M1 + M2) at the time of follicle aspiration, as detected following hyaluronidase treatment of cumulus-oocyte complex.

[3] Cells were stained immunocytochemically for progesterone receptor (PR) and also incubated in vitro for 24 h to assess P production (ng/mL/8 × 10^4 cells).

[4] Interval of progesterone levels above baseline or from day 10 until menses.

from baseline (11 ng/mL) to >400 ng/mL within 1–2 h; multiple injections of GnRH or GnRHa extended the interval of the LH surge to 8 and >14 h, respectively. When follicles were aspirated 27 h after the hCG injection, 86% of the collected oocytes had re-entered meiosis (metaphase I or II). In contrast, few of the oocytes collected 27 h after the initial GnRH/GnRHa injections exhibited meiotic activity (with the exception of those from one monkey in the GnRH × 3 group). Many of the granulosa cells in follicular aspirates of hCG-treated monkeys stained positively via immunocytochemistry for progesterone receptor (PR). However, cells from only one animal in the GnRH/GnRHa groups exhibited detectable PR staining. During 24-h culture, basal progesterone production by granulosa cells from hCG-treated monkeys was higher than that by cells from GnRH/GnRHa groups. Finally, hCG treatment increased circulating progesterone to peak levels of 30-40 ng/mL and elicited functional luteal phases of 11–12 days. In contrast, only one animal in the GnRH/GnRHa groups displayed elevated progesterone levels in the luteal phase.

Collectively, the data indicate that LH exposure reminiscent of gonadotropin surges in rodents or domestic animals is insufficient to routinely reinitiate meiotic maturation of oocytes or to support the development/

function of the corpus luteum in primates. Whereas the hCG treatment used in these studies will induce ovulation (9), it is unlikely that the GnRH/GnRHa regimens will achieve follicle rupture. There is evidence that attenuated LH surges of 24–38 h will induce ovulatory changes in follicles during artificial IVF cycles in women (10), but further studies titrating the LH requirements for oocyte maturation, ovulation, and luteal development are needed. An emerging question is why the primate follicle requires such prolonged exposure to LH for ovulatory events. Does folliculogenesis in primates yield a dominant follicle that is relatively insensitive or unresponsive to LH?

Cellular Composition of the Corpus Luteum

The origins, dynamics, and specific functions of the cellular components within the primate corpus luteum remain obscure. Development of the corpus luteum is believed to involve *(a)* the conversion of granulosa cells to luteal cells and *(b)* the migration of vascular elements into the luteinizing granulosa layer, but *(c)* the fate and function of theca cells from the antecedent follicle remains controversial. The primate corpus luteum differs from that of many species in that two cell types, so-called luteal and paraluteal cells, are compartmentalized. Foci of paraluteal cells around the periphery and in deep folds of the luteal gland led some researchers to propose that these cells originate from the theca layer of the follicle. Others speculated that their presence is related to the ability of the primate corpus luteum to synthesize estrogens. Recently Sasano et al. (11) immunocytochemically localized the 17α-hydroxylase and aromatase P-450s in human ovaries, noting a distinct compartmentalization in both the large preovulatory follicle and the corpus luteum. The 17α-hydroxylase staining was confined to the theca interna of the follicle and paraluteal cells of the corpus luteum, whereas the aromatase was detected in granulosa cells of the follicle and luteal cells in the parenchyma of the corpus luteum. These novel findings are consistent with the concepts that *(a)* paraluteal and luteal cells are derived from theca and granulosa cells, respectively, of the follicle, and *(b)* a two-cell model for estrogen production, similar to that proposed for the follicle, may be retained in the primate corpus luteum.

The discovery that corpora lutea of domestic animals consist of at least two morphologically distinct subpopulations of luteal cells with important functional and regulatory differences has dramatically revised theories on the control of luteal function (12, 13). Recent studies on monkeys and women also suggest that luteal cells differ markedly in their size, steroidogenic capacity, and ability to respond to luteotropic factors. We reported (14) that the size distribution of steroidogenic cells (as judged by histochemical staining for 3β-hydroxysteroid dehydrogenase) enzymatically dispersed from the macaque corpus luteum exhibited three distinct regions, defined as small (≤15-μm diameter), medium (16–20 μm), and large (>20 μm) luteal cells. Highly enriched subpopulations of small and large cells were separated by flow cytometry, based upon their light scatter properties. When incubated in vitro, large cells secreted up to 30-fold more progesterone than small cells (14, 15). Under basal conditions, neither cell subpopulation produced appreciable estrogen, but large cells converted 12-fold more exogenous androstenedione to estrogens than did small cells. The current data suggest that the large luteal cells are more steroidogenic and are the major source of estrogens, as compared to small cells. Whether the medium-sized cells are intermediate or similar to small or large luteal cells is unknown. Also the cellular sources of other hormones (e.g., relaxin and inhibin) and local factors (e.g., prostaglandins and growth factors) await further study. Such substances could originate from steroidogenic or nonsteroidogenic cells in the corpus luteum.

Brannian and coworkers (15) recently reported that the agonist responsiveness of small and large luteal cell populations obtained from the macaque corpus luteum varied during the luteal phase of the menstrual cycle. Human chorionic gonadotropin (hCG), prostaglandin E_2 (PGE_2) and dibutyryl (db) cAMP stimulated in vitro progesterone production by both small and large cells from the early luteal phase (days 3–5). But by mid-luteal phase (days 7–8), none of these agonists stimulated progesterone production by small cells. Although large cells became unresponsive to PGE_2 by mid-late luteal phase (days 11–12), hCG and db-cAMP continued to stimulate steroidogenesis in large cells even at late luteal phase (days 14–15). Although not specifically designed to examine the phenomenon, this study (15) and others (16) suggest that luteal cell subpopulations are demographically dynamic. There is a progressive decrease in steroidogenic cell density and in the large:small cell ratio in dispersed cell preparations as the primate corpus luteum ages in the menstrual cycle.

The differential decline in sensitivity to endocrine and paracrine factors acting via cAMP-mediated pathways, together with reduced cell numbers, in luteal cell subpopulations may play a role in controlling the function and/or lifespan of the corpus luteum in the menstrual cycle. However, large cells remain responsive to hCG even at mid-to-late luteal phase, suggesting that this cell type is a target for CG action during rescue of the corpus luteum in early pregnancy. As models are proposed for the function and regulation of luteal cell types in various species (Fig. 1), common and distinctive features are emerging. Whereas large luteal cells invariably produce greater amounts of progesterone than small cells, the responsiveness of these cell preparations to agonists, such as gonadotropins, may vary. For example, there are reports that LH and cAMP stimulate progesterone production exclusively by small

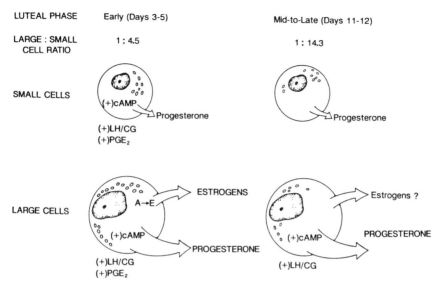

FIGURE 1. Features of steroidogenesis and agonist regulation of small and large luteal cell preparations from the rhesus monkey at specific stages of the menstrual cycle. The corpus luteum is developing during the early luteal phase (3–5 days after the LH surge), but on the verge of regression or CG rescue by days 11–12 of the luteal phase in nonfertile or fertile cycles, respectively. See text for details. (Derived from data in references 14, 15.)

luteal cells in the sheep (13), whereas large luteal cells in the rat respond primarily to these substances (17). The differences in responsiveness between cell subpopulations may reflect species differences. Alternatively, they may be due in part to differences between laboratories in the techniques for dispersing and isolating cell populations and in the criteria for classifying large and small cells. As reported above, responses of cell subpopulations may also vary during the lifespan of the corpus luteum. Novel approaches are needed to discern the origins, activities, regulation, and interactions of different cell groups within the corpus luteum of women and nonhuman primates, as well as other mammalian species.

Endocrine Regulators of the Macaque Corpus Luteum

The importance of the anterior pituitary, and particularly the secretion of LH, in the regulation of the corpus luteum of the menstrual cycle has been recognized since the 1960s (18, for review). Although reports by Asch and associates dispute this view, extensive work employing anti-LH antisera, GnRH antagonists, and hypothalamic-clamped monkeys indicate that the low levels of LH circulating during the luteal phase are essential for the normal steroidogenic function and typical lifespan of the corpus luteum. The recent discovery that deglycosylated (degly) preparations of LH and CG exhibit significant antagonism of gonadotropin-stimulated cAMP (19) and steroid (20) production offered a novel tool for testing LH control of luteal function. If LH and CG play important luteotropic roles during the menstrual cycle and early pregnancy, respectively, then administration of degly hCG should suppress circulating progesterone levels and cause luteolysis. However, Patton and coworkers report that 24-h systemic infusion of degly hCG into women (21) and chronic infusion of up to 72-μg degly hCG/day directly into the corpus luteum of monkeys (22) failed to alter luteal function. Notably, intraluteal infusion of degly hCG did not prevent the rise in serum progesterone levels produced by small doses of hCG administered peripherally to monkeys. Whereas degly hCG/hLH are promising tools for studying gonadotropin action in vitro, these studies and others in male macaques (23) disappointingly suggest that degly preparations are not easily applied to in vivo studies on the roles of gonadotropins in the primate gonads.

The discovery that LH is secreted in a pulsatile manner that changes markedly as the menstrual cycle advances has led to new insight into LH's luteotropic role. As progesterone secretion commences during luteal development, LH pulse frequency decreases. Moreover, the slowing of LH pulses is associated at least initially with a rise in pulse amplitude. Pulsatile progesterone secretion is evident by mid-luteal phase, which often correlates with LH pulses (24). Thus, the methods of rapid, repetitive blood sampling employed in these studies confirm the acute steroidogenic action of LH on the mature corpus luteum of the cycle. The declining frequency of LH pulses during the luteal phase led researchers to speculate that this phenomenon played a role in initiating timely luteolysis. However, elegant studies by Hutchison and Zeleznik (25) in hypothalamic-clamped monkeys indicated that (a) prevention of the decline in LH pulse frequency during the luteal phase, (b) premature reduction of LH pulse frequency in the early luteal phase to that observed at luteal regression, and (c) reduction of LH pulse amplitude failed to alter mean levels of circulating progesterone and/or the length of the luteal phase. These authors conclude that the reduction in LH pulse frequency as occurs in the spontaneous menstrual cycle is not sufficient to promote luteal regression. It may, however, provide a gonadotropic milieu that facilitates luteolysis or other activities in extraluteal ovarian compartments.

Experimental data indicate that the functional lifespan of the corpus luteum is prolonged in early pregnancy by CG, a glycoprotein hormone produced by the syncytiotrophoblast of the implanting blastocyst (18, for review). However, the cellular actions of CG that are essential for extension of the luteal lifespan remain undefined. An unanswered question is why the corpus luteum is rescued by an additional LH-like hormone (i.e., CG) in the face of continued LH support from the pituitary. It is unclear whether CG prevents a luteolytic signal from occurring in the fertile cycle or overcomes the existing signal by a quantum increase in luteotropic support. Due to differences in secretion patterns and circulating half-lives of LH and CG, there are quantitative and qualitative differences in the gonadotropin milieu in early pregnancy. Compared to the intermittent pulses of LH circulating in the luteal phase, the switch to continuous, increasing levels of CG may be sufficient to rescue the corpus luteum (26). Alternatively, there may be critical differences in the cellular actions of placental CG versus pituitary LH that facilitate rescue of the corpus luteum.

Both LH and CG are believed to share the same receptor sites, and both hormones stimulate cAMP and steroid production in primate luteal cells (27, 19). But there are reports that the duration of CG action is longer than that of LH in terms of enhanced steroidogenesis, which correlates with differences in the rate of receptor movement or turnover in cell membranes following binding of CG versus LH (28). However, these studies were performed in nonprimates comparing species-heterologous hormones (e.g., human CG versus ovine LH). Molskness and coworkers (29) recently performed analogous experiments examining the duration of the steroidogenic response of luteinized granulosa cells from monkeys to hLH, hCG, and oLH. There were no differences in the patterns of progesterone production during acute (15–30 min) or chronic (6 h) exposure to hLH or hCG at any hormone concentration (1–100 ng/mL). Compared to control conditions, acute or chronic exposure to as little as 1-ng/mL hLH or hCG caused a rapid and sustained increase in cell steroidogenesis. In contrast, acute exposure to up to 50-μg/mL oLH caused a transient simulation of progesterone production, with activity diminishing immediately following 15–30 min exposure. This study failed to extend the concept of disparate actions of gonadotropins to primates where both LH and CG are endogenous hormones. Indeed, the results suggest that earlier reports reflect species differences in LH, as opposed to differences between primate pituitary and placental gonadotropins. Nevertheless, further studies are needed to determine whether actions of hLH and hCG differ and contribute to the rescue of the primate corpus luteum in early pregnancy.

Paracrine and Autocrine Regulators of the Corpus Luteum

Steroids

After the discovery that the corpus luteum of the menstrual cycle was independent of uterine control, investigators hypothesized that local factors synthesized within the corpus luteum or ovary regulated luteal function and lifespan in primates. Citing evidence that systemic or intraluteal injections of estrogen induce premature luteolysis in women and monkeys, Knobil (30) proposed that estrogens produced by the corpus luteum initiate a self-destruct mechanism at the end of the cycle. Conversely, Rothchild (31) drew upon a collection of findings to propose that progesterone is a "universal luteotropin," promoting its own secretion in many species, including primates. Since evidence suggests that ovarian androgens act locally to modulate follicular function, it is possible that this class of steroids also acts on the subsequent corpus luteum. In collaboration with Dr. Robert Brenner at ORPRC, we tested the hypothesis that if progesterone, androgens, or estrogens regulate the corpus luteum via classical mechanisms of steroid hormone action, then luteal tissue contains specific receptors for these steroids.

Ovaries from throughout the follicular and luteal phase of the menstrual cycle were collected from macaque monkeys and processed for immunocytochemical detection of receptors using specific monoclonal antibodies against the human estrogen receptor (ER), progesterone receptor (PR), and androgen receptor (AR). Although ER was detected in "control" estrogen-responsive tissues (i.e., the macaque oviduct and the rabbit corpus luteum) and in the surface epithelium of the macaque ovary, ER was *not* detected in any cells of developing follicles or within the corpus luteum at any stage of the cycle (2). Despite the absence of ER, PR staining was detected in the nuclei of thecal and stromal cells around growing follicles, luteinizing granulosa cells in the periovulatory follicle, and luteal cells of the functional corpus luteum (2). Notably, luteal cells that produced progesterone, as judged by histochemical staining for 3β-hydroxysteroid dehydrogenase, also contained immunoreactive PR. Furthermore, the percentage of PR-positive cells within the corpus luteum correlated with the levels of circulating progesterone: rising during luteal development and diminishing during luteolysis. Most recently (32), AR was detected in theca and granulosa cells of growing follicles and within many luteal cells throughout the lifespan of the corpus luteum in the menstrual cycle. Sucrose gradient analyses with radiolabeled progestin or androgen demonstrated a shift in the binding peak in monkey ovarian tissue upon addition of PR or AR antibodies, supporting the presence of specific steroid receptors.

These data do not support the concept of a local receptor-mediated role for estrogen in the regulation of folliculogenesis or luteal function in primates. Other reports, for example by Hutchison and Zeleznik (25), also question whether the luteolytic action of estrogen is directly on the corpus luteum; they conclude that estrogen administered systemically or intraluteally induces luteolysis via an indirect mechanism involving feedback inhibition of pituitary LH secretion. Ellinwood and Resko's work (33) implies that endogenous estrogen is not a primary regulator of luteolysis in the menstrual cycle. Although estrogen levels within the corpus luteum were effectively diminished (80–90%) by administering an aromatase inhibitor to monkeys during the luteal phase, luteolysis occurred at the expected time. Thus, much of the evidence accumulated in the 1980s does not support the hypothesis of a direct luteolytic action of estrogen within the corpus luteum of the menstrual cycle. The absence or a very low concentration of ER does not preclude receptor-independent or nonclassical effects of estrogen in the corpus luteum, such as direct inhibition of 3β-hydroxysteroid dehydrogenase activity. Investigators have reported direct effects of estrogens on primate luteal cells, particularly inhibition of gonadotropin-stimulated steroidogenesis (18). The high concentrations of estrogens and acute conditions employed in these studies may favor nonreceptor-mediated actions of steroids.

The data are consistent with receptor-mediated autocrine or paracrine roles for progesterone and androgens in folliculogenesis, as well as during the development and function of the corpus luteum in the menstrual cycle. Specific actions of these steroids on luteal cells await investigation. Progesterone may be promoting its own production (31) or the synthesis of other substances. To the author's knowledge, there is only one report suggesting androgen action in primate luteal tissue, as inferred from the modulation of inhibin production in cultures of luteinized granulosa cells (34). As summarized in Table 2, the distribution of PR and AR varies during the lifespan of the corpus luteum: Notably, PR is markedly diminished, whereas AR is retained in regressing luteal tissue. If the presence of immunoreactive R equates with luteal cell sensitivity, it is tempting to speculate that the loss of progesterone action and/or continuation of androgen action plays a role in luteolysis during the menstrual cycle. The factors controlling the dynamics of PR and AR expression in the follicle and corpus luteum also remain unclear. In classical target tissues, such as the uterus, estrogen induces the formation of PR. However, if the primate follicle and corpus luteum are devoid of ER, then induction and maintenance of PR must involve other regulators, such as gonadotropins (see earlier section, The LH Surge).

TABLE 2. Immunocytochemical detection of steroid receptors in the macaque ovary.

Receptor	Preovulatory Follicle[*]		Corpus Luteum		
	Granulosa	Theca	Early	Mid	Late
Estrogen	−	−	−	−	−
Progesterone	−	+	+	+	−
Androgen	+	+	+	+	+

Source: Adapted from references 2 and 32.
[*]Prior to the midcycle LH surge.

Prostaglandins

In many nonprimate species, prostaglandin $F_{2\alpha}$ from the uterus is the leading candidate as the luteolytic hormone. Although the uterus is not regarded as a source of luteolysin in primates (35), the effects of exogenous $PGF_{2\alpha}$ and its analogs on the corpus luteum in vivo received considerable attention through the 1970s with results varying from no effect to initiation of premature luteolysis (18, for review). The equivocal results may be due to many variables, including *(a)* difficulty in getting sufficient $PGF_{2\alpha}$ to luteal tissue, particularly since PGs are rapidly metabolized by the pulmonary system, and *(b)* endogenous PGs produced by luteal tissue limit further response to exogenous $PGF_{2\alpha}$. Notably, researchers administering $PGF_{2\alpha}$ locally into the corpus luteum succeeded in causing premature luteolysis in women and monkeys (35).

Nevertheless, the physiologic role of endogenous PGs in regulating the function or lifespan of the primate corpus luteum remains unsubstantiated. If the predominant action of $PGF_{2\alpha}$ is to cause luteal regression, then suppressing its synthesis or action could prolong the lifespan of the corpus luteum in the menstrual cycle. Unfortunately, specific inhibitors of $PGF_{2\alpha}$ synthesis or action are not available. Therefore, we administered a general (cyclooxygenase) inhibitor of PG synthesis, sodium meclofenamate, directly into the corpus luteum of rhesus monkeys for 7 days beginning at mid-luteal phase of the menstrual cycle (36). Compared to controls (saline infusion into the corpus luteum or meclofenamate infusion systemically), intraluteal infusion of the PG synthesis inhibitor caused premature luteolysis. Although nonspecific or PG antagonist actions of meclofenamate cannot be ruled out (36, 37), this study by Sargent and colleagues offers the first in vivo evidence that local PGs may have an obligatory luteotropic role during the menstrual cycle.

Subsequent studies (38, 39) identified PGs of the D, E, and I series (ranked in order of potency) that acutely stimulate cAMP and progesterone production by macaque luteal tissue in vitro. In contrast, PGA_2 had antigonadotropic activities similar to that reported earlier for $PGF_{2\alpha}$; it prevented hCG-stimulated cAMP and progesterone production by luteal cells. To determine if steroidogenic PGs could modulate macaque luteal function in vivo, Zelinski-Wooten and associates (39) infused PGD_2, E_2, or I_2 analog directly into the corpus luteum for up to 14 days, beginning at mid-luteal phase of the cycle. Doses of 300- to 500-ng/h typically failed to alter the function (as monitored by daily levels of serum progesterone) or lifespan of the corpus luteum. However, co-infusion of PGD_2 or E_2 (and to a lesser extent, I_2 analog) with $PGF_{2\alpha}$ maintained progesterone levels and prevented premature menses seen with infusion of $PGF_{2\alpha}$ alone. These studies established the specificity of exogenous $PGF_{2\alpha}$ in causing luteolysis in macaques during the menstrual cycle. Although PGs that were steroidogenic in vitro did not chronically alter luteal function in vivo, they did prevent the luteolytic action of exogenous $PGF_{2\alpha}$. It is possible that local regulation of the primate corpus luteum is influenced by the balance between production/action of stimulatory and inhibitory PGs, and possibly other products of recently elucidated pathways of arachidonate metabolism (40).

Challenge for the 1990s

Despite important advances, our understanding of the processes underlying the formation and regression of the corpus luteum in the menstrual cycle, or its further differentiation and delayed demise in early pregnancy is superficial. Current research suggests that the primate corpus luteum consists of subpopulations of luteal cells that differ in endocrine activity, plus other cell types that may influence luteal cell function (Fig. 2). In addition to classical hormones, the number of substances that the corpus luteum produces with

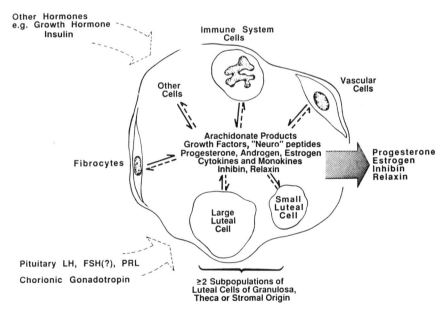

FIGURE 2. Summary of the cell populations within the primate corpus luteum and their many products that may serve as local (autocrine or paracrine) regulators of luteal function or as classical hormones. Solid arrows denote secretion, whereas dotted arrows denote action on target cells. Hormones from the pituitary, placenta, or other endocrine glands that may act on the corpus luteum to regulate function or lifespan are also represented. (From Stouffer RL, Corpus luteum function and dysfunction, Clin Obstet Gynecol 1990;33, with permission.)

putative local actions is becoming astronomical. These include endocrine products (e.g., progesterone), prostaglandins, and other derivatives of arachidonate metabolism, neurohormones or analogs (e.g., oxytocin), growth factors, and the latest group, the cytokines and monokines (e.g., tumor necrosis factor). New techniques must be applied to identify various cell types, their functions, and their endocrine, paracrine, and autocrine regulation within the corpus luteum. Discerning the population dynamics of cell types and interactions between cell groups will lead to an understanding of how cells combine to produce the normal activity and lifespan of the primate corpus luteum in the menstrual cycle and early pregnancy.

Acknowledgments. The author thanks the talented and industrious group of graduate students, postdoctoral fellows, and clinical researchers that performed the studies described in this chapter. A special thanks to Drs. Robert Brenner, Miles Novy, Phil Patton, Stan Shiigi, and Don Wolf for their collaborative interactions at ORPRC. This is ORPRC Publication No. 1722. Research in the author's laboratory was supported by NIH grants RR-00163, HD-18185, HD-20869, and HD-22408.

References

1. Wolf DP, VandeVoort CA, Meyer-Haas GR, et al. In vitro fertilization and embryo transfer in the rhesus monkey. Biol Reprod 1989;41:335-46.
2. Hild-Petito S, Stouffer RL, Brenner RM. Immunocytochemical localization of estradiol and progesterone receptors in the monkey ovary throughout the menstrual cycle. Endocrinology 1988;123:2896-2905.
3. Aladin Y, Yu Q, Brenner RM, Molskness TA, Stouffer RL. Novel action of the gonadotropin surge in primates: Induction of progesterone receptors in granulosa cells [Abstract]. Biol Reprod 1989;40(suppl 1):91.
4. Weick RF, Dierschke DJ, Karsch FJ, Butler WR, Hotchkiss J, Knobil E. Periovulatory time courses of circulating gonadotropic and ovarian hormones in the rhesus monkey. Endocrinology 1973;93:1140-7.
5. Fink G. Gonadotropin secretion and its control. In: Knobil E, Neill J, eds. The physiology of reproduction. New York: Raven Press, 1988:1349-77.
6. Baird DT, Swanston IA, McNeilly AS. Relationship between LH, FSH, and prolactin concentration and the secretion of androgens and estrogens by the preovulatory follicle in the ewe. Biol Reprod 1981;24:1013-25.
7. Zelinski-Wooten MB, Lanzendorf SE, Wolf DP, Stouffer RL. Titrating luteinizing hormone (LH) surge requirements for ovulatory changes in primate follicles, I. Oocyte maturation and corpus luteum function [Abstract]. VIII Ovarian Workshop: Regulatory Processes and Gene Expression in the Ovary. Serono Symposia, USA, Maryville, TN, 1990.
8. Aladin Chandrasekher Y, Brenner RM, Molskness TA, Stouffer RL. Titrating

luteinizing hormone (LH) surge requirements for ovulatory changes in primate follicles, II. Progesterone receptor expression in luteinizing granulosa cells [Abstract]. VIII Ovarian Workshop: Regulatory Processes and Gene Expression in the Ovary. Serono Symposia, USA, Maryville, TN, 1990.

9. VandeVoort CA, Baughman WL, Stouffer RL. Comparison of different regimens of human gonadotropins for superovulation of rhesus monkeys: Ovulatory response and subsequent luteal function. J In Vitro Fert Embryo Transfer 1989; 6:85-91.

10. Messinis IE, Templeton A. The effect of pulsatile follicle stimulating hormone on the endogenous luteinizing hormone surge in women. Clin Endocrinol 1986; 25:633-40.

11. Sasano H, Okamoto M, Mason JI, et al. Immunolocalization of aromatase, 17α-hydroxylase and side-chain-cleavage cytochromes P-450 in the human ovary. J Reprod Fertil 1989;85:163-9.

12. Koos RD, Hansen W. The large and small cells of the bovine corpus luteum: Ultrastructural and functional differences. In: Schwartz NB, Hunziker-Dunn M, eds. Dynamics of ovarian function. New York: Raven Press, 1981:197-203.

13. Niswender GD, Schwall RH, Fitz TA, Farin CE, Sawyer HR. Regulation of luteal function in domestic ruminants: New concepts. Recent Prog Horm Res 1985; 41:101-51.

14. Hild-Petito SA, Shiigi SM, Stouffer RL. Isolation and characterization of cell subpopulations from the monkey corpus luteum of the menstrual cycle. Biol Reprod 1989;40:1075-85.

15. Brannian JD, Stouffer RL. Changes in agonist-responsiveness of subpopulations of monkey luteal cells during the menstrual cycle [Abstract]. Biol Reprod 1990;42(suppl 1):117.

16. Fisch B, Margara RA, Winston RML, Hillier SG. Cellular basis of luteal steroidogenesis in the human ovary. J Endocrinol 1989;122:303-11.

17. Nelson S, Khan I. Estradiol biosynthesis in the corpus luteum of the pregnant rat involves two different luteal cell populations [Abstract]. Endocrinology 1987;120(suppl):216.

18. Stouffer RL. Perspectives on the corpus luteum of the menstrual cycle and early pregnancy. Semin Reprod Endocrinol 1988;6:103-13.

19. Eyster KM, Stouffer RL. Adenylate cyclase in the corpus luteum of the rhesus monkey, II. Sensitivity to nucleotides, gonadotropins, catecholamines, and non-hormonal activators. Endocrinology 1985;116:1552-8.

20. Richardson MC, Masson GM, Sairam MR. Inhibitory action of chemically deglycosylated human chorionic gonadotropin on hormone-induced steroid production by dispersed cells from human corpus luteum. J Endocrinol 1984; 101:327-32.

21. Patton PE, Calvo FO, Fujimoto VY, Bergert ER, Kempers RD, Ryan RJ. The effect of deglycosylated human chorionic gonadotropin on corpora luteal function in healthy women. Fertil Steril 1988;49:620-5.

22. Patton PE, Stouffer RL, Zelinski-Wooten MB. The effect of intraluteal infusion of deglycosylated human chorionic gonadotropin on the corpus luteum in rhesus monkeys. J Clin Endocrinol Metab 1990;70:1213-8.

23. Liu L, Southers JL, Banks SM, et al. Stimulation of testosterone production in the cynomolgus monkey in vivo by deglycosylated and desialylated human choriogonadotropin. Endocrinology 1989;124:175-80.

24. Ellinwood WE, Norman RL, Spies HG. Changing frequency of pulsatile luteinizing hormone and progesterone secretion during the luteal phase of the menstrual cycle of rhesus monkeys. Biol Reprod 1984;31:714-22.

25. Zeleznik AJ, Hutchison J. Luteotropic actions of LH on the macaque corpus luteum. In: Stouffer RL, ed. The primate ovary. New York: Plenum Press, 1987:163-74.

26. Monfort SL, Hess DL, Hendricks AG, Lasley BL. Absence of regular pulsatile gonadotropin secretion during implantation in the rhesus macaque. Endocrinology 1989;125:1766-73.

27. Cameron JL, Stouffer RL. Gonadotropin receptors of the primate corpus luteum, I. Characterization of ^{125}I-labeled human luteinizing hormone and human chorionic gonadotropin binding to luteal membranes from the rhesus monkey. Endocrinology 1982;110:2059-67.

28. Niswender GD, Roess DA, Barisas BG. Receptor-mediated differences in the actions of ovine luteinizing hormone vs. human chorionic gonadotropin. In: Stouffer RL, ed. The primate ovary. New York: Plenum Press, 1987:237-48.

29. Molskness TA, Zelinski-Wooten MB, Hild-Petito SA, Stouffer RL. Comparison of the actions of luteinizing hormone (LH) and chorionic gonadotropin (CG) in primate ovarian cells [Abstract]. International Symposium on Glycoprotein Hormones. Serono Symposia, USA, Newport Beach, CA, 1989.

30. Knobil E. On the regulation of the primate corpus luteum. Biol Reprod 1973;8:246-58.

31. Rothchild I. The regulation of the mammalian corpus luteum. Recent Prog Horm Res 1981;37:183-298.

32. Hild-Petito S, West NB, Brenner RM, Stouffer RL. Localization of androgen receptors in follicular and luteal tissue of the monkey ovary during the menstrual cycle [Abstract]. Biol Reprod 1990;42(suppl 1):109.

33. Ellinwood WE, Resko JA. Effect of inhibition of estrogen synthesis during the luteal phase on function of the corpus luteum in rhesus monkeys. Biol Reprod 1983;28:636-44.

34. Tsonis CG, Hillier SG, Baird DT. Production of inhibin bioactivity by human granulosa-lutein cells: Stimulation by LH and testosterone in vitro. J Endocrinol 1987;112:R11-4.

35. Auletta FJ, Flint AP. Mechanisms controlling corpus luteum function in sheep, cows, nonhuman primates, and women especially in relation to the time of luteolysis. Endocr Rev 1988;9:88-105.

36. Sargent EL, Baughman WL, Novy MJ, Stouffer RL. Intraluteal infusion of a prostaglandin synthesis inhibitor, sodium meclofenamate, causes premature luteolysis in rhesus monkeys. Endocrinology 1988;123:2261-9.

37. Zelinski-Wooten MB, Sargent EL, Molskness TA, Stouffer RL. Disparate effects of the prostaglandin synthesis inhibitors, meclofenamate, and flurbiprofen on monkey luteal tissue *in vitro*. Endocrinology 1990;126:1380-7.

38. Molskness TA, VandeVoort CA, Stouffer RL. Effects of prostaglandins on the

gonadotropin-sensitive adenylate cyclase in the primate (*Macaca mulatta*) corpus luteum of the menstrual cycle. Prostaglandins 1987;34:279-90.
39. Zelinski-Wooten MB, Stouffer RL. Intraluteal infusions of prostaglandins of the E, D, I and A series prevent $PGF_{2\alpha}$-induced, but not spontaneous, luteal regression in rhesus monkeys. Biol Reprod (in press).
40. Ichikawa F, Yoshimura Y, Oda T, et al. The effects of lipoxygenase products on progesterone and prostaglandin production by human corpora lutea. J Clin Endocrinol Metab 1990;70:849-55.
41. Stouffer RL. Corpus luteum function and dysfunction. Clin Obstet Gynecol 1990;33.

7

Steroid Signaling in the Follicular Paracrine System

S.G. HILLIER AND I.M. TURNER

Locally produced regulatory factors co-ordinate gonadotropin-dependent theca/granulosa cell interaction during preovulatory follicular development. In this chapter, we review evidence that steroids act as essential paracrine signals in ovarian follicles and speculate on the functional significance of steroids as modulators of regulatory protein (inhibin and activin) production by developing granulosa cells.

Regulatory Steroid Action

The two-cell, two-gonadotropin model of estrogen synthesis in the preovulatory follicle provided the first satisfactory explanation of the cellular basis of estrogen synthesis and laid the foundations for modern concepts of a follicular paracrine system (1). Estrogens had long been recognized as intrafollicular organizers that promote granulosa cell development and responsiveness to gonadotropins in vivo (2–5), and locally produced androgens were implicated in the control of follicular atresia (6). Towards the end of the 1970s, increased use of primary granulosa cell culture systems to study androgen action in vitro revealed unexpected abilities of aromatizable and nonaromatizable androgens to act alone (7, 8) and synergistically with FSH (9, 10) to stimulate progesterone synthesis and aromatase activity (11, 12). With the demonstration that granulosa cells possess androgen receptors (13) that mediate androgenic augmentation of FSH-induced granulosa cell differentiation (14), it was suggested that LH-induced thecal androgens, besides serving as aromatase substrates, might function as "intercellular (theca or granulosa) regulators that mediate certain follicular requirements for stimulation by LH" (15). Regulatory roles in the follicular paracrine system for androgens along with estrogens, other steroids, and diverse nonsteroidal factors are now widely accepted (16–18).

Androgen

Androgens produced by thecal cells cross the lamina basalis, penetrate the granulosa cell layer and accumulate in follicular fluid (19, 20). There is experimental evidence for involvement of androgens in follicular atresia (see below), but androgen levels in follicular fluid of atretic follicles do not differ markedly from those in healthy follicles of a comparable size (21, 22). Depending on the stage of development (controlled by FSH), granulosa cells express enzymes that interconvert androstenedione and other steroids with potential regulatory functions in the follicle wall, including testosterone (via 17-ketoreductase [23]), 5α-reduced androgens (via 5α-reductase [24]), estradiol (via aromatase [24]), and catechol estrogens (via estrogen hydroxylase [25]).

For several mammalian species, including a nonhuman primate (26), it has been shown that FSH-induced differentiation of cultured granulosa cells is modulated by the presence of androgens at concentrations found in follicular fluid (16, 17). Androgens active in this regard include testosterone, androstenedione, and their nonaromatizable 5α-reduced congeners. Receptor-mediated androgen action in granulosa cells leads to increased generation of cAMP and expression of genes encoding FSH-inducible proteins, including steroidogenic cyctochrome P-450s and inhibin/activin subunits (Fig. 1). The

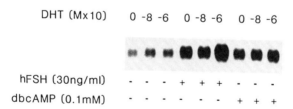

DHT (Mx10)   0 -8 -6   0 -8 -6   0 -8 -6

hFSH (30ng/ml)   - - -   + + +   - - -
dbcAMP (0.1mM)   - - -   - - -   + + +

FIGURE 1. Androgenic augmentation of hFSH/cAMP-stimulated inhibin α-subunit mRNA expression in rat granulosa cells. Granulosa cells from estrogen-primed immature female rat ovaries were cultured for 48 h with and without submaximal stimulatory concentrations of hFSH (30 ng/mL) or dibutyryl cAMP (100 μM), in the presence and absence of 10^{-8} or 10^{-6}M 5α-dihydrotestosterone (DHT). Total RNA (10 μg) from cells receiving each treatment was separated by electrophoresis on an agarose formaldehyde gel and transferred to a nylon membrane, which was hybridized with a ^{32}P-labeled rat inhibin α-subunit cDNA probe. The autoradiographic signal given by the ~1.6-kb inhibin α-subunit mRNA is shown. (I.M. Turner and S.G. Hillier, unpublished data.)

net effect is enhanced sensitivity to FSH, consistent with a role for locally produced androgens in modulating follicular threshold requirements for stimulation by FSH.

Degree of exposure to FSH and stage of preovulatory development determine how granulosa cells respond to androgen. Experiments in vivo using estrogen-primed hypophysectomized immature rats have shown that in the absence of FSH, treatment with LH/hCG (stimulates ovarian androgen production [6]) or androgen (27) inhibits granulosa cell proliferation and promotes follicular atresia. On the other hand, joint treatment with FSH and androgen promotes preovulatory follicular growth and estrogen secretion (28). Whether androgens exert specific regulatory actions in granulosa cells at advanced stages of FSH-induced differentiation is uncertain since such cells convert aromatizable androgens to estradiol and may also produce androgen metabolites that are competitive aromatase inhibitors (29). Exposure of mature granulosa cells to excessive amounts of androgen is generally associated with reduced steroid secretion and increased follicular atresia (30–32).

Estrogen

Estrogen is a putative intrafollicular autocrine regulator. Treatment of hypophysectomized immature female rats with exogenous estrogen stimulates granulosa cell mitosis, raises gonadotropin receptor levels and amplifies follicular responsiveness to exogenously administered gonadotropin (4, 5, 33, 34). At the subcellular level, estrogen augments FSH-induced expression of the regulatory subunit RIIβ of type II cAMP-dependent protein kinase, as well as the aromatase and cholesterol side-chain cleavage cytochrome P-450s (5, 33–35). Estrogen also stimulates expression of inhibin α- and β_B-subunit mRNAs (36) (see Fig. 2) and augments FSH-induced production of inhibin protein(s) by cultured rat granulosa cells (37).

Regulatory actions of estrogen in granulosa cells are presumed to be mediated by binding of the steroid to receptor(s) that regulate rates of transcription from estrogen responsive genes (5). A protein with the physicochemical properties of an estrogen receptor has been detected by ligand-binding assays in nuclei and cytosol from whole ovaries and granulosa cells (38–40). However, at least one other estrogen-binding species is present in rat granulosa cells, which could also participate in estrogen action (41). The finding that mouse ovaries express at least two mRNA species that cross-hybridize with RNA probes complementary to the steroid-binding domain of the mouse estrogen receptor provides further evidence that steroid binding sites other than that of the classic estrogen receptor might mediate autocrine estrogen action in the ovaries (42).

Whether estrogens exert physiologically significant regulatory effects in

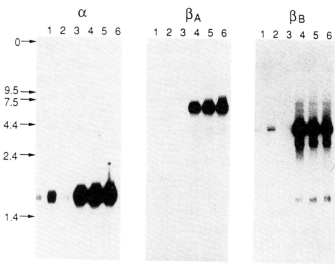

FIGURE 2. Stimulatory effects of hFSH and estrogen on expression of inhibin subunit mRNAs in rat granulosa cells. Granulosa cells from estrogen-primed immature female rat ovaries were cultured for 48 h with and without a maximal stimulatory dose of steroid (10^{-6}M) and/or hFSH (100 ng/mL) (1 = control; 2 = estradiol alone; 3 = 5α-dihydrotestosterone alone; 4 = hFSH alone; 5 = hFSH plus estradiol; 6 = hFSH plus 5α-dihydrotestosterone.) Total RNA (5 μg) from cells receiving each treatment was separated by electrophoresis on an agarose formaldehyde gel and transferred to a nylon membrane, which was sequentially hybridized with each ^{32}P-labeled rat inhibin cDNA probe (*left panel* = α-subunit; *center panel* = β_A-subunit; *right panel* = β_B subunit.) Numbers on the left denote approximate mRNA sizes (kb). The ~1.6-kb hybridization signal in the right-hand panel is a residual inhibin α-subunit probe that was incompletely stripped from the membrane before reprobing. (From Turner IM, Saunders PTK, Shimasaki S, Hillier SG, Regulation of inhibin subunit gene expression by FSH and estradiol in cultured rat granulosa cells, Endocrinology 1989;125:2790-2, with permission.)

human granulosa cells is less certain, the only relevant data having come from nonhuman primate models. In an immunocytochemical study of monkey ovaries, granulosa cells stained negatively for the estrogen receptor, whereas intense positive staining occurred in the ovarian surface epithelium (43). Treatment of cultured marmoset granulosa cells with estradiol augmented FSH-inducible inhibin production without enhancing steroidogenesis (44).

The raised follicular fluid estrogen level in the preovulatory follicle is widely believed to contribute to the intrafollicular mechanism whereby a single preovulatory follicle is selected to ovulate in the human menstrual cycle. There is no direct evidence to support regulatory estrogen action in human granulosa cells, but both aromatase activity (45) and follicular fluid estradiol levels (20, 46) increase during preovulatory follicular development and correlate positively with follicular "health" (16). Once selected (see above), the preovulatory follicle is presumed to be developmentally favored through the activation of a local positive feedback loop in which the estrogen it produces stimulates granulosa cell proliferation as well as augmenting cellular responsiveness to gonadotropins, thereby causing further increases in estrogen formation and so on (20, 34, 47). As discussed below, follicular androgens and nonsteroidal factors, such as inhibins and activins, may also participate in this local feedback interaction.

Granulosa-derived estrogen is also implicated as a paracrine regulator of thecal cell function (48) and may be involved in the suppression of thecal androgen synthesis in response to the mid-cycle LH surge (49).

Assessment of direct estrogen action in isolated granulosa cell systems may be complicated by the fact that preovulatory granulosa cells acquire increased capacity to metabolize estradiol to catechol estrogens (25). Catechol estrogens have been identified in ovarian follicular fluid (50) and have been shown to augment FSH-induced steroid synthesis and inhibit granulosa cell proliferation in vitro (51, 52). Thus, this class of estrogen might also serve regulatory functions in vivo.

Steroids and Regulatory Protein Action: Inhibins and Activins

Neither FSH nor estrogen are granulosa cell mitogens in vitro although they are when administered in vivo (53). This raises the question of whether locally produced growth factors co-ordinate mitogenic and differentiative actions of gonadotropins and sex steroids. Candidates for such roles include insulin-like growth factors, epidermal growth factor, transforming growth factors, inhibins and activins, heparin-binding growth factors, and cytokines. Here, we focus on the inhibin/activin family of regulatory proteins.

Inhibins and Activins

Mature inhibin is a 32-kDa glycoprotein that has been isolated from ovarian follicular fluid as two distinct forms composed of a common α-subunit and one of two β-subunits, β_A and β_B (54–59). Treatment of pituitary cell cultures with inhibin suppresses FSH secretion, whereas treatment with the homodimeric β_A (β_A form of inhibin, termed activin-A [60] or FSH-releasing protein [61]) stimulates FSH release. These properties are likely to reflect physiological functions of inhibin and activin in the human endocrine system, notably during the luteal phase of the menstrual cycle when inhibin is secreted in large amounts by the corpus luteum (62).

The human preovulatory follicle does not appear to secrete important amounts of inhibin until the mid-cycle LH surge begins (62). However, inhibin and activin are both believed to serve local regulatory functions within developing ovarian follicles (63). Interest in the putative intragonadal function(s) of these factors is fueled by the high degree of structural homology (30–40%) that exists between them and the members of a family of growth factors, which are synthesized from precursors of high molecular weight and expressed during embryogenesis and organogenesis across a wide range of animal phyla (58, 64). Members of this gene family include TGF β, mullerian duct inhibiting substance (causes mullerian duct regression in males), decapentaplegic gene complex (active during insect embryogenesis), and vg1 protein (a mesoderm-inducing factor in frog embryos). Bone marrow expresses inhibin β_A mRNA and human lukaemic cells produce activin (65). Moreover, treatment with activin in vitro stimulates erythroid differentiation (haemoglobin accumulation) in human erythrolukaemic cell cultures and this effect is inhibited by co-treatment with inhibin (66). Thus it seems increasingly likely that inhibins and activins and/or their component subunits play fundamental roles in tissue growth and differentiation.

Control of Inhibin/Activin Gene Expression

Secretion of inhibin protein by rat (37, 67–70), bovine (71), human (72, 73) and nonhuman primate granulosa cells (44) is regulated by gonadotropins and sex steroids in vitro. The three inhibin subunits are encoded by separate genes (74–78) whose expression in granulosa cells is developmentally regulated and inducible by FSH (79, 80) (Fig. 2). Interestingly, expression of the α- and β_B-subunit mRNAs (which jointly encode inhibin) in cultured rat granulosa cells is enhanced by treatment with estradiol in vitro, whereas the β_A-subunit mRNA (which encodes activin-A) shows no discernible response to estradiol under identical experimental conditions (36) (Fig. 2). This suggests to us a mechanism whereby locally produced estrogen could influence relative rates of granulosa cell inhibin and activin synthesis during follicular development in vivo.

Intrafollicular Regulatory Functions of Inhibins and Activins

Specific regulatory functions of inhibin, activin, their precursors, or free subunits in ovarian follicles have yet to be defined. In rat thecal cell cultures, inhibin was shown to augment LH-stimulated production of androstenedione, whereas activin was inhibitory (81). In rat granulosa cell cultures, inhibin purified from porcine (82) but not bovine (83) follicular fluid inhibited aromatase activity. Reasons for the discrepancy are uncertain but may reside in the specific forms of inhibin and experimental conditions used. Activin enhanced FSH-stimulated aromatase activity in rat granulosa cells but inhibited progesterone production (83). Activin also inhibited the growth of chinese hamster ovary cells in culture. Treatment with inhibin alone had no significant effect on ovarian cell growth, although it partially overcame the inhibitory effect of activin (84).

Functional Interplay Between Androgen and Inhibin

The forgoing evidence suggests that the androgen/estrogen and inhibin/activin axes of the follicular paracrine system might be functionally interlinked. In continuing in vitro studies of development-dependent human granulosa cell function, we find that the presence of testosterone or 5α-dihydrotestosterone in culture medium markedly augments FSH-stimulated inhibin production by cells harvested from immature antral follicles (73, and unpublished data) (Fig. 3). Similar augmentative effects of androgens on

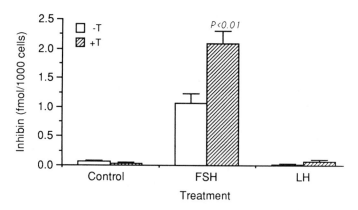

FIGURE 3. Androgenic augmentation of hFSH-induced production of inhibin by human granulosa cells. Granulosa cells were pooled from four 5-mm diameter follicles in a human ovary and cultured (15,000 cells/0.5 mL medium) for 96 h (medium change at 48 h) in serum-free medium 199 containing no additions, testosterone (T) (10^{-6}M), gonadotropin (hFSH or hLH, 30 ng/mL), or gonadotropin plus T, as indicated. Inhibin levels in the medium (radioimmunoassay using porcine Iα(1-26)-Gly^{27}-Tyr^{28} as immunogen, tracer, and standard (see reference 44) are shown as means (± SEM) of incubations in triplicate. Note the response to hFSH, which is increased ~2-fold by the presence of T. The lack of response to hLH is consistent with the functional immaturity of the cells studied. (S.G. Hillier, S.G. Wickings, I.M. Turner, P. Illingworth, E.L. Yong, L.E. Reichert, Jr., A.S. McNeilly, and D.T. Baird, unpublished data.)

FSH-responsive inhibin production have been reported using bovine (71), rat (37, 68), and marmoset monkey granulosa cell cultures (44), suggesting broad relevance to mammalian granulosa cell function. Interestingly, we find that inhibin production by FSH-treated human granulosa cell cultures is refractory to treatment with estradiol (73, and unpublished data). Such an androgen-specific effect on human granulosa cells contrasts with the situation for rat and marmoset monkey granulosa cells where both androgen and estrogen synergize with FSH to promote inhibin production in vitro. Rats and marmoset monkeys are both polyovulatory, whereas human beings are monovulators (37, 44). This raises the question if androgen-responsive inhibin production has particular functional significance for monovulatory species, including humans. Evidence from animal experiments suggests that androgen potentiates FSH-induced granulosa cell inhibin production, whereas inhibin augments LH responsive thecal/interstitial androgen production. It has yet to be established if inhibin augments human thecal androgen production. However, such functional interplay between androgen and inhibin would have special relevance to follicular selection and development in women, since it could provide the basis of a paracrine mechanism for setting the responsiveness of individual follicles to FSH and LH.

Acknowledgments. The research reported in this chapter was supported by grants from the Wellcome Trust and Medical Research Council.

References

1. Armstrong DT, Dorrington JH. Estrogen biosynthesis in the ovaries and testes. In: Thomas A, Singhal RL, eds. Regulatory mechanisms affecting gonadal hormone action; vol 2. Baltimore: University Park Press, 1979:217-58.
2. Gaarenstroom JH, de Jongh SE. A contribution to the knowledge of the influence of gonadotropic and sex hormones on the gonads of rats. In: Houwink R, Ketelaar JAAA, eds. Monographs on the progress of research in Holland during the war, vol. 7. Amsterdam: Elsevier, 1946:59-164.
3. Hisaw FL. Development of the Graafian follicle and ovulation. Physiol Rev 1947;27:95-119.
4. Goldenberg RL, Reiter EO, Ross GT. Follicle response to exogenous gonadotropins: An estrogen-mediated phenomenon. Fertil Steril 1973;24:121-125.
5. Richards JS. Maturation of ovarian follicles: Actions and interaction of pituitary and ovarian hormones on follicular differentiation. Physiol Rev 1980;60:51-89.
6. Louvet J-P, Harman SM, Schreiber JR, Ross GT. Evidence for a role of androgens in follicular maturation. Endocrinology 1975;97:366-72.
7. Schomberg DW, Stouffer RL, Tyrey, L. Modulation of progestin secretion in ovarian cells by 17β-hydroxy-5α-androstan-3-one (dihydrotestosterone): A direct demonstration in monolayer culture. Biochem Biophys Res Commun 1976; 68:77-85.

8. Lucky AW, Schreiber JR, Hillier SG, Schulman JD, Ross GT. Progesterone production by cultured granulosa cells: Stimulation by androgens. Endocrinology 1977;100:128-33.

9. Armstrong DT, Dorrington JH. Androgens augment FSH-induced progesterone secretion by cultured rat granulosa cells. Endocrinology 1976;99:1411-4.

10. Nimrod A, Lindner HR. A synergistic effect of androgen on the stimulation of progesterone secretion by FSH in cultured rat granulosa cells. Mol Cell Endocrinol 1976;5:315-20.

11. Daniel SAJ, Armstrong DT. Enhancement of follicle-stimulating hormone induced aromatase activity by androgen in cultured rat granulosa cells. Endocrinology 1980;107:1027-33.

12. Hillier SG, de Zwart FA. Evidence that induction/activation of granulosa cell aromatase activity by follicle-stimulating hormone is an androgen receptor-regulated process in vitro. Endocrinology 1981;109:1303-5.

13. Schreiber JR, Ross GT. Further characterization of a rat ovarian testosterone receptor with evidence for nuclear translocation. Endocrinology 1976;99:590-6.

14. Hillier SG, Knazek RA, Ross GT. Androgenic stimulation of progesterone production by granulosa cells from preantral ovarian follicles: Further in vitro studies using replicate cell cultures. Endocrinology 1977;100:1539-49.

15. Hillier SG, van Hall EV, van den Boogaard AJM, de Zwart FA, Keyzer R. Activation and modulation of the granulosa cell aromatase system: Experimental studies with rat and human ovaries. In: Rolland R, van Hall EV, Hillier SG, McNatty KP, Schoemaker J, eds. Follicular maturation and ovulation. Amsterdam: Excerpta Medica, 1982:51-70.

16. Hillier SG. Sex steroid metabolism and follicular development in the ovaries. Oxf Rev Reprod Biol 1985;7:168-222.

17. Daniel SAJ, Armstrong DT. Androgens in the ovarian microenvironment. Semin Reprod Endocrinol 1986;4:89-100.

18. Tonetta ST, DiZerega GS. Intragonadal regulation of follicular maturation. Endocr Rev 1989;10:205-29.

19. Tsang BK, Moon YS, Simpson CW, Armstrong DT. Androgen biosynthesis in human ovarian follicles: Cellular source, gonadotropic control, and adenosine 3',5'-monophosphate mediation. J Clin Endocrinol Metab 1979;48:153-8.

20. McNatty KP. Hormonal correlates of follicular development in the human ovary. Aust J Biol Sci 1981;34:249-68.

21. Brailly S, Gougeon A, Milgrom E, Bomsel-Helmreich O, Papiernik E. Androgens and progestins in the human ovarian follicles: Differences in the evolution of preovulatory, healthy nonovulatory, and atretic follicles. J Clin Endocrinol Metab 1981;53:128-34.

22. Westergaard L, Christensen IJ, McNatty KP. Steroid levels in ovarian follicular fluid related to follicle size and health status during the normal menstrual cycle in women. Hum Reprod 1986;1:227.

23. Bjersing L. On the morphology and endocrine functions of granulosa cells in ovarian follicles and corpora lutea. Biochemical, histochemical, and ultrastructural studies on the porcine ovary with special reference to steroid hormone synthesis. Acta Endocrinol [Suppl] (Copenh) 1967;125.

24. McNatty KP, Reinhold VN, DeGrazia C, Osathanondh R, Ryan K. Metabolism

of androstenedione by human ovarian tissue in vitro with particular reference to reductase and aromatase activity. Steroids 1979;34:429-43.

25. Hammond JM, Hersey RM, Walega MA, Weisz J. Catecholestrogen production by porcine ovarian cells. Endocrinology 1986;118:2292-9.

26. Harlow CR, Hillier SG, Hodges JK. Androgen modulation of follicle-stimulating hormone-induced granulosa cell steroidogenesis in the primate ovary. Endocrinology 1986;119:1403-5.

27. Hillier SG, Ross GT. Effects of exogenous testosterone on ovarian weight, follicular morphology and intraovarian progesterone concentration in estrogen-primed, hypophysectomized immature female rats. Biol Reprod 1979;20:261-8.

28. Armstrong DT, Papkoff H. Stimulation of aromatization of exogenous and endogenous androgens in ovaries of hypophysectomized rats in vivo by follicle stimulating hormone. Endocrinology 1976;99:1144-51.

29. Hillier SG, van den Boogaard AJM, Reichert LE, Jr, van Hall EV. Intraovarian sex steroid hormone interactions and the control of follicular maturation: Aromatization of androgens by human granulosa cells in vitro. J Clin Endocrinol Metab 1980;50: 640-7.

30. Harlow CR, Shaw HJ, Hillier SG, Hodges JK. Factors influencing FSH-induced steroidogenesis in marmoset granulosa cells: Effects of androgens and stages of follicular development. Endocrinology 1988;122:2780-7.

31. Armstrong DT, Siuda A, Opavsky MA, Chandrasekhara Y. Bimodal effects of luteinizing hormone and role of androgens in modifying superovulatory responses of rats to infusion with purified follicle-stimulating hormone. Biol Reprod 1989;40:54-62.

32. Opavsky MA, Armstrong DT. Effects of luteinizing hormone on superovulatory and steroidogenic responses of rat ovaries to infusion with follicle-stimulating hormone. Biol Reprod 1989;40:12-25.

33. Richards JS, Jahnsen T, Hedin L, et al. Ovarian follicular development: From physiology to molecular biology. Recent Prog Horm Res 1987;43:231-70.

34. Hsueh AJW, Adashi EY, Jones PBC, Welsh TJ, Jr. Hormonal regulation of the differentiation of cultured granulosa cells. Endocr Rev 1984;5:76-126.

35. Toaff ME, Strauss JF, Hammond JM. Regulation of cytochrome P-450scc in immature porcine granulosa cells by FSH and estradiol. Endocrinology 1983; 112:1156-8.

36. Turner IM, Saunders PTK, Shimasaki S, Hillier SG. Regulation of inhibin subunit gene expression by FSH and estradiol in cultured rat granulosa cells. Endocrinology 1989;125:2790-2.

37. Bicsak T, Cajander SB, Vale W, Hsueh AJW. Inhibin: Studies of stored and secreted forms by biosynthetic labelling and immunodetection in cultured rat granulosa cells. Endocrinology 1988;122:741-8.

38. Richards JS. Estradiol receptor content in rat granulosa cells during follicular development: Modification by estradiol and gonadotropins. Endocrinology 1975;97:1174-84.

39. Saiduddin S, Zassenhaus HP. Estradiol-17β receptors in the immature rat ovary. Steroids 1977;29:97-213.

40. Kudolo GB, Elder MG, Myatt L. A novel oestrogen binding species in rat granulosa cells. J Endocrinol 1984;102:83-91.

41. Kudolo GB, Elder MG, Myatt L. Further characterization of the second oestrogen-binding species of the rat granulosa cell. J Endocrinol 1984;102: 93-102.
42. Hillier SG, Saunders PTK, White R, Parker MG. Oestrogen receptor mRNA and a related RNA transcript in mouse ovaries. J Mol Endocrinol 1989;2:39-45.
43. Hild-Petito S, Stouffer RL, Brenner RM. Immunocytochemical localization of estradiol and progesterone receptors in the monkey ovary throughout the menstrual cycle. Endocrinology 1988;123:2896-905.
44. Hillier SG, Wickings EJ, Saunders PTK, Shimisaki S, Reichert LE, Jr, McNeilly AS. Hormonal control of inhibin production by primate granulosa cells. J Endocrinol 1989;123:65-73.
45. Hillier SG. Reichert LE, Jr, van Hall EV. Control of preovulatory follicular estrogen biosynthesis in the human ovary. J Clin Endocrinol Metab 1981;52: 847-56.
46. Bomsel-Helmreich O, Gougeon A, Thebault A, Salterelli D, Milgrom E, Frydman R, Papiernik E. Healthy and atretic human follicles in the preovulatory phase: Differences in evolution of follicular morphology and steroid content of follicular fluid. J Clin Endocrinol Metab 1979;48:686-94.
47. Hillier SG. Regulation of follicular oestrogen biosynthesis: A survey of current concepts. J Endocrinol 1981;89(suppl):3P-19P.
48. Leung PCK, Armstrong DT. Interactions of steroids and gonadotrophins in the control of steroidogenesis in the ovarian follicle. Annu Rev Physiol 1980;42: 71-82.
49. Erickson GF, Magoffin DA, Dyer CA, Hofeditz C. The ovarian androgen producing cells: A review of structure/function relationships. Endocr Rev 1985; 6:371-99.
50. Dehennin L, Blacker C, Reifsteck A, Scholler R. Estrogen 2-, 4-, 6- or 16-hydroxylation by human follicles shown by gas chromatography associated with stable isotope dilution. J Steroid Biochem 1984;20:465-71.
51. Hudson KE, Hillier SG. Catechol oestradiol control of FSH-stimulated granulosa cell steroidogenesis. J Endocrinol 1985;106:R1-R3.
52. Spicer LJ, Hammond JM. Catechol estrogens inhibit proliferation and DNA synthesis in porcine granulosa cells in vitro: Comparison with estradiol, 5α-dihydrotestosterone, gonadotropins and catecholamines. Mol Cell Endocrinol 1989;64:119-26.
53. Hammond JM, English HF. Regulation of deoxyribonucleic acid synthesis in cultured porcine granulosa cells by growth factors and hormones. Endocrinology 1987;120:1039-46.
54. Ling N, Ying S-Y, Ueno N, Esch F, Denoroy L, Guillemin R. Isolation and partial characterization of a Mr 32,000 protein with inhibin activity from porcine follicular fluid. Proc Natl Acad Sci USA 1985;82:7217-21.
55. Rivier J, Spiess J, McClintock R, Vaughan J, Vale W. Purification and partial characterization of inhibin from porcine follicular fluid. Biochem Biophys Res Commun 1985;133:120-7.
56. Miyamoto K, Hasegawa Y, Fukuda M, et al. Isolation of porcine follicular fluid inhibin of 32K daltons. Biochem Biophys Res Commun 1985;129:396-403.
57. Robertson DM, Foulds LM, Leversha L, et al. Isolation of inhibin from bovine follicular fluid. Biochem Biophys Res Commun 1985;126:220-6.

58. Vale W, Rivier C, Hsueh A, et al. Chemical and biological characterization of the inhibin family of protein hormones. Recent Prog Horm Res 1988;44:1-30.
59. Ying S-Y. Inhibins, activins, and follistatins: Gonadal proteins modulating the secretion of follicle-stimulating hormone. Endocr Rev 1988;9:267-93.
60. Vale W, Rivier J, Vaughan J, et al. Purification and characterization of an FSH releasing protein from porcine ovarian follicular fluid. Nature 1986;321:776-9.
61. Ling N, Ying S-Y, Ueno N, et al. Pituitary FSH is released by a heterodimer of the β-subunits from the two forms of inhibin. Nature 1986;321:779-82.
62. McLachlan RI, Cohen NL, Dahl KD, Bremner WL, Soules MR. Serum inhibin levels during the periovulatory interval in normal women: Relationship with sex steroid and gonadotrophin levels. Clin Endocrinol (Oxf);32:39-48.
63. de Jong FH. Inhibin. Physiol Rev 1988;68:555-607.
64. Roberts AB, Flanders KC, Kondaiah P, et al. Transforming growth factor β: Biochemistry and roles in embryogenesis, tissue repair and remodeling, and carcinogenesis. Recent Prog Horm Res 1988;44:157-93.
65. Eto Y, Tsuji Y, Takezawa M, Takano S, Yokogawa Y, Shibai H. Purification and characterization of erythroid differentiation factor (EDF) isolated from human luekemia cell line THP-1. Biophys Biochem Res Commun 1987;142:1095-103.
66. Yu J, Shao L, Lemas V, et al. Importance of FSH-releasing protein and inhibin in erythroid differentiation. Nature 1987;330: 765-7.
67. Erickson GF, Hsueh AJW. Secretion of inhibin by rat granulosa cells in vitro. Endocrinology 1978;103:1960-3.
68. Suzuki T, Miyamoto K, Hasegawa Y, et al. Regulation of inhibin production by rat granulosa cells. Mol Cell Endocrinol 1987;54:185-95.
69. Bicsak TA, Hsueh AJW. Recent advances in inhibin research. In: Stouffer RL. ed. The primate ovary. New York: Plenum Press, 1988:35-47.
70. Zhang Z, Lee VWK, Carson RS, Burger HG. Selective control of rat granulosa cell inhibin production by FSH and LH in vitro. Mol Cell Endocrinol 1988; 56:35-40.
71. Henderson KM, Franchimont P. Inhibin production by bovine ovarian tissues in vitro and its regulation by androgens. J Reprod Fertil 1983;67:291-8.
72. Tsonis CG, Hillier SG, Baird DT. Production of inhibin bioactivity by human granulosa-lutein cells: Stimulation by LH and testosterone in vitro. J Endocrinol 1987;112:R11-R14.
73. Hillier SG, Wickings EJ, McNeilly AS, Reichert LE, Jr, Illingworth P, Baird DT. Hormone-dependent production of inhibin by cultured human granulosa cells [Abstract]. J Endocrinol 1990;124(suppl):69.
74. Mason AJ, Hayflick JS, Ling N, et al. Complementary DNA sequences of ovarian follicular fluid inhibin show precursor structure and homology with transforming growth factor-β. Nature 1985;318:659-63.
75. Mason AJ, Niall HD, Seeburg PH. Structure of two human ovarian inhibins. Biochem Biophys Res Commun 1986;135:957-64.
76. Forage RG, Ring JW, Brown RW, et al. Cloning and sequence analysis of cDNA species coding for the two subunits of inhibin from bovine follicular fluid. Proc Natl Acad Sci USA 1986;83:3091-5.
77. Mayo KE, Cerelli GM, Spiess J, et al. Inhibin A-subunit cDNAs from porcine ovary and human placenta. Proc Natl Acad Sci USA 1986;83:5849-53.
78. Esch FS, Shimasaki S, Cooksey K, et al. Complementary deoxyribonucleic acid

(cDNA) cloning and DNA sequence analysis of rat ovarian inhibins. Mol Endocrinol 1987;1:388-96.

79. Woodruff T, Meunier H, Jones PB, Hsueh AJW, Mayo KE. Rat inhibin: Molecular cloning of α- and β-subunit complementary deoxyribonucleic acids and expression in the ovary. Mol Endocrinol 1987;1:561-9.

80. Woodruff TK, D'Agostino JB, Schwartz NB, Mayo KE. Dynamic changes in inhibin messenger RNAs in rat ovarian follicles during the reproductive cycle. Science 1988;239:1296-9.

81. Hsueh AJW, Dahl KD, Vaughan J, et al. Heterodimers and homodimers of inhibin subunits have different paracrine action in the modulation of luteinizing hormone-stimulated androgen biosynthesis. Proc Natl Acad Sci USA 1987; 84:5082-6.

82. Ying S-Y, Becker A, Ling N, Ueno N, Guillemin R. Inhibin and beta type transforming growth factor (TGFβ) have opposite modulating effects on the follicle stimulating hormone (FSH)-induced aromatase activity of cultured rat granulosa cells. Biochem Biophys Res Commun 1986;136:969-75.

83. Hutchison LA, Findlay JK, de Vos FL, Robertson DM. Effects of bovine inhibin, transforming growth factor-β and bovine activin-A on granulosa cell differentiation. Biochem Biophys Res Commun 1987;146:1405-12.

84. Gonzalez-Manchon C, Vale W. Activin-A, inhibin and transforming growth factor-β modulate growth of two gonadal cell lines. Endocrinology 1989; 125:1666-72.

Part III

Hormonal Control and Gene Expression in the Ovary

8

Regulation of Inhibin and Activin Genes in the Rat Ovary

JOANNA C. DYKEMA, JASON O. RAHAL, AND KELLY E. MAYO

The gonadotropins, luteinizing hormone (LH) and follicle stimulating hormone (FSH), play major roles in regulating the mammalian reproductive cycle by influencing the gametogenic and steroidogenic functions of the gonads (1, 2). The simultaneous release of LH and FSH from anterior pituitary gonadotrophs is known to be positively regulated by the hypothalamic decapeptide GnRH (3, 4). More recently, several gonadal peptides that specifically modulate FSH synthesis and secretion have been isolated and characterized. These include the inhibins, activins, and follistatin (5–12).

The multiple forms of inhibin and activin are related molecules derived from the combinatorial assembly of three polypeptide chains termed α (18 kDa), β_A (14 kDa), and β_B (14 kDa). Inhibins are 32-kDa $\alpha\beta$-dimers, whereas activins are 28-kDa $\beta\beta$-dimers. Despite their structural similarities, the effects of inhibin and activin on FSH secretion are functionally antagonistic; inhibin suppresses FSH secretion, while activin stimulates FSH secretion and synthesis (5–10). Follistatin is a structurally distinct 35-kDa single-chain polypeptide that, like inhibin, decreases FSH release from cultured pituitary cells. In addition, follistatin has been shown to be an activin binding protein (13).

To explore the expression and regulation of the inhibin and activin genes, we have isolated α, β_A, and β_B cDNA clones from the rat ovary (14, J.C. Dykema and K.E. Mayo, unpublished). Using these cDNA probes, we have examined the localization and regulation of the inhibin and activin mRNAs in various reproductive tissues. This chapter describes the expression of the inhibin and activin α and β_A mRNAs in the rat ovary throughout the reproductive cycle.

In Situ Hybridization to Detect Inhibin and Activin mRNAs

In order to examine ovarian expression of the α and β_A mRNAs, in situ hybridization was utilized. This technique is summarized in Figure 1. Briefly, it entails removal and quick freezing of the tissues of interest, preparation of

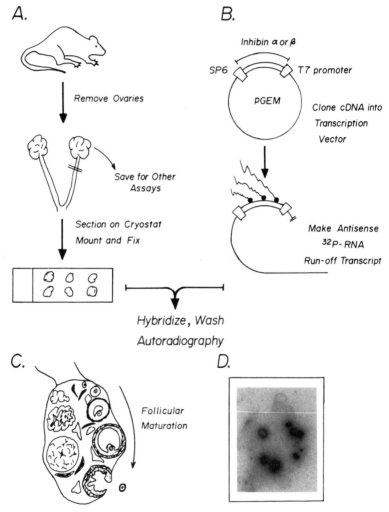

FIGURE 1. The use of in situ hybridization to localize inhibin and activin mRNAs in the rat ovary. *A* and *B* schematically depict the preparation of tissue and probe for hybridization. In *C*, a sketch of a rat ovary shows the morphological changes that occur as a follicle is recruited, matures, ovulates, and differentiates into luteal tissue. *D* is the autoradiographic detection of probe hybridizing to maturing follicles in an ovarian section.

Northern RNA Blot   *In Situ* **Hybridization**

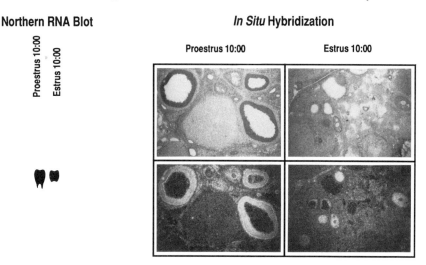

FIGURE 2. Detection of inhibin α-chain mRNA in the rat ovary using RNA blotting and in situ hybridization. Ovaries were removed at the cycle times indicated. Total ovarian RNA (10 μg) was loaded in each lane of a denaturing agarose gel, the RNA was transferred to a nylon membrane, and the membrane was probed with a ^{32}P-labeled α-inhibin cDNA. In situ hybridization was performed as indicated in the text using a ^{35}S-labeled riboprobe, and exposure was for 2 weeks. Sections were stained with hematoxylin/eosin. The upper photomicrographs were taken using bright field optics; the lower photomicrographs were taken using darkfield optics.

20-μ tissue sections on a cryostat, mounting of sections onto microscope slides, tissue fixation, hybridization with [32]P- or ^{35}S-labeled antisense riboprobes specific for the α- or β_A-chains, and, finally, liquid emulsion autoradiography to visualize the hybridizing probe. In situ hybridization is a particularly powerful technique because it allows estimation of mRNA abundance as well as localization of the mRNAs to individual cells. This is a distinct advantage over RNA blotting, which is useful for quantitating changes in mRNA levels, but does not allow differentiation between the various ovarian cell types. For example, Figure 2 compares RNA blotting and in situ hybridization for analyzing α-chain gene expression at two times during the estrous cycle (proestrous and estrous morning). While α mRNA levels do not change dramatically, in situ hybridization reveals localization of the α mRNA to large preovulatory follicles in the proestrous ovary and small newly recruited follicles in the estrous ovary. To ensure that any mRNA expression detected by in situ hybridization is specific, two controls are included in each experiment: The appropriate sense-strand probes are hybridized to ovarian tissue, and antisense probes are hybridized to a tissue that does not express the inhibin and activin genes (for example, liver). Both of these controls were performed for all experiments reported here (not shown).

Results

Inhibin and Activin mRNA Expression Changes Throughout the Estrous Cycle

Recent efforts in our laboratory have been aimed at refining and expanding previous studies in which in situ hybridization was used to examine inhibin and activin mRNA expression in the rat ovary throughout the estrous cycle (14, 15). Two approaches have been taken to accomplish this. First, the riboprobes used for in situ hybridization have been labeled with [^{35}S]UTP rather than the [^{32}P]UTP used in earlier experiments. This change results in greater sensitivity and enhanced resolution of the hybridization signal. Second, ovaries were collected more frequently throughout the estrous cycle, particularly during the physiologically significant times surrounding the gonadotropin surges and ovulation, thus giving a more complete view of changes in α and β_A mRNA expression. The rats used for these experiments

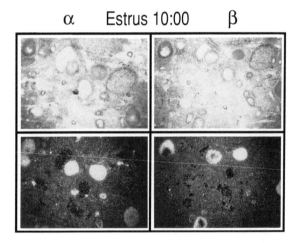

α Estrus 10:00 β

FIGURE 3. Recruited follicles (>350-μ mean diameter) expressing α and β_A mRNAs on estrous morning. The top panels are brightfield views of adjacent hematoxylin/ eosin stained ovarian sections. The bottom panels are the same fields photographed using darkfield optics to show the autoradiographic silver grains indicative of probe hybridization. The left section was hybridized with an α-chain probe; the right section, with a β_A-chain probe. Expression of both the α and β_A mRNAs is detected in small newly recruited follicles at this time in the estrous cycle.

(Sprague-Dawley, Charles River) were housed in 14 h:10 h light:dark conditions, and exhibited regular 4-day estrous cycles. Cycle stages were determined by daily cytological examination of vaginal smears, and only animals exhibiting at least 2 consecutive 4-day cycles were used. Serum samples were collected and measured for LH and FSH by radioimmunoassay. All animals exhibited appropriate proestrous gonadotropin surges (data not shown). All in situ hybridizations shown here were performed simultaneously using a single batch of α- or β_A-antisense riboprobes so that direct comparison of α and β_A mRNA levels between animals could be made.

The results of these experiments support our previous findings that both α and β_A mRNAs are localized predominantly to the granulosa cells of maturing follicles. At 1000 h estrous morning, small follicles newly recruited by the secondary FSH surge can be seen expressing both α and β_A mRNAs (Fig. 3). mRNA levels increase as these follicles grow during metestrus, diestrus, and proestrus (Figs. 4–6). Expression peaks in mature follicles at approximately 1600 h proestrus and then begins to decline at about 1830 h proestrus in follicles showing signs of gonadotropin stimulation (Fig. 7). By 2100 h proestrus, α mRNA expression is substantially reduced, and β_A mRNA is nearly undetectable in large gonadotropin-stimulated follicles (Fig. 8). At 0200 h estrus, both α and β_A mRNA levels are extremely low in follicles that are about to be ovulated (Fig. 9). Increased expression of the α and β_A mRNAs is observed in newly recruited small follicles on estrous morning (Figs. 9–10).

α Metestrus 10:00 β

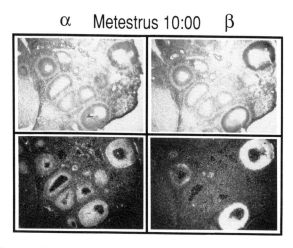

FIGURE 4. Maturing follicles continuing to express α and β_A mRNAs on metestrous morning. In situ hybridization and photography of these and all of the following rat ovarian sections were as described in Figure 3. The smaller follicles expressing only α mRNA are most likely early atretic follicles.

α   Diestrus 10:00   β

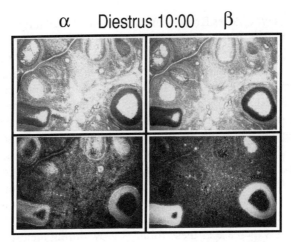

FIGURE 5. Highly expressed α and β$_A$ mRNAs in growing follicles on diestrous morning. Several healthy follicles (~500-μ mean diameter) that express both α and β$_A$ mRNAs are observed. A few atretic follicles expressing only low levels of α-chain mRNA can also be seen (*left panels*).

α   Proestrus 10:00   β

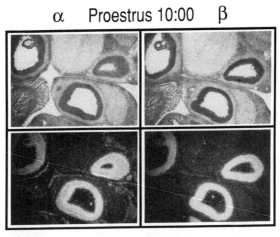

FIGURE 6. Inhibin and activin α- and β$_A$-chain mRNAs co-localized to the granulosa cells of large mature follicles on proestrous morning. Note the absence of atretic follicles expressing only the α-chain mRNA seen in Figures 4–5. An aging corpus luteum that does not express either α or β$_A$ mRNA can be seen in the upper part of each photomicrograph.

α   Proestrus 18:30   β

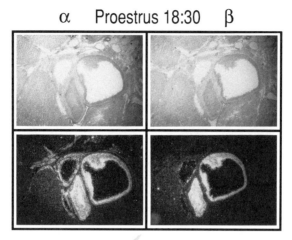

FIGURE 7. Expression of the α- and β_A-chain mRNAs beginning to decline in large follicles that show early signs of gonadotropin stimulation. At 1830 h proestrus, following the onset of the primary LH surge, α and β_A mRNAs begin to decline from the peak levels observed on proestrous afternoon. Note the thinning of the follicle wall and expansion of the antrum in the large expressing follicle.

α   Proestrus 21:00   β

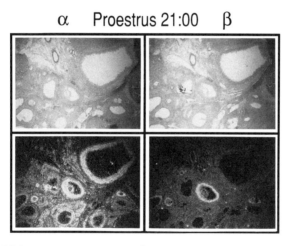

FIGURE 8. Inhibin and activin α- and β_A-chain mRNA expression dramatically decreased in large gonadotropin-stimulated preovulatory follicles on proestrous evening. The single large follicle shown continues to express low levels of α mRNA, while β_A mRNA is not detected. Expression of the α and β_A mRNAs in a smaller nonovulatory follicle and of α mRNA in interstitial gland can also be observed.

α   Estrus 02:00   β

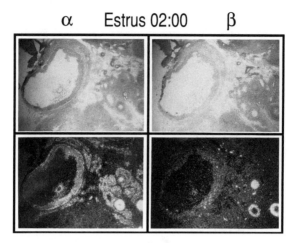

FIGURE 9. Expression of α and β$_A$ mRNAs in large preovulatory follicles early on estrous morning. The large follicle shown (>800-μ mean diameter) contains very low levels of α and β$_A$ mRNA just prior to ovulation. Also note the expression of both α and β$_A$ mRNA in small newly recruited follicles and the presence of α mRNA in interstitial gland.

α   Estrus 04:00   β

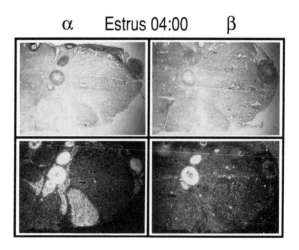

FIGURE 10. The newly formed corpus luteum expressing α but not β$_A$ mRNA on estrous morning. A newly formed corpus luteum expressing α mRNA is observed in the lower, central part of each photomicrograph. To its right is an older corpus luteum that does not express either the α- or β$_A$-chain mRNAs. Newly recruited follicles (>350-μ mean diameter) expressing both α and β$_A$ mRNAs can also be seen.

It should be noted that although Figures 3–10 show only α and β_A mRNA hybridization results, a rat β_B cDNA has been used to examine β_B mRNA expression in more recent experiments. These preliminary data indicate that ovarian β_A and β_B mRNA expression are quite similar, although the β_B mRNA is less abundant than the β_A mRNA.

Differences in Expression of the α and β_A mRNAs

Although the patterns of α and β_A mRNA expression described in the previous section are generally similar, there are instances when the expression patterns clearly diverge. One notable example is the expression of α mRNA, but not β_A mRNA in follicles observed on metestrous and diestrous morning (Figs. 4–5). Histological examination indicates that these are follicles in the earliest stages of atresia, suggesting that β_A mRNA expression is more rapidly lost than α mRNA expression as these follicles cease normal development. In a similar fashion, β_A mRNA decline more rapidly than α mRNA in gonadotropin-stimulated preovulatory follicles. By 2100 h proestrus (Fig. 8), β_A mRNA is nearly undetectable, while α mRNA persists at reduced levels in large follicles. α-chain mRNA levels further decline by 2400 h on proestrus (15, and data not shown). Even at later times on proestrous evening and estrous morning, low levels of α mRNA are found in preovulatory follicles in the absence of β_A mRNA (Fig. 9, and additional times not shown).

A second example of divergent expression is apparent in examining the ovarian cell types that express the α- and β_A-chain mRNAs. While both mRNAs are predominantly found in the granulosa cells of maturing follicles, the α mRNA is somewhat more broadly distributed and is found in interstitial cells (Figs. 8–9) and in newly differentiated luteal cells (Fig. 10). The expression observed in the corpus luteum appears to be transient, as no α mRNA is observed in older corpora lutea (Figs. 6 and 10). We can not eliminate the possibility that the β_A mRNA is also expressed in these cell types at levels below the detection limits of the in situ hybridization assay employed.

Discussion

The data presented in this chapter indicate that in situ hybridization is an extremely powerful approach for examining dynamic patterns of gene expression in heterogeneous tissues such as the ovary. While levels of the inhibin and activin mRNAs in whole ovary do change during the estrous cycle, as determined by RNAse protection and RNA blotting assays (15, and K.E. Mayo unpublished), in situ hybridization reveals that the most dramatic changes in inhibin and activin gene expression are confined to healthy, maturing follicles. We find that both the α and β_A mRNAs are initially expressed in small newly recruited follicles early on estrous morning, increase in growing follicles during metestrus and diestrus, and peak in large, mature follicles on proestrous afternoon. Subsequently, expression of both the α- and β_A-chain mRNAs declines in gonadotropin-stimulated follicles on proestrous evening. Similar results obtained using in situ hybridization have been reported by Meunier and coworkers (16). Although localization and measurement of the α and β_A mRNAs does not provide information on the actual hormones produced and secreted from the ovary (inhibin versus activin), serum inhibin levels during the rat estrous cycle generally parallel the changes reported here for α and β_A mRNAs (17).

Extensive in vivo and in vitro evidence suggests that inhibin modulates FSH secretion and is in turn regulated by the gonadotropins (18–21). Consistent with this idea, the α- and β_A-chain mRNAs are initially expressed in follicles newly recruited by the secondary FSH surge and increase in growing follicles under the influence of basal FSH levels during much of the estrous cycle. An intriguing observation made in this and in previous in situ hybridization studies (15, 16) is that expression of the α- and β_A-chain mRNAs dramatically decreases in preovulatory follicles at the time of the primary gonadotropin surges. By using a specific GnRH antagonist to block the endogenous gonadotropin surges, we have previously demonstrated that the preovulatory gonadotropin surges are required for the decline in inhibin and activin gene expression that normally occurs on proestrous evening (22). Replacement of these antagonist-treated animals with either exogenous FSH or LH restores appropriate regulation of the α and β_A mRNAs, suggesting that these hormones work by a common cAMP-mediated mechanism to modulate inhibin and activin gene expression in preovulatory follicles. The dual nature of gonadotropin regulation of α- and β_A-gene expression observed in these studies is similar to that seen for other gonadotropin-regulated genes expressed in the ovary, including the type II regulatory subunit of cAMP-dependent protein kinase and several of the cytochrome P-450 steroidogenic enzymes (23–24).

We have found that the patterns of α- and β_A-gene expression in the rat ovary are generally similar, but that they are not identical. Expression of the β_A mRNA appears to be more tightly regulated than expression of the α mRNA. β_A mRNA levels decline more rapidly in atretic follicles and in gonadotropin-stimulated preovulatory follicles than do α-chain mRNA levels. In stimulated preovulatory follicles, β_A mRNA decreases to undetectable levels, while the α mRNA continues to be expressed at low levels. These differences could simply reflect a shorter half-life of the β_A mRNA, or they might be a consequence of divergent transcriptional regulation of the two genes. The α-chain mRNA appears to be more broadly expressed than the

β_A-chain mRNA in the ovary. In addition to the transient expression in interstitial cells and luteal cells described here, we have previously found that the α mRNA is expressed at low levels in small follicles prior to recruitment, while the β_A mRNA is undetectable (25). Interestingly, the β_A mRNA is widely expressed in nongonadal tissues, while the α-chain mRNA exhibits a more restricted pattern of expression (26, and J.O. Rahal and K.E. Mayo, unpublished). Consistent with these divergent patterns of expression of α and β mRNAs, recent analysis of the α- and β_B-genes suggests that their putative promoter regions are structurally quite distinct (27, and J.C. Dykema and K.E. Mayo, unpublished).

Based on the changes in α- and β_A-gene expression observed during the estrous cycle in these and other experiments, we have proposed a model for the interactions between ovarian inhibin expression and pituitary FSH secretion (28). On estrous morning, the secondary FSH surge likely plays an important role in signaling the initial expression of the α and β_A mRNAs in newly recruited follicles (25). The inhibin produced by these follicles is proposed to act on the pituitary to return FSH secretion to basal levels. Throughout much of the estrous cycle, growing follicles secrete inhibin that functions to maintain low basal FSH secretion. On proestrous afternoon, the primary LH and FSH surges act to suppress inhibin gene expression in large preovulatory follicles; presumably, this decline in inhibin production would be permissive for continued elevated FSH secretion, resulting in the secondary FSH surge on estrous morning. Our future challenges lie in developing appropriate physiological models to further test these ideas and in deciphering the molecular mechanisms by which the inhibin and activin genes are regulated during the reproductive cycle.

References

1. Pierce GP, Parsons TF. Glycoprotein hormones: Structure and function. Annu Rev Biochem 1981;50:465-95.
2. Dorrington JH, Armstrong DT. Effects of FSH on gonadal functions. Recent Prog Horm Res 1979;35:301-42.
3. Amoss M, Burgus R, Blackwell R, Vale W, Fellows R, Guillemin R. Purification, amino acid composition and amino-terminus of the hypothalamic luteinizing hormone releasing factor (LRF) of ovine origin. Biochem Biophys Res Commun 1971;44:205-10.
4. Schally AV, Arimura A, Baba Y, et al. Isolation and properties of the FSH and LH-releasing hormone. Biochem Biophys Res Commun 1971;43:393-9.
5. Robertson DM, Foulds LM, Leversha L, et al. Isolation of inhibin from bovine follicular fluid. Biochem Biophys Res Commun 1985;126:220-6.
6. Miyamoto K, Hasegawa Y, Fukuda M, et al. Isolation of porcine follicular fluid inhibin of about 32 kDa. Biochem Biophys Res Commun 1985;129:396-403.
7. Ling N, Ying S-Y, Ueno N, Esch F, Denoroy L, Guillemin R. Isolation and

partial characterization of a M_r 32,000 protein with inhibin activity from porcine ovarian follicular fluid. Proc Natl Acad Sci USA 1985;82:7217-21.

8. Rivier J, Spiess J, McClintock R, Vaughan J, Vale W. Purification and partial characterization of inhibin from porcine follicular fluid. Biochem Biophys Res Commun 1985;133:120-7.

9. Vale W, Rivier J, Vaughan J, et al. Purification and characterization of an FSH-releasing protein from porcine ovarian follicular fluid. Nature 1986;321:776-9.

10. Ling N, Ying S-Y, Ueno N, et al. Pituitary FSH is released by a heterodimer of the β-subunits from the two forms of inhibin. Nature 1986;321:779-82.

11. Ueno N, Ling N, Ying S-Y, Esch F, Shimasaki S, Guillemin R. Isolation and partial characterization of follistatin: A single-chain M_r 35,000 monomeric protein that inhibits the release of follicle-stimulating hormone. Proc Natl Acad Sci USA 1987;84:8282-6.

12. Esch F, Shimasaki S, Mercado M, et al. Structural characterization of follistatin: A novel follicle-stimulating hormone release-inhibiting polypeptide from the gonad. Mol Endocrinol 1987;1:849-55.

13. Nakamura T, Takio K, Eto Y, Shibai H, Titani K, Sugino H. Activin-binding protein from rat ovary is follistatin. Science 1990;247:836-8.

14. Woodruff TK, Meunier H, Jones PBC, Hsueh AJW, Mayo KE. Rat inhibin: Molecular cloning of α- and β-subunit complementary deoxyribonucleic acids and expression in the ovary. Mol Endocrinol 1987;1:561-8.

15. Woodruff TK, D'Agostino J, Schwartz NB, Mayo KE. Dynamic changes in inhibin messenger RNAs in rat ovarian follicles during the reproductive cycle. Science 1988;239:1296-9.

16. Meunier H, Cajander SB, Roberts VJ, et al. Rapid changes in the expression of inhibin α-, $β_A$- and $β_B$-subunits in ovarian cell types during the rat estrous cycle. Mol Endocrinol 1988;2:1352-63.

17. Hasegawa Y. Changes in serum concentrations of inhibin during the estrous cycle of the rat, pig, and cow. In: Burger HG, de Krester DM, Findlay JK, Igarushi M, eds. Inhibin-non-steroidal regulation of follicle stimulating hormone secretion. New York: Raven Press, 1987:119-33.

18. Rivier C, Rivier J, Vale W. Inhibin-mediated feedback control of follicle-stimulating hormone secretion in the female rat. Science 1986;234:205-8.

19. Davis SR, Burger HG, Robertson DM, Farnworth PG, Carson RS, Krozowski Z. Pregnant mare's serum gonadotropin stimulates inhibin subunit gene expression in the immature rat ovary: Dose response characteristics and relationships to serum gonadotropins, inhibin, and ovarian steroid content. Endocrinology 1988; 123:2399-407.

20. Rivier C, Roberts V, Vale W. Possible role of luteinizing hormone and follicle-stimulating hormone in modulating inhibin secretion and expression during the estrous cycle of the rat. Endocrinology 1989;125:876-82.

21. LaPolt PS, Piquette GN, Soto D, Sincich C, Hsueh AJW. Regulation of inhibin subunit messenger ribonucleic acid levels by gonadotropins, growth factors, and gonadotropin-releasing hormone in cultured rat granulosa cells. Endocrinology 1990;127:823-31.

22. Woodruff TK, D'Agostino J, Schwartz NB, Mayo KE. Decreased inhibin gene expression in preovulatory follicles requires primary gonadotropin surges. Endocrinology 1989;124:1-7.

23. Richards JS, Jahnsen T, Hedin L, et al. Ovarian follicular development: From physiology to molecular biology. Rec Prog Horm Res 1987;43:231-76.
24. Richards JS, Hedin L. Molecular aspects of hormone action in ovarian follicular development, ovulation, and luteinization. Annu Rev Physiol 1988;50:441-63.
25. D'Agostino J, Woodruff TK, Mayo KE, Schwartz NB. Unilateral ovariectomy increases inhibin messenger ribonucleic acid levels in newly recruited follicles. Endocrinology 1989;124:310-7.
26. Meunier H, Rivier C, Evans RM, Vale W. Gonadal and extragonadal expression of inhibin α, β_A, and β_B subunits in various tissues predicts diverse functions. Proc Natl Acad Sci USA 1988;85:247-51.
27. Feng Z-M, Li Y-P, Chen C-L C. Analysis of the 5' flanking regions of rat inhibin α- and β_B-subunit genes suggests two different regulatory mechanisms. Mol Endocrinol 1989;3:1914-25.
28. Woodruff TK, Mayo KE. Regulation of inhibin synthesis in the rat ovary. Annu Rev Physiol 1990;52:807-21.

9

mos Proto-Oncogene Product and Cytostatic Factor

NICHOLAS SCHULZ AND GEORGE F. VANDE WOUDE

The *mos* oncogene has been useful for studying oncogene/proto-oncogene function and has provided unique insight into the molecular basis of neoplastic transformation. Like many other oncogenes, *mos* was discovered as part of the acute transforming retrovirus Moloney murine sarcoma virus (Mo-MSV). Mo-MSV is a replication-defective virus that causes fibrosarcomas in mice, rats, and hamsters (1–3). Reviews of the properties of Mo-MSV have been published (4, 5). Early studies with Mo-MSV (6) described what is now referred to as the toxicity of acute infection. A large percentage of fibroblasts infected with Mo-MSV round up and show evidence for premature chromatin condensation, ring chromosome formation, and chromosome pulverization (7). The floating cells do not proliferate, while the cells that remain attached typically develop as foci of disoriented spindle-shaped transformed cells (8). These transformed cells are anchorage independent, grow in semisolid media to high saturation density, and show a disruption of the cytoskeleton, all of which are changes observed with other transformed cells and transforming genes. Papkoff et al. (9) demonstrated that cells acutely infected with Mo-MSV express a 30- to 100-fold higher level of *mos* product than stably transformed cell populations (10, 11). The recent discovery that the *mos* proto-oncogene product is cytostatic factor (CSF) suggests that toxicity during acute infection is due to CSF activity caused by high levels of Mo-MSV *mos* product (12). The mouse *mos* oncogene product expressed in transformed cells represents only 0.0005% of the total cellular protein (10, 11), indicating that it is extraordinarily efficient and has a high specific activity as an oncoprotein. The toxicity displayed at high levels of *mos* product expression and transforming properties at lower levels are quantitative properties that must be explained in order to understand the molecular basis of transformation.

TABLE 1. Properties of the *mos* proto-oncogene.

Property	Reference
Constitutive expression in somatic cells results in morphological transformation.	50
Upstream sequences influence activation as an oncogene (primates–amphibians).	15–17
Intronless (primates and amphibians).	11, 14, 23
c-*mos* RNA expression is	
Low in brain, kidney, mammary gland, placenta, epididymis, heart and lung; high in embryos;	20, 22, 28
Highest in germ cells;	22, 25–27
Not detected in liver, skin, intestine, and spleen.	20, 22
c-*mos* is required for oocyte maturation in mouse and *Xenopus* oocytes; product is CSF or a component of it.	12, 42

A summary of the properties of the *mos* proto-oncogene is shown in Table 1. The *mos* proto-oncogene isolated from the mouse genome was the first cellular proto-oncogene shown to have transforming activity (13). A proviral LTR linked to the *mos* proto-oncogene locus was as efficient as v-*mos* in transforming potential (14), which led to the conclusion that constitutive expression of the *mos* gene in somatic cells results in expression of the transformed phenotype. Upstream sequences in the genomic locus have been shown to influence activation of the *mos* proto-oncogene locus as an oncogene. In different species, these sequences range from open reading frames that overlap the initiating ATG of the *mos* proto-oncogene (15, 16) to sequences in the mouse locus that are transcription attenuation signals (17, 18). We have found that in order to activate the proto-oncogene locus by an LTR, it is necessary to either inactivate overlapping open reading frames or interrupt the transcription attenuation signal (16, 17, 19, 20). Moreover, *mos* proto-oncogene RNA transcripts do not contain these regulatory regions, and the normal function of these upstream sequences may be only to prevent RNA expression or translation, which could be deleterious to cell function (16). Compared to most other proto-oncogenes, the *mos* gene is intronless, and from primates through amphibians, the transcripts from the locus are direct copies of the genome (21, 22–24). The only post-transcriptional modification detected is polyadenylation (23).

The development of a sensitive RNA detection assay (23) was key in identifying *mos* transcripts in a variety of tissues (Table 1). These studies also revealed that *mos* expression was high in gonadal tissue and in early embryos (22, 23). This was followed by the demonstration that the *mos* proto-oncogene is expressed specifically in germ cells (22, 25–27) and is required for germ cell development in both mouse (7, 28) and *Xenopus* (25) oocytes and, therefore, in vertebrates. More importantly, the product, p39^{mos}, is CSF or the active component of it (12), an activity responsible for arresting vertebrate oocytes at metaphase II (29–32).

The *mos* proto-oncogene is expressed in germ cells during maturation, and its expression in maturing mouse oocytes demonstrates that it is a member of maternally inherited messenger RNAs (33). By in situ hybridization, expression was detected in growing and maturing oocytes, persisting through ovulation (Fig. 1), but expression was not evident in fertilized eggs (25). This

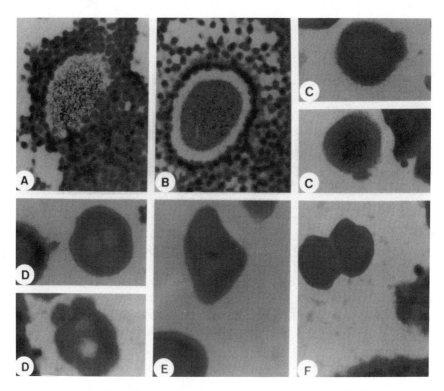

FIGURE 1. In situ hybridization demonstrating expression of *mos* RNA throughout meiotic maturation, ovulation, fertilization, and first cleavage (excerpted from reference 26). The number of silver grains is proportional to amount of *mos* RNA present. *A* and *B*: Sections of an ovary at 0 h and 7 h after treatment with human chorionic gonadotropin (post-hCG), respectively. Note cumulus cells compacted around the oocyte in *A* and expanded away from the oocyte in *B*. *C*: Oviduct section at 21 h post-hCG obtained from an unmated female, showing hybridization to the oocyte and the presence of first polar body. *D*: Sections through oviducts obtained from a mated mouse at 21 h post-hCG, showing male and female pronuclei and polar bodies. *E* and *F*: Sections of oviduct obtained from a mated mouse at 30 h post-hCG, showing the zygote with chromosomes condensed (*E*) or undergoing cleavage (*F*). All sections (shown at 125×) were processed in the same manner, hybridized at the same time, and exposed for 10 days.

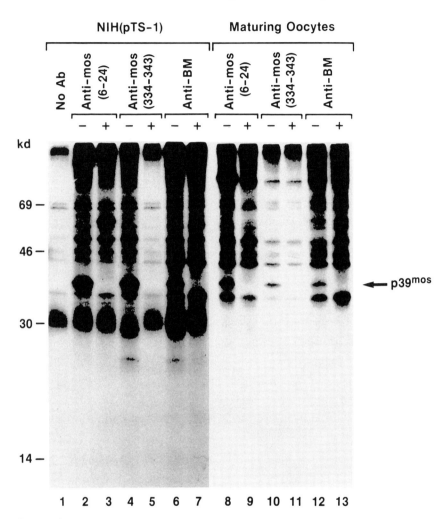

FIGURE 2. Immunoprecipitation analyses of *mos*-encoded protein from *mos*-transformed NIH/3T3 cells and meiotic mouse oocytes (excerpted from reference 7). Cells were metabolically labeled with [^{35}S]methionine and [^{35}S]cysteine for 1 h [NIH(pTS-1) cells] or 3 h (maturing oocytes). Aliquots of clarified lysates, either in the absence (–) or presence (+) of competing antigen, were subjected to immunoprecipitation analyses using 3 different *mos*-specific antibodies: anti-*mos*-(6-24), anti-*mos*-(334-343), or anti-BM. The arrow points to the protein specifically precipitated by all 3 *mos*-specific antisera from *mos*-transformed NIH/3T3 cells [NIH(pTS-1)] or maturing mouse oocytes.

provided the first opportunity to test whether the *mos* oncogene and proto-oncogene products were the same, evidence that was needed to support the hypothesis that constitutive expression of *mos* product in somatic cells was responsible for its transformed phenotype (Table 1). NIH/3T3 cells transformed with a recombinant DNA molecule containing the Mo-MSV LTR transcription control element fused to the mouse c-*mos* locus (pTS1) express a 39,000-Da product, p39^{mos} (Fig. 2). The same size product is found in maturing mouse oocytes (Fig. 2) and provides unequivocal evidence that expression of the proto-oncogene product in somatic cells is responsible for the transformed phenotype (7).

The expression of *mos* during oocyte maturation provided the first opportunity to test whether *mos* was required for this developmental process. Sense and antisense oligodeoxyribonucleotides or phosphothioate derivatives corresponding to regions of the *mos* RNA transcript were microinjected directly into maturing mouse oocytes in vitro (Fig. 3). Only the antisense

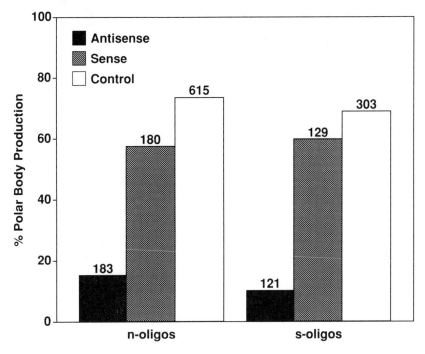

FIGURE 3. Blockage of PB emission by *mos* oligonucleotides (excerpted from reference 7). Cumulus cell-enclosed oocytes blocked at the GV stage in IBMX-containing medium were microinjected with a mixture of 3 different antisense or sense oligodeoxyribonucleotides (n-oligos) or phosphothioate oligodeoxyribonucleotides (s-oligos) and allowed to mature overnight. Control microinjected oocytes were examined in each experiment. Numbers over columns refer to the number of oocytes examined per group in at least 4 separate experiments.

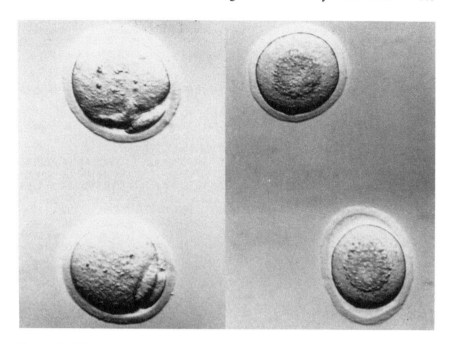

FIGURE 4. Mouse oocytes injected with *mos* oligonucleotides (excerpted from reference. 7). Cumulus cell-enclosed oocytes blocked at the GV stage in IBMX-containing medium and microinjected with a mixture of sense or antisense oligodeoxyribonucleotides were allowed to mature overnight. Nomarski optics of sense-injected oocytes (*left panel*) show polar body emission and organelles distributed throughout the cytoplasm. Antisense-injected oocytes (*right panel*) show organelles clustered in the pericentral region.

molecules inhibited polar body emission and therefore blocked meiotic maturation.

The morphology of the antisense-treated oocytes interrupted in maturation was quite dramatic (Fig. 4). Sense-injected oocytes underwent normal maturation and polar body production (Fig. 4). The antisense-injected oocytes underwent germinal vesicle breakdown (GVBD) and metaphase chromosome condensation (5), but were arrested at a stage when cytoplasmic particulates and mitochondria had migrated over the nucleus during GVBD. Normally after GVBD, these particulates redistribute to the cytoplasm. This demonstrates that the depletion of *mos* during maturation interrupts this developmental process at a specific stage of cytoskeletal morphogenesis.

While the mammalian mouse system has provided unique insight into *mos* proto-oncogene function, the amphibian *Xenopus laevis* system provides many more advantages for studying function during the stages of early development. First, these stages are well characterized biologically, and large numbers of oocytes are easily obtained and manipulated in vitro:

```
Xl    1    MPSPIPVERFLPRDLSPSIDLRPCSSPLELSHR--KLPGGLPACSGRRRLLPPRLAWCSIDWEQV
Ch    1         FNS   LE   A              VVIPGKDG AFL G-TP P T R                DRL
Mu    1         LSLC Y  E    V S S    I   VAPRKAG  FL --TTPP APG  R       F
Hu    1         LALRPY RSEF  V A          S  P---A  LL --  TLP APR  R

Xl   64    LLLEPLGSGGFGSVYRATYRGETVALKKVKRSTKNSLASKQSFWAELNAARLRHPHVVRVVAASA
Ch   65    C  Q         A K    H V    V Q  K S R   R          V   Q DN             T
Mu   64    C MHR        K     H VP  I Q NKC DLR  QR            I     DNI            T
Hu   61    C  QR  A     K      QVP  I Q NKC   R   RR           V     DNI            T

Xl  129    SCPGDPGCPGTIIMEYTGTGTLHQRIYG--RS-P------PLGA-------EICMRYARHVADGL
Ch  130    CA ASQNSL     V NV    HV   -T DAWRQGEEEEG CGRKALSMAEAVC SCDIVT
Mu  129    RT E SNSL     FG NV   V    AT  - E-----   SC-REQLSLGK LK SLD VN
Hu  126    RT AGSNSL     FG NV   V    AAGH- EGDAGE HCRTGGQLSLGK LK SLD VN

Xl  178    RFLHRDGVVHLDLKPANVLLAPGDLCKIGDFGCSQRLREGDEAAGGEPCCTQLRHVGGTYTHRAP
Ch  194    A    SQ I        I ITEHGA              E   ------LSQSHHVCQQ
Mu  187    L    SQSIL       I ISEQ V  S           K QDL------RCRQASPH I        Q
Hu  190    L    SQSI        I ISEQ V  S           EK EDL------LCFQ PSYPL

Xl  243    ELLKGEPVTAKADIYSFAITLWQMVSRELPYTGDRQCVLYAVVAYDLRPEM-GPLFSHTEEGRAA
Ch  253         R               I M Q  L E  Y        N     PLAAAI HESAV QRL
Mu  246    I    IA P       G        TT V  S EP Y Q     N     SLA AV TASLT KTL
Hu  249         G P               TTKQA S E  HI               SLSAAV EDSLP QRL

Xl  307    RTIVQSCWAARPQERPNAEQLLERLEQECAMCTGGPPSCSPESNAPPPLGTGL* (359)
Ch  318    S ISC  K DVE  LS A     PS RALKENL* (349)
Mu  311    QN I     E  ALQ  G  L QRD KAFRGALG* (343)
Hu  314    GDVI R   RPSAAQ  S RL    VD TSLK ELG* (346)
```

FIGURE 5. Amino acid sequence comparison of vertebrate c-*mos* genes (excerpted from reference 21). Complete amino-acid sequence of c-*mos*[xe] (Xl) is aligned with the chicken (Ch), mouse (Mu), and human (Hu) c-*mos* amino acid sequences. The amino acid sequence for chicken, mouse, or human is included only when it differs from that at *Xenopus mos*. Among the amino acids in common, those that are conserved among members of the *src* kinase family are identified by closed circles.

Specific protein products can be expressed by injection of mRNA, and it is possible to interrupt the function of exogenously added or endogenous RNA by microinjection of antisense oligodeoxyribonucleotides.

The amino acid sequence of *Xenopus mos* compared to human, mouse, and chicken *mos* reveals that it is less well conserved between species than other proto-oncogenes (Fig. 5). For example, between chicken and human the *src* proto-oncogene shares 90% homology, while the *mos* proto-oncogene shares approximately 60% (24). Most of the conserved regions are in the sequences shared among the *src* kinase family members (21).

The expression of *mos* RNA in specific *Xenopus* tissues is similar to other vertebrates (21), and high levels are expressed in adult oocytes. The analysis of its expression pattern during early development (Fig. 6) shows that as in mammals, *mos* mRNA is part of the maternally inherited messenger RNA

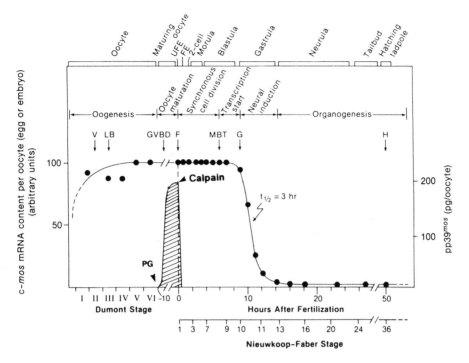

FIGURE 6. Expression of c-*mos* RNA and *mos* protein (p39^{mos}) during early development of *Xenopus laevis* (excerpted from reference 12). (F = fertilization; FE = fertilized egg; G = gastrulation; GVBD = germinal vesicle breakdown; H = hatching tadpole; LB = lampbrush stage; MBT = mid-blastula transition; PG = progesterone; UFE = unfertilized egg; V = start of vitellogenesis.)

pool. It is present at the earliest stage of oocyte development and persists through the late blastula stage, when the transcript disappears with a half-life of 3.5 h. The presence of the RNA after fertilization is different from that found in mouse oocytes (25).

The availability of large numbers of *Xenopus* oocytes at each developmental stage provided the opportunity to determine when the *mos* product is expressed. Surprisingly, the *mos* protein, p39^{mos}, was only present during progesterone-induced oocyte maturation (Fig. 7), even though *mos* mRNA was present throughout oogenesis and early embryonic development (Fig. 6). This demonstrated that very special controls regulate *mos* RNA translation, but the most important aspect of this discovery is that p39^{mos} is expressed only during maturation. The only developmental program that occurs during this period is MPF-mediated re-entry into meiosis, meiosis I, and arrest at metaphase II of meiosis, suggesting that p39^{mos} was involved in meiosis. MPF (32, 34) is the universal regulator of meiosis and mitosis and consists of two components, p34^{cdc2} and cyclin (35, 36). In *Xenopus*, oocyte maturation

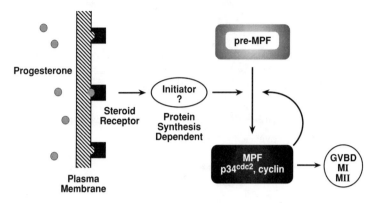

FIGURE 7. Maturation in *Xenopus* oocytes. In *Xenopus*, fully grown oocytes arrested at the G_2/M border of prophase are induced to mature with progesterone. This leads to the translation of *initiator* product(s) required for activation of pre-MPF to MPF. MPF is an active kinase complex consisting of p34^{cdc2}, and cyclin and is responsible for germinal vesicle (or nuclear) breakdown (GVBD) and chromosome condensation. MPF is autocatalytic and cycles during meiosis and is present at high levels in mature oocytes arrested at metaphase of meiosis II.

in vivo as well as in vitro is induced by progesterone (Fig. 7). As with mouse oocytes (7) (Figs. 2, 3), p39^{mos} is also required for *Xenopus* oocyte maturation, and injection of fully grown oocytes with *mos* antisense oligo-deoxyribonucleotides blocks GVBD induced by progesterone (21) (Fig. 8). One important difference between mouse and *Xenopus* is that mouse oocyte maturation proceeds past GVBD (Fig. 4). GVBD and chromosome condensation are characteristics that have been attributed to MPF activity (37). The differences between mouse and *Xenopus* provided the first suggestion that *mos* is required not only at the beginning of maturation, but also at later stages of meiosis.

Another very important result obtained from these assays was that antisense depletion of *mos* also prevented insulin-induced oocyte maturation (21). Endogenous p21^{ras} functions through the insulin-induced maturation pathway (38, 39) but not the progesterone-induced pathway, indicating that in the endogenous and normal developmental pathway, *mos* function is downstream from, but in the same pathway as, endogenous p21^{ras} function (Fig. 9). A similar conclusion, that *ras* is upstream from *mos*, has been reported by Stacey and his colleagues (40). We have emphasized the importance of understanding normal function in order to understand transforming activity. The *Xenopus* system is powerful for determining how these endogenous proto-oncogene products interact. The major question we have addressed in this system, however, is what role *mos* might play in maturation as well as what might be its relationship to MPF.

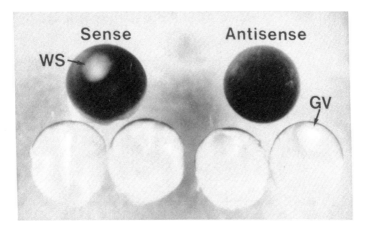

FIGURE 8. Effects of *mos* sense and antisense oligodeoxyribonucleotides on *Xenopus* oocyte GVBD (excerpted from reference 21). Oocytes microinjected with antisense oligodeoxyribonucleotides failed to produce a white spot (WS) and undergo GVBD.

It has been known since the mid-1970s from the work of Wasserman and Masui (41) that early stages of progesterone-induced maturation are sensitive to protein synthesis inhibitors (Fig. 7). At later stages, maturation becomes protein synthesis independent, and this corresponds to the activation of MPF from pre-MPF (41). Thus, addition of MPF directly to oocytes abrogates the protein synthesis requirement. This led Wasserman and Masui to conclude that de novo synthesis of an *initiator* was required to start maturation. The expression of p39^{mos} only during maturation (Fig. 6) suggested that it was a candidate initiator. Indeed, there is a rapid increase in p39^{mos} synthesis after progesterone treatment (Fig. 10), which precedes the time when oocyte maturation became protein synthesis independent or MPF is activated (42).

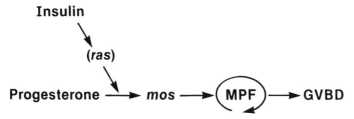

FIGURE 9. Interrelationship of endogenous *ras* and *mos* products. Oocyte maturation induced by insulin but not progesterone occurs via endogenous p21^{ras}. Depletion of endogenous *mos* prevents maturation by either inducer and *mos* product is downstream.

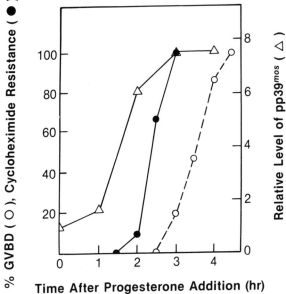

FIGURE 10. The level of pp39^mos in oocytes before and after progesterone treatment and kinetics of GVBD and pre-MPF activation (excerpted from reference 42). *Top*: Maturation of fully grown stage VI oocytes was induced by progesterone and labeled with [^{35}S]methionine at 1-h intervals before and after progesterone treatment. Oocyte extracts were subjected to immunoprecipitation analysis with either monoclonal antibody (termed 5S) raised against the *Xenopus* c-*mos* product *(a)* (42) or a peptide antiserum C232 *(b)* (21) in the presence (+) or absence (–) of the peptide antigen. *Bottom*: Oocytes of the same batch described in the top panel were scored for GVBD every 30 min after progesterone addition or were treated with cycloheximide at 30-min intervals after progesterone addition. After 12 h, oocytes were examined for percent of GVBD (open circles) or cycloheximide resistance of GVBD (closed circles). Densitometric measurements of autoradiographs as shown in the top panel and performed in parallel are shown (open triangles).

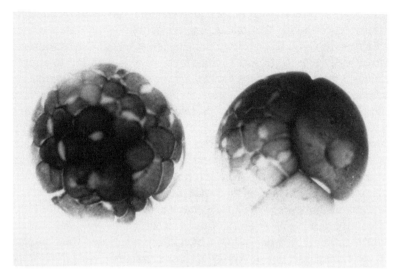

FIGURE 11. Morphology of embryos in *mos* RNA-arrested embryos (excerpted from reference 12). Animal-pole view of embryos injected with either 5'-capped truncated (*left*) or 5'-capped normal (*right*) *mos* RNA. Synthetic *mos* RNA was injected into one blastomere (right half) of a 2-cell embryo. Cleavage arrest is observed only when injected with intact *mos* RNA (*right*).

By injecting *mos* RNA directly into fully grown oocytes, it was possible to demonstrate that overexpression of p39^{mos} induced maturation. However, the kinetics were slower than with progesterone, suggesting that other protein products (e.g., cyclin) or perhaps biochemical changes that occur during maturation, such as decrease in levels of cAMP, were required (42).

Studies by Watanabe et al. (43) indicated that even though the *mos* product was stable in unfertilized mature oocytes (Fig. 6), within 30 min after fertilization, all p39^{mos} disappeared, explaining why the product was not detected in fertilized eggs (21). The rapid disappearance of *mos* after egg activation with a calcium ionophore (a process akin to fertilization) (43) was ultimately explained by showing that *mos* is specifically degraded by calcium-dependent calpain protease (Fig. 6).

The properties of calcium sensitivity and absence of product after fertilization in cleaving embryos are consistent with the properties of the long-known activity CSF (44). This activity is believed to be responsible for arresting vertebrate oocytes at metaphase II of meiosis. CSF was first characterized by Masui and Markert and is also associated with mature oocytes (32). Masui and Clarke showed that CSF injected into a blastomere of a cleaving embryo arrests it at metaphase of mitosis (29). The similar characteristics of p39^{mos}

and CSF led Sagata et al. (12) to question whether p39^{mos} was responsible for CSF activity. In these experiments, one blastomere of a 2-cell embryo injected with *mos* RNA was arrested in cleavage at metaphase of mitosis and displayed CSF activity (Fig. 11). Moreover, it was possible to show that antibodies directed against *mos* could neutralize CSF activity extracted from mature oocytes. Thus, p39^{mos} is responsible for arresting oocytes at metaphase II of meiosis. This activity is also required for the stabilization of MPF (12).

More recently, to determine the function of p39^{mos}, we have attempted to characterize what CSF/*mos* might be. It was known from cytological examination that CSF-arrested mitotic cells have larger-than-normal spindles (45). Also, taxol, a drug that binds to and stabilizes microtubules and spindles, can arrest cleaving embryos at metaphase and thus resembles CSF/*mos* in activity (46). Moreover, p39^{mos} appears to be specifically degraded by calpain after fertilization (43), a point from which eggs are released from metaphase II and enter anaphase and chromosomes move poleward via spindle depolymerization (47, 48). This raised the question whether p39^{mos}, as a serine kinase (43), may be associated with tubulin. Preliminary evidence indicates that p39^{mos} associates with tubulin in vitro, and α- and β-tubulin are major substrates of *mos* kinase phosphorylation in vitro (49). Thus, CSF/*mos* product associates with tubulin, and we believe it may interact or influence the formation and stability of microtubule as spindles. The dramatic interruption of the movement of cytoplasmic particulates observed in maturing mouse oocytes depleted of *mos* would be consistent with the *mos* product functioning directly or indirectly in microtubule assembly (Fig. 4).

If this is the normal function of p39^{mos}, then the major question to be addressed is how *mos* expression in somatic cells can result in transformation. The *mos* product may only function during meiosis/mitosis, and we have proposed that unscheduled, constitutive expression of p39^{mos} in somatic cells causes the expression of the mitotic phenotype during interphase (12, 21). Because microtubule polymerization/depolymerization is dynamic (47), in transformed cells, a low level of p39^{mos} may influence modification of microtubule. The identification of tubulin as a potential *mos* target suggests a mechanism for transformation (49). Since CSF/*mos* stabilizes MPF (12), a proportional amount of MPF may also be stabilized. At high levels, MPF induces GVBD and chromosome condensation (29). Altered cellular and nuclear morphology (Table 2) could be a derivative of mitotic cell rounding and GVBD. The loss of contact inhibition is more difficult to explain, but we believe that this could correspond to a phenotype that may normally occur during cytokinesis. Thus, daughter cells cannot growth arrest when they are in contact during cytokinesis. This phenotype, expressed during interphase, could be responsible for loss of contact inhibition of tumor cells. Perhaps the most important characteristic that this model can provide is

TABLE 2. Characteristics of the transformed phenotype.

Characteristic	Reference
Cellular morphology	
Nuclear Structure	51
Cytoskeleton	52, 53
Growth characteristics and cell metabolism	54, 55
Anchorage independence and loss of contact inhibition	56
Changes in extracellular matrix	57–59
Growth factor independence	60, 61
Genetic instability	62, 63

an explanation for genetic instability in tumor cells. The constitutive maintenance of MPF during late S phase could result in premature chromosome condensation events. This would generate free ends in DNA and such structures in lower eukaryotes are highly recombinogenic. This could explain the high frequency of chromosomal translocations observed in tumor cells.

Acknowledgment. This chapter has been excerpted with permission from a chapter entitled "The Molecular Basis of Neoplastic Disease" by Schulz and Vande Woude, which will be published by Williams & Wilkins in a book entitled *Molecular Foundations in Oncology* edited by Samuel Broder.

References

1. Berman LD. Comparative morphologic study of the virus-induced solid tumors of Syrian hamsters. JNCI 1967;252:456-9.
2. Huebner RJ, Hartley JW, Roure WP, Lane WT, Capps WI. Rescue of the defective genome of Moloney virus from a noninfectious hamster tumor and the production of pseudotype sarcoma viruses with various murine leukemia viruses. Proc Natl Acad Sci USA 1966;56:1164-9.
3. Levy JP, Leclerc JC. The murine sarcoma virus-induced tumor: Exception or general model in tumor immunology. Adv Cancer Res 1977;24:1-66.
4. Seth A, Vande Woude GF. The *mos* oncogene. In: Reddy EP, Skalka AM, Curran T, eds. The oncogene handbook. Amsterdam: Elsevier, 1988:195-211.
5. Weiss R, Teich N, Varmus H, Coffin J, eds. Molecular biology of tumor viruses. 2nd ed. Cold Spring Harbor, NY: Cold Spring Harbor Laboratory, 1982.
6. Fischinger PJ, Haapala DK. Quantitative interactions of feline leukaemia virus and its pseudotype of murine sarcoma virus in cat cells: Requirement for DNA synthesis. J Gen Virol 1971;13:203-14.
7. Paules RS, Buccione R, Moschel RC, Vande Woude GF, Eppig JJ. Mouse *mos* protooncogene product is present and functions during oogenesis. Proc Natl Acad Sci USA 1989;86:5395-9.

8. Hartley JW, Rowe JP. Production of altered cell foci in tissue culture by defective Moloney sarcoma virus particles. Proc Natl Acad Sci USA 1966;55:780-5.

9. Papkoff J, Hunter T, Beemon K. In vitro translation of virion RNA from Moloney murine sarcoma virus. Virology 1980;101:91-103.

10. Papkoff J, Lai MH, Hunter T, Verma IM. Analysis of transforming gene products from Moloney murine sarcoma virus. Cell 1981;27:109-19.

11. Papkoff J, Nigg EA, Hunter T. The transforming protein of Moloney murine sarcoma virus is a soluble cytoplasm protein. Cell 1983;33:161-72.

12. Sagata N, Watanabe N, Vande Woude GF, Ikawa Y. The c-*mos* proto-oncogene product is a cytostatic factor responsible for meiotic arrest in vertebrate eggs. Nature 1989;342:512-8.

13. Oskarsson M, McClements WL, Blair DG, Maizel JV, Vande Woude GF. Properties of a normal mouse cell DNA sequence (*sarc*) homologous to the *src* sequence of Moloney sarcoma virus. Science 1980;207:1222-4.

14. Blair DG, McClements W, Oskarsson M, Fischinger P, Vande Woude GF. Biological activity of cloned Moloney sarcoma virus DNA: Terminally redundant sequences may enhance transformation efficiency. Proc Natl Acad Sci USA 1980;77:3504-8.

15. Watson R, Oskarsson M, Vande Woude GF. Human DNA sequence homologous to the transforming gene (*mos*) of Moloney murine sarcoma virus. Proc Natl Acad Sci USA 1982;79:4078-82.

16. Paules RS, Propst F, Dunn KJ, et al. Primate c-*mos* proto-oncogene structure and expression: Transcription initiation both upstream and within the gene in a tissue-specific manner. Oncogene 1988;3:59-68.

17. Wood TG, McGeady ML, Baroudy B, Blair DG, Vande Woude GF. Mouse c-*mos* oncogene activation is prevented by upstream sequences. Proc Natl Acad Sci USA 1984;81:7817-21.

18. McGeady ML, Wood TG, Maizel JV, Vande Woude GF. Sequence upstream to the mouse c-*mos* oncogene may function as a transcription termination signal. DNA 1986;5:289-98.

19. Blair DG, Oskarsson MK, Seth A, et al. Analysis of the transforming potential of the human homolog of *mos*. Cell 1986;46:785-94.

20. Yew N, Oskarsson M, Daar I, Blair DG, Vande Woude GF. *mos* gene transforming efficiencies correlate with oocyte maturation and cytostatic factor activities. Submitted.

21. Sagata N, Oskarsson M, Copeland T, Brumbaugh J, Vande Woude GF. Function of c-*mos* proto-oncogene product in meiotic maturation in *Xenopus* oocytes. Nature 1988;335:519-25.

22. Propst F, Rosenberg MP, Iyer A, Kaul K, Vande Woude GF. c-*mos* proto-oncogene RNA transcripts in mouse tissues: Structural features, developmental regulation and localization in specific cell types. Mol Cell Biol 1987;7:1629-37.

23. Propst F, Vande Woude GF. c-*mos* proto-oncogene transcripts are expressed in mouse tissues. Nature 1985;315:516-8.

24. Schmidt M, Oskarsson MK, Dunn JK, et al. Chicken homolog of the *mos* proto-oncogene. Mol Cell Biol 1988;8:923-9.

25. Goldman DS, Kiessling AA, Cooper GM. Post-transcriptional processing sug-

gests that c-*mos* functions as a maternal message in mouse eggs. Oncogene 1988; 3:159-62.

26. Keshet E, Rosenberg M, Mercer JA, et al. Developmental regulation of ovarian-specific *mos* expression. Oncogene 1988;2:235-40.
27. Goldman DS, Kiessling AA, Millette CF, Cooper GM. Expression of c-*mos* RNA in germ cells of male and female mice. Proc Natl Acad Sci USA 1987;84:4509-13.
28. Mutter GL, Wolgemuth DJ. Distinct developmental patterns of c-*mos* protooncogene expression in female and male mouse germ cells. Proc Natl Acad Sci USA 1987;84:5301-5.
29. Masui Y, Clarke AJ. Oocyte maturation. J Int Rev Cytol 1979;57:185-282.
30. Ford CC. Maturation promoting factor and cell cycle regulation. J Embryol Exp Morphol 1985;89:271-84.
31. Maller JL. Regulation of amphibian oocyte maturation. Cell Differ 1985;16: 211-21.
32. Masui Y, Markert CL. Cytoplasmic control of nuclear behavior during meiotic maturation of frog oocytes. J Exp Zool 1971;177:129-46.
33. O'Keefe SJ, Wolfes H, Hiessling AA, Cooper GM. Microinjection of antisense c-*mos* oligonucleotides prevents meiosis II in the maturing mouse egg. Proc Natl Acad Sci USA 1989;86:7038-42.
34. Smith LD, Ecker RE. The interaction of steroids with Rana pipiens oocytes in the induction of maturation. Dev Biol 1971;25:232-47.
35. Lohka MJ, Hayes MK, Maller JL. Purification of maturation-promoting factor, an intracellular regulator of early mitotic events. Proc Natl Acad Sci USA 1988; 85:3009-13.
36. Gautier J, Minshull J, Lohka M, Glotzer M, Hunt T, Maller JL. Cyclin is a component of maturation-promoting factor from *Xenopus*. Cell 1990;60:487-94.
37. Murray AW, Kirschner MW. Dominoes and clocks: The union of two views of the cell cycle. Science 1989;246:614-21.
38. Korn LJ, Siebel CW, McCormick F, Roth RA. *Ras* p21 as a potential mediator of insulin action in *Xenopus* oocytes. Science 1987;236:840-3.
39. Deshpande AK, Kung H-F. Insulin induction of *Xenopus laevis* oocyte maturation is inhibited by monoclonal antibody against p21 *ras* proteins. Mol Cell Biol 1987;7:1285-8.
40. Smith MR, DeGudicibus SJ, Stacey DW. Requirement for c-*ras* proteins during viral oncogene transformation. Nature 1986;320:540-3.
41. Wasserman WJ, Masui Y. A cytoplasmic factor promoting ooctye maturation: Its extraction and preliminary characterization. Science 1976;191:1266-8.
42. Sagata N, Daar I, Oskarsson M, Showalter SD, Vande Woude GF. The product of the *mos* proto-oncogene as a candidate "initiator" for oocyte maturation. Science 1989;245:643-6.
43. Watanabe N, Vande Woude GF, Ikawa Y, Sagata N. Specific proteolysis of the c-*mos* proto-oncogene product by calpain upon fertilization of *Xenopus* eggs. Nature 1989;342:505-11.
44. Meyerhof PG, Masui Y. Ca^{++} and Mg^{++} control of cytostatic factors from Rana pipiens oocytes which cause metaphase and cleavage arrest. Dev Biol 1977; 61:214-29.

45. Masui Y. A cytostatic factor in amphibian oocytes: Its extraction and partial characterization. J Exp Zool 1974;187:141-7.
46. Heidemann SR, Gallas PT. The effect of taxol on living eggs of *Xenopus laevis*. Dev Biol 1980;80:489-94.
47. Kirschner M, Mitchison T. Beyond self-assembly: From microtubules to morphogenesis. Cell 1986;45:329-42.
48. Koshland DE, Mitchison TJ, Kirschner MW. Polewards chromosome movement driven by microtubule depolymerization in vitro. Nature 1988;331:499-504.
49. Zhou R, Oskarsson M, Paules RS, Schulz N, Vande Woude GF. The c-*mos* protooncogene product polymerizes with and phosphorylates tubulin. Submitted.
50. Blair DG, McClements W, Oskarsson M, Fischinger P, Vande Woude GF. Biological activity of cloned Moloney sarcoma virus DNA: Terminally redundant sequences may enhance transformation efficiency. Proc Natl Acad Sci USA 1980;77:3504-8.
51. Smith HS, Springer EL, Hackett AJ. Nuclear ultrastructure of epithelial cell lines derived from human carcinomas and nonmalignant tissues. Cancer Res 1979;39:332-44.
52. Hynes RO. Cell surface proteins and malignant transformation. Biochem Biophys Acta 1976;458:73-107.
53. Tucker RW, Sanford KK, Frankel FR. Tubulin and actin in paired nonneoplastic and spontaneously tranformed neoplastic cell lines in vitro: Fluorescent antibody studies. Cell 1978;13:629-42.
54. Weinhouse S. Metabolism and isozyme alterations in experimental hepatomas. Fed Proc 1973;32:2162-7.
55. Racker E. Resolution and reconstitution of biological pathways from 1919 to 1984. Fed Proc 1983;42:2899-909.
56. Abercrombie M. Contact inhibition and malignancy. Nature 1979;281:259-62.
57. Folkman J, Moscana A. Role of cell shape in growth control. Nature 1978;273:345-9.
58. Burger MM. Cell surfaces in neoplastic transformation. In: Horecker BL, Stadtman ER, eds. Current topics in cellular regulation; vol 3. New York: Academic Press, 1971:135-93.
59. Hynes RO, Fox CF, eds. Tumor cell surfaces and malignancy. New York: Alan R. Liss, 1980.
60. Cherington PV, Smith BL, Pardee AB. Loss of epidermal growth factor requirement and malignant transformation. Proc Natl Acad Sci USA 1979;76:3937-41.
61. Bartholomew JC, Yokoto H, Ross P. Effect of serum on the growth of BALB 3T3 A31 mouse fibroblasts and an SV40-transformed derivative. J Cell Physiol 1976;88:277-86.
62. Rowley JD, Testa JR. Chromosome abnormalities in malignant hematologic diseases. Adv Cancer Res 1982;36:103-48.
63. Yunis JJ. The chromosomal basis of human neoplasia. Science 1983;221:227-35.

10

Regulation of Genes Encoding Steroidogenic Enzymes in the Ovary

MARKUS LAUBER, MICHELLE DEMETER, DAVID STIRLING,
RAYMOND RODGERS, MICHAEL R. WATERMAN,
AND EVAN R. SIMPSON

The pattern of steroid hormone biosynthesis in the ovary occurs in a highly coordinated and episodic fashion that is determined in part by the pattern of gonadotropin secretion. In the case of the bovine ovary, a dramatic switch in the pattern of steroid secretion occurs at the time of ovulation. Following the gonadotropin surge, there is a marked increase in the secretion of progesterone by the developing corpus luteum, and at the same time, there is an equally dramatic decline in the secretion of androgens and estrogens. With the development of antibodies against the various steroidogenic enzymes and the isolation and cloning of cDNA inserts complementary to mRNA species encoding these enzymes, it became possible to analyze the molecular mechanisms underlying these differential switches in steroid hormone secretion.

Northern and Western Analyses

Follicles and corpora lutea were collected from bovine ovaries throughout the cycle and aliquots of the protein were submitted to Western blotting analysis utilizing antibodies raised against purified bovine side-chain cleavage cytochrome P-450 (P-450$_{SCC}$), 17α-hydroxylase cytochrome P-450 (P-450$_{17\alpha}$), and adrenodoxin (1). It was observed that the expression of P-450$_{SCC}$ and adrenodoxin was low in follicles but increased abruptly and dramatically following the onset of luteinization. With the subsequent onset of luteolysis, there was precipitous decline in the levels of both of these proteins. By contrast, the expression of P-450$_{17\alpha}$ was readily detectable in follicles, but following ovulation, it declined abruptly to undetectable levels. On the other hand, the expression of control enzymes NADPH-cytochrome c

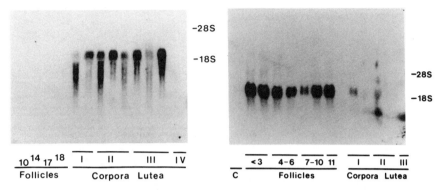

FIGURE 1. *Left:* Relative levels of P-450$_{SCC}$ mRNA in bovine follicles and corpora lutea as determined by Northern blotting analysis of total RNA (20 µg) from individual follicles of differing diameter (10, 14, 17, and 18 mm) and individual corpora lutea of differing stages of development (I, II, III, and IV). Positions of 18S and 28S ribosomal RNA are indicated. *Right:* Relative levels of P-450$_{17\alpha}$ mRNA in bovine follicles and corpora lutea as determined by Northern blotting analysis of poly*(A)*$^+$ RNA (5 µg) from ovarian cortex *(c)* and individual (11 mm) and pools (<3 mm, 4–6 mm, and 7–10 mm) of follicles and individual corpora lutea of differing stages of development (I, II, and III). (From Ireland JJ, Murphee RL, Coulson PB, Acccuracy of predicting stages of bovine estrous cycle by gross appearance of the corpus luteum, J Dairy Sci 1980;63:155–63.)

reductase, a microsomal marker, and F1-ATPase, a mitochondrial marker, changed much less dramatically. Thus, it is clear that the differential expression of steroid biosynthesis throughout the bovine ovarian cycle can be explained, in part, by the differential expression of the enzymes responsible for their biosynthesis.

In order to investigate whether the levels of these enzymes were in turn a reflection of the levels of the mRNA species encoding these enzymes, Northern analysis (2) was conducted on RNA extracted from follicles and corpora lutea throughout the bovine ovarian cycle, using as probes cDNAs complementary to mRNAs encoding P-450$_{SCC}$, P-450$_{17\alpha}$, adrenodoxin, and the LDL receptor. It was found that the levels of mRNA encoding P-450$_{SCC}$, adrenodoxin (Fig. 1), and the LDL receptor were low in follicles, increased dramatically following ovulation, and then decreased equally abruptly with the onset of luteolysis. Thus, the pattern of expression of all three of these proteins, which are intimately involved in progesterone biosynthesis, follows very closely the pattern of progesterone secretion throughout the bovine ovarian cycle. The activity of HMG CoA reductase was also determined and, again, closely paralleled that of these proteins. Thus, it appears that the pattern of secretion of progesterone is explicable, in large part, by the pattern of expression of the enzymes responsible for its biosynthesis, together with the proteins required to optimize the supply of cholesterol to the steroidogenic machinery required for progesterone biosynthesis. By contrast, when the levels of mRNA encoding P-450$_{17\alpha}$ were determined (Fig. 1, *left*), they were found to be detectable in follicles, but then promptly disappeared with the onset of ovulation and were undetectable following luteinization, thus again mimicking the pattern of androgen secretion in the bovine ovary.

Factors Regulating Expression of Steroidogenic Enzymes in the Ovary

Based on these results, we can conclude that the pattern of steroid hormone secretion throughout the ovarian cycle is explicable, in large part, on the basis of the differential expression of the various enzymes involved in the steroidogenic pathway. The next problem that arises is determining what is responsible for regulating the expression of these enzymes and, in particular, the mRNA levels encoding these enzymes. Like others, we have been interested in the possibility that a number of growth factors and cytokines produced locally within the ovary—some in response to gonadotropins—may differentially regulate the expression of steroidogenic enzymes in either a paracrine or autocrine fashion. In particular, in the case of 17α-hydroxylase expression by thecal cells, it has been established in our laboratory using cultures of human thecal cells (J.M. McAllister, unpublished) as well as bovine thecal cells (M. Demeter, unpublished) that a number of growth factors are inhibitory of 17α-hydroxylase activity. These include bFGF, TGF β, EGF, as well as the phorbol ester, TPA. Because the presence of bFGF has previously been characterized in the bovine ovary (3), particularly in the corpus luteum, we decided to examine the expression of this growth factor in the bovine ovary. Using a riboprobe technique and RNA extracted from follicles and corpora lutea from bovine ovaries throughout the ovarian cycle, it was established that the expression of bFGF was undetectable in follicles, but that it was expressed to a high level in corpora lutea throughout the luteal phase of the cycle (Fig. 2) and in fact was also expressed even in corpora lutea undergoing luteolysis (4). This result suggested that the expression of bFGF in the bovine ovary might be in response to gonadotropins.

Consequently, bovine luteal cells were placed in primary culture, and the expression of bFGF by these cells was examined. It was found that the expression was extremely low in control cells but was induced markedly in the presence of either hCG, LH, or dibutyryl cAMP (4, 5). Thus, it is possible to present a reasonably coherent hypothesis that bFGF formed in luteinizing cells as a consequence of the gonadotropin surge serves not only as an angiogenic factor, but also to suppress the expression of 17α-hydroxylase

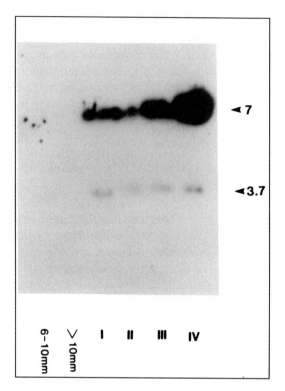

FIGURE 2. Expression of mRNA encoding bFGF in ovarian tissue. Poly*(A)*⁺ RNA
(25 µg per lane) was prepared from medium and large follicles, and corpora lutea of
the various stages of luteal phase as defined by Ireland et al. (9) and subjected to
Northern analysis.

and thus contribute to the differential expression of the steroidogenic enzymes that occurs at the time of ovulation in the bovine ovary.

Regulation of the Genes Encoding Steroidogenic Enzymes

Of course, bFGF is only one of many locally produced factors that might
regulate the expression of the steroidogenic enzymes, and such experiments
do not necessarily provide information as to which may be the most important physiologically. A different approach, then, to understanding the regulation of these enzymes is to examine the factors influencing the transcription
of the genes encoding these enzymes with the hope that definition of the cis-
acting and trans-acting elements responsible for the regulation will not only

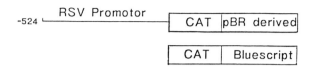

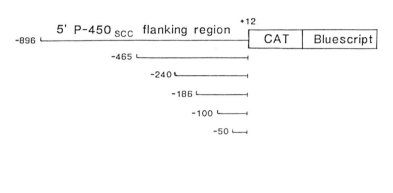

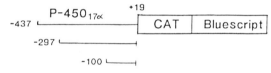

FIGURE 3. Schematic diagram of reporter genes used in transient transfection. Sequences of the 5' regulatory regions have been fused to the CAT reporter gene (see references 8 and 9). These constructs contain the respective putative P-450$_{SCC}$ and P-450$_{17\alpha}$ TATA boxes and start sites of transcription. The RSV-CAT construct was used as a positive control and contains part of the Rous sarcoma virus, leading to constitutive high expression. The CAT construct lacks specific promotor sequences and was used to monitor nonspecific CAT activity.

provide important information in its own right, but will eventually lead back to the cell surface and a complete picture of the regulatory pathway. To this end (Fig. 3), a series of chimeric constructs containing fragments of the 5'-end of the bovine P-450$_{SCC}$ and P-450$_{17\alpha}$ genes fused upstream of the chloramphenicol acetyl transferase (CAT) gene were prepared (6, 7). These were transfected into bovine luteal cells and bovine thecal cells by means of the technique of electroporation (8). When the series of P-450$_{SCC}$ constructs was transfected into bovine luteal cells, it was observed that deletion from −186 to −100 drastically reduced both the basal and forskolin-stimulated

TABLE 1. Relative expression of CAT reporter gene constructs after transfection into bovine luteal and thecal cells in primary culture.

DNA Construct	CAT activity (% conversion)		Cell Type
	−Forskolin	+Forskolin	
RSV-CAT	98.5	98.7	Luteal
CAT	8.8	9.5	Luteal
SCC-896	8.3	14.3	Luteal
SCC-465	15.2	26.7	Luteal
SCC-240	47.3	53.5	Luteal
SCC-186	15.0	56.8	Luteal
SCC-100	2.4	3.9	Luteal
SCC-50	4.4	3.1	Luteal
17α-437	2.0	4.8	Luteal
17α-297	4.1	4.2	Luteal
17α-100	2.5	2.4	Luteal
RSV-CAT	71.9	67.2	Thecal
CAT	1.7	4.9	Thecal
SCC-186	9.8	24.8	Thecal
17α-297	25.5	34.8	Thecal

Note: Numbers represent % conversion of [^{14}C]chloramphenicol to acetylated products and are calculated from one single experiment. Similar relative CAT reporter gene expression has been obtained in two other independent experiments. Conditions for electrophoration and for determination of CAT activity are described in reference 10.

activity (Table 1), indicating that this region contained perhaps a basal enhancer and a cAMP-responsive element. A feature of these steroidogenic genes, however, is that no classical cAMP-responsive element, such as TGACGTCA, has been detected. An identical pattern of expression has been observed when this set of constructs was transfected into mouse Y1 adrenal tumor cells (6), indicating that the regulation of the P-450$_{SCC}$ gene in adrenal cells and luteal cells appears to occur via similar mechanisms. Interestingly, however, when the corresponding P-450$_{17\alpha}$ constructs were transfected into bovine luteal cells, no expression of CAT was observed either in the presence or absence of forskolin (Table 1). Thus, the expression of the transfected constructs appears to follow that of the endogenous expression. On the other hand, when the P-450$_{SCC}$ (−186 to +12 bp) and P-450$_{17\alpha}$ (−297 to +19 bp) constructs were transfected into bovine thecal cells in culture, both of these were expressed, and the expression appeared to be stimulated by forskolin (10). Thus again, in these cells the expression of the transfected constructs parallels closely that of the endogenous expression.

Conclusions

It appears, therefore, that primary bovine luteal and thecal cells in culture provide a model system to study the differential expression of the genes encoding $P-450_{SCC}$ and $P-450_{17\alpha}$. In particular, the failure of the luteal cells to express constructs containing the 5' end of the $P-450_{17\alpha}$ gene, strongly indicates that during the process of luteinization, either a positive transcription factor required for expression of $P-450_{17\alpha}$ has been lost, or else a negative transcription factor shutting off the expression of $P-450_{17\alpha}$ has been expressed. Use of these cells, therefore, should provide the means of defining the trans-acting elements responsible for the differential expression of these two genes and thus, ultimately, the mechanism underlying the dramatic switch in the steroidogenic profile that takes place in the bovine ovary at the time of ovulation.

Acknowledgments. This work was supported in part by USPHS grants HD-13234 and DK-28350, as well as by grant 32.25326.88 from the Swiss National Foundation for Scientific Research. M. D. was supported in part by USPHS training grant T32-HD-07190.

References

1. Rodgers RJ, Waterman MR, Simpson ER. Cytochromes $P-450_{SCC}$, $P-450_{17\alpha}$, adrenodoxin and reduced nicotinamide adenine dinucleotide phosphate cytochrome P-450 reductase in bovine follicles and corpora lutea. Changes in specific contents during the ovarian cycle. Endocrinology 1986;118:1366-74.
2. Rodgers RJ, Waterman MR, Simpson ER. Levels of messenger ribonucleic acid encoding cholesterol side-chain cleavage cytochrome P450, 17α-hydroxylase P450, adrenodoxin and low density lipoprotein receptor in bovine follicles and corpora lutea throughout the ovarian cycle. Mol Endocrinol 1987;1:274-9.
3. Gospodarowicz D, Massoglia S, Cheng J, Fujii DK. Effect of fibroblast growth factor and lipoproteins on the proliferation of endothelial cells derived from bovine adrenal cortex, brain cortex and corpus luteum capillaries. J Cell Physiol 1986;127:121-36.
4. Stirling D, Waterman MR, Simpson ER. Expression of mRNA encoding basic fibroblast growth factor in bovine corpora lutea and cultured luteal cells. J Reprod Fertil (in press).
5. Stirling D, Magness RR, Stone R, Waterman MR, Simpson ER. Angiotensin II inhibits luteinizing hormone-stimulated cholesterol side-chain cleavage expression and stimulates basic fibroblast growth factor expression in bovine luteal cells in primary culture. J Biol Chem 1990;265:5-8.
6. Ahlgren R, Simpson ER, Waterman MR, Lund J. Characterization of the pro-

moter-regulatory region of the bovine CYP11A (P450$_{SCC}$) expression. J Biol Chem 1990;265:3313-9.

7. Lund J, Ahlgren R, Wu D, Kagimoto M, Simpson ER, Waterman MR. Transcriptional regulation of the bovine CYP17 (P450$_{17\alpha}$) gene. Identification of two cAMP regulatory regions lacking the consensus CRE. J Biol Chem 1990; 265:3304-12.

8. Lauber ME, Waterman MR, Simpson ER. Expression of genes encoding steroidogenic enzymes in the bovine corpus luteum. J Reprod Fertil (in press).

9. Ireland JJ, Murphee RL, Coulson PB. Acccuracy of predicting stages of bovine estrous cycle by gross appearance of the corpus luteum. J Dairy Sci 1980;63: 155-63.

10. Lauber M, Demeter M, Waterman MR, Simpson ER. Regulation of expression of the genes encoding P450$_{SCC}$ and P450$_{17\alpha}$ throughout the bovine ovarian cycle [Abstract]. VIII Ovarian Workshop. Serono Symposia, USA, Maryville, TN, 1990. (*See* Chapter 10, this volume.)

11

Oxysterols: Regulation of Biosynthesis and Role in Controlling Cellular Cholesterol Homeostasis in Ovarian Cells

JEROME F. STRAUSS, III, HANNAH RENNERT,
RITSU YAMAMOTO, LEE-CHUAN KAO,
AND JUAN G. ALVAREZ

Steroid-producing cells obtain cholesterol for use in hormone synthesis by de novo synthesis from acetyl co-enzyme A or through accumulation of cholesterol from circulating lipoproteins. Tropic hormones, which augment steroidogenesis (e.g., pituitary gonadotropins acting on ovarian cells), increase both de novo sterol synthesis and lipoprotein cholesterol uptake. Recent review articles summarize the various observations documenting this regulation (1–4).

The mechanisms by which tropic hormones control proteins involved in cholesterol synthesis and lipoprotein uptake have not been fully elucidated. Nonetheless, it appears that one of the primary ways in which cellular sterol homeostasis is modulated is by negative feedback by sterols. The genes encoding key enzymes in the biosynthetic pathway of cholesterol including 3-hydroxy-3-methylglutaryl co-enzyme A synthase (HMG-CoA synthase) and HMG-CoA reductase contain sequences in their 5'-flanking regions, which confer sterol regulation of gene transcription (5). These octameric sequences, called sterol regulatory elements (SREs), are also found in the 5'-flanking DNA of the human LDL receptor gene.

The SREs, which have a consensus sequence of 5'-CACC CC/GT AC-3', are known to bind nuclear proteins that are the presumed trans-factors that mediate effects on gene transcription. The SREs seem to be conditional positive elements that function with other DNA sequences to enhance transcription in the absence of sterol. In the presence of sterol, the positive transcriptional activities of the SREs are lost. Although the SREs in the HMG-CoA reductase and LDL receptor genes appear to be similar, additional different positive transcription factors seem to be involved in the control of these genes, accounting for the divergent expression observed under certain circumstances (6).

Oxysterols as Effectors of Cellular Cholesterol Regulation

Although an increase in cell cholesterol relative to metabolic needs results in reduced transcription of genes with SREs, there is evidence that cholesterol per se is not the effector responsible for the changes in gene transcription. Cholesterol is not a particularly effective suppressor of either de novo sterol synthesis or LDL receptor expression (7). In contrast, hydroxysterols, particularly sterol molecules with hydroxylated side chains (e.g., 25-hydroxycholesterol) are up to 100 times more potent inhibitors of both cholesterol synthesis and LDL receptor levels than pure cholesterol. These observations led to the hypothesis that a hydroxysterol, generated from cholesterol, is the true effector of transcriptional control of genes involved in cellular cholesterol homeostasis.

The mechanism(s) by which hydroxysterols might act to control cholesterol homeostasis remain obscure. Hydroxysterol-binding proteins have been detected in a variety of cells (8). There is a correlation between binding of various oxysterols to the putative receptor and capacity to suppress HMG-CoA reductase activity. The oxysterol-binding proteins are ~97 kDa in size, and one has been purified to homogeneity and its cDNA sequenced, revealing a potential leucine zipper (9). Rajavashisth et al. (10) reported the cloning of a cDNA for a 19-kDa protein with 7 zinc fingers that binds to the SRE octameric DNA sequence. This factor might participate with the putative oxysterol receptor in controlling gene transcription.

Evidence for Enzymatic Generation of an Effector Molecule from Cholesterol

Ketoconazole is an antifungal agent known to inhibit a number of cytochrome P-450 enzymes involved in cholesterol biosynthesis (e.g., 14α-demethylase) and metabolism, including cytochrome P-450$_{SCC}$ (11). We hypothesized that ketoconazole might also inhibit an enzyme required for formation of the regulatory sterol molecule from cholesterol. To test this notion, we treated JEG-3 choriocarcinoma cells, a trophoblastic steroidogenic cell line, with various concentrations of ketoconazole and found that [^{14}C]acetate flux through the pathway of de novo sterol synthesis was increased when the drug was added at a concentration of 50 μM (12). This suggested that ketoconazole was blocking the formation of an inhibitory factor.

Fusion gene constructs consisting of 6500 base pairs of the human LDL receptor gene 5'-flanking DNA, containing the known SREs, coupled to the bacterial gene for the enzyme chloramphenicol acetyl transferase (CAT) were introduced into JEG-3 cells in transient expression assays and CAT activity measured when cells were exposed to serum lipoproteins or 25-hydroxycholesterol in the absence or presence of ketoconazole. Serum lipoproteins reduced CAT activity in the absence of ketoconazole, but in the presence of the drug, serum or LDL were unable to reduce CAT expression. However, ketoconazole had no effect on 25-hydroxycholesterol-mediated suppression of CAT activity. Since ketoconazole was found not to interfere with LDL uptake, it was concluded that the drug was acting by blocking formation of a regulatory compound, presumably as a P-450 enzyme inhibitor.

Gupta et al. (13) reported that ketoconazole prevented the suppression of HMG-CoA reductase activity in rat intestinal epithelial cells exposed to LDL. These authors also found that ketoconazole did not affect LDL uptake and concluded that it was acting to block formation of a regulator of HMG-CoA reductase.

Cholesterol Hydroxylases

Hydroxysterols are produced as intermediates in biosynthetic pathways including bile acid synthesis in the liver and possibly in steroid hormone synthesis (Fig. 1). The enzymatic synthesis of some of these compounds, such as 7α-hydroxycholesterol, seems to be restricted to specific tissues like the liver, whereas 24-hydroxycholesterol and 26-hydroxycholesterol appear to be made by a variety of cell types. It is not yet known whether 25-hydroxycholesterol is derived by an enzymatic reaction or by oxidation.

Relatively little has been known until recently about the enzyme systems that generate hydroxysterols. Cholesterol 24-hydroxylase is believed to be a microsomal enzyme (14), whereas the enzyme-generating 26-hydroxycholesterol is mitochondrial and utilizes reducing equivalents generated through NADPH and the ferredoxin reductase/ferredoxin electron transport system (15). Of interest is the fact that individuals with the rare disease, *cerebrotendinous xanthomatosis*, which is associated with increased de novo

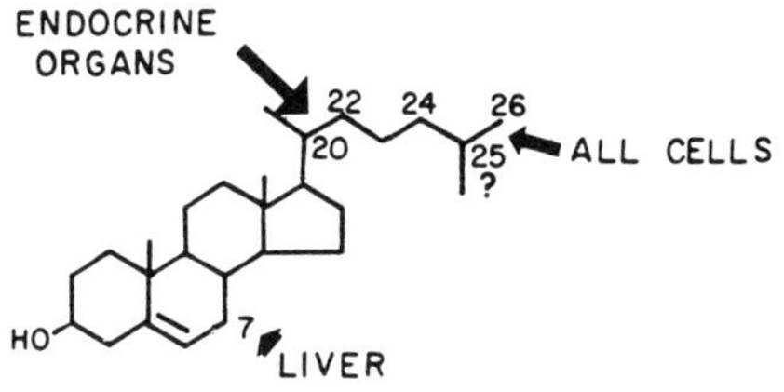

FIGURE 1. Hydroxysterols derived from cholesterol. These are potential regulators of cellular cholesterol homeostasis.

sterol synthesis, have low levels of 26-hydroxycholesterol in their blood and have a deficiency in 26-hydroxylase in their cells (16). The latter observations make 26-hydroxycholesterol an attractive candidate for the regulatory oxysterol.

26-Hydroxycholesterol Regulation of Ovarian Cell Cholesterol Synthesis

It has previously been documented that 25-hydroxycholesterol is a potent inhibitor of rat ovarian cell de novo sterol synthesis (17). Utilizing cultured human granulosa cells, we found that exogenous 26-hydroxycholesterol causes a profound inhibition of [^{14}C]acetate incorporation into both cellular sterols and secreted progestin (Fig. 2). In contrast, the amount of progesterone produced by the cells in the presence of 26-hydroxycholesterol is increased, presumably reflecting the utilization of 26-hydroxycholesterol as a substrate by the cholesterol side-chain cleavage enzyme. Others have shown that exogenous 26-hydroxycholesterol inhibits HMG/CoA reductase and LDL uptake in cultured human fibroblasts, L-cells, and Chinese hamster ovary cells (Table 1). These findings are all consistent with the idea that 26-hydroxycholesterol could be an endogenous regulator of cellular sterol homeostasis.

26-Hydroxylase Activity in Ovarian Cells

Utilizing the ovaries of pregnant mare's serum gonadotropin (PMSG)/hCG-primed immature rats, we demonstrated that isolated mitochondria convert

TABLE 1. 26-hydroxycholesterol as a regulator of cellular cholesterol metabolism.

Cell Type	Activity	Reference
Chinese hamster ovary cells	Inhibition of HMG-CoA reductase	Esterman et al., J Lipid Res 24:1304, 1983.
	Inhibition of D$_2$O incorporation into sterols	Esterman et al., J Lipid Res 26:950, 1985.
L-cells	Inhibition of HMG-CoA reductase	Taylor et al., J Biol Chem 259:12382, 1984.
Human granulosa cells	Inhibition of [^{14}C]acetate incorporation into sterol and progestins	Rennert et al., Endocrinology, 1990.
Human fibroblasts	Inhibition of uptake and degradation of LDL	Lorenzo et al., FEBS Lett 218:77, 1987.

[³H]cholesterol to [³H]26-hydroxycholesterol (Fig. 3). 26-hydroxylase activity was localized to the mitochondrial subcellular fraction of the ovary, and it was inhibited in a dose-dependent manner by ketoconazole (18). The identity of the reaction product was established by chromatography in several thin-layer chromatographic systems, HPLC, and by recrystallization of labeled product to constant specific activity. Accumulation of 26-hydroxycholesterol in the reaction mixture was stimulated in the presence of aminoglutethimide, which was added to prevent metabolism of the hydroxysterol by the cholesterol side-chain cleavage enzyme system (18). The production of 26-hydroxycholesterol by isolated mitochondria was also stimulated by calcium.

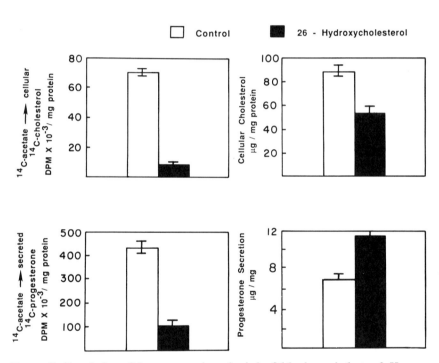

FIGURE 2. Regulation of de novo sterol synthesis by 26-hydroxycholesterol. Human granulosa cells were cultured for 6 days in serum containing medium, followed by 48 h in serum-free medium. 26-hydroxycholesterol (5 µg/mL) was added to some cultures for an 18-h period. During the last 5 h of incubation, [¹⁴C]acetate (40 µCi) was added. Cell lipid extracts and medium were processed for analysis of cholesterol and progesterone and incorporation of [¹⁴C]acetate into these compounds. Values presented are means I±SE of triplicate cultures in each treatment group. (From Rennert H, Fischer RJ, Alvarez JG, Trzaskos JM, Strauss JF, III, Generation of regulatory oxysterols: 26-hydroxylation of cholesterol by ovarian mitochrondria, Endocrinology 1990;127:738–46, with permission.)

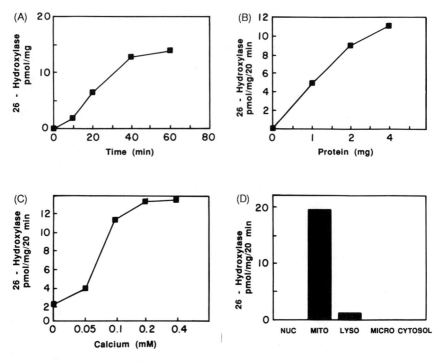

Figure 3. Characterization of 26-hydroxylase in rat ovaries. *A*: 26-hydroxy-cholesterol formation with respect to incubation time. Mitochondria (2 mg/protein) were incubated for up to 60 min. Values are means of at least triplicate determinations at each time point. *B*: Relationship between 26-hydroxycholesterol formation and mitochondrial protein. Varying quantities of mitochondrial protein were incubated for 20 min. Values presented are means of duplicate determinations at each protein concentration. *C*: Effect of calcium on 26-hydroxycholesterol formation. Mitochondria (2 mg/protein) were incubated with the indicated concentration of calcium added to the assay buffer for 20 min. Values presented are means of triplicate determinations. *D*: Subcellular distribution of 26-hydroxylase activity. The indicated subcellular fractions (2 mg/protein) were incubated for 20 min under standard conditions. Values presented are means of triplicate determinations. (From Rennert H, Fischer RJ, Alvarez JG, Trzaskos JM, Strauss JF, III, Generation of regulatory oxysterols: 26-hydroxylation of cholesterol by ovarian mitochrondria, Endocrinology 1990;127:738–46, with permission.)

26-hydroxylase activity in isolated mitochondria is relatively unstable upon freezing. Activity in stored mitochrondia decayed completely over a 37-day period in contrast to cholesterol side-chain cleavage activity, which declined 20% during the same time (Fig. 4).

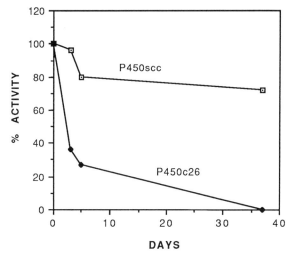

FIGURE 4. Stability of 26-hydroxylase (P-45$_{c26}$) and P-450$_{SCC}$ activity to storage at –80°C.

These observations establish that 26-hydroxylase is present in ovarian cells and that it is a ketoconazole-sensitive enzyme with several characteristics that distinguish it from P-450$_{SCC}$. Thus, at least two cholesterol-metabolizing enzymes exist in ovarian mitochondria, although the level of 26-hydroxylase activity is far less than that of cholesterol side-chain cleavage enzyme.

Cloning of a cDNA Homologous to 26-Hydroxylase

Andersson et al. (19) recently cloned the cDNA for rabbit cholesterol 26-hydroxylase from a liver library. The deduced amino acid sequence revealed a protein with a structure consistent with a cytochrome P-450 enzyme, including a leader sequence with characteristics of a mitochondrial import peptide and a conserved heme binding domain near the carboxy terminus of the protein. Expression of this cDNA in COS cells resulted in significant 26-hydroxylase activity.

Utilizing this rabbit cDNA, we cloned a homologous 1.9-Kb cDNA from a rat liver library, which encodes a protein with 533 amino acid residues. The deduced amino acid sequence is 73% identical to the rabbit 26-hydroxylase sequence (Fig. 5). The protein has a 32 amino acid amino-terminal sequence characteristic of a mitochondrial import sequence that is rich in basic and hydrophobic residues. There is significant identity at the amino acid level in the heme-binding and putative sterol-binding domains between rat 26-

M A V L S R M R L R W A L L D T R V M G H G L C P Q G A R A L A*A I

P A A L   R D H E S T   E G P G T G Q D R P R L P S L A E L P G P G T L R

F L F Q L F L R G Y V L H L H E L Q A L N K A K Y G P M W   T   T T F G

T R T N Y N L A S A P   L   L E Q V M R Q E G K Y P I R D S M E Q W K E

H R D H K G L S Y G I   F I T Q G P Q W   Y H L R H S L N Q R M L K P A

E A A L Y T D A L N E   V I S D F   I   A R L D Q V R T E S A S G D Q V P D

V A H L L Y H L A L E A   I   C Y I L F E K R V G C L E P S I P E D T A T F

I R S V G L M F K N S V Y V T F L P K W S R P L L P F W K R Y M N N

W D N I F S F G E K M I H Q K V Q E I E A Q L Q A A G P D G V Q V S G

Y L H F   L L T K E L L S P Q E T V G T F P E L I L A G V D T T S N T L T

W A L Y H L S K N P E   I Q E A L H   K E V T G V V P F G K V P Q N K D
       p l l k a   s i k e t l r l   hp
F A H M<u>P L L K A V   I K E T L R L Y P</u>V V P T N S R I   I T E K E T E I N

G F L F P K N T Q F V L C H Y V V S   R D P S V F P E P E S F Q P H R W
              f g wg vr qc l g r r i a e i
L R K R E D D N S G I   Q H P F G S V P<u>F G Y G V R S C L G R R I A E L</u>
e m tif l
<u>E M Q L L L</u>S R L I   Q   K Y E V V L   S P G M G E V K S V S R I V L V P S

K K V S L R F L Q R Q

FIGURE 5. Deduced amino acid sequence (single letter code) of rat 26-hydroxylase. Underlined regions denote the putative substrate-binding domain (double lines) and heme-binding domain (single line). The corresponding amino acid sequence of rat P-450_{SCC} is given in small letters with bold type indicating differences. The asterisk indicates the proposed cleavage site yielding the mature enzyme.

hydroxylase and rat P-450_{SCC}, but other regions of the proteins are not similar (20). These observations suggest these two cholesterol hydroxylating enzymes are derived from a common but perhaps distant ancestor.

Genomic Southern blot analysis revealed that the 26-hydroxylase gene is present in low copy numbers and that there is probably a unique gene for the enzyme. Although 26-hydroxylase mRNA is most abundant in the liver, where the enzyme functions in bile acid synthesis, we found mRNA for the enzyme in a variety of other tissues. The rat 26-hydroxylase cDNA hybridized with mRNA species of 2.1 and 2.3 Kb in luteinized (PMSG/hCG-primed) rat ovaries. A single 2.3-Kb mRNA was found in liver. The estimated relative abundance of P-450_{26} mRNA compared to P-450_{SCC} mRNA was approximately 1:20, consistent with the differences in measured enzyme activity. These findings corroborate the expression of the 26-hydroxylase gene in rat ovarian cells. Northern blot analysis of total RNA from human granulosa cells also revealed the presence of 26-hydroxylase mRNA in these cells (18).

Because the overall nucleotide sequence position identity between the 26-hydroxylase and P-450$_{SCC}$ cDNAs is relatively low, it is unlikely that the 26-hydroxylase cDNA hybridizes with P-450$_{SCC}$ mRNA in hybridizations performed under high stringency.

Regulation of Ovarian 26-Hydroxylase Activity and mRNA Levels

26-hydroxylase activity measured in the presence of aminoglutethimide was inhibited by addition of pregnenolone or progesterone in a dose-dependent fashion (18). Significant inhibition was found with concentrations of steroid on the order of 1–10 μM, concentrations that are within the physiological range. These observations suggest that the observed stimulation of 26-hydroxylase by aminoglutethimide may be due to suppression of cholesterol side-chain cleavage enzyme and hence formation of pregnenolone and progesterone. These observations also raise the novel possibility that 26-hydroxycholesterol formation is regulated by steroidogenic activity. When steroidogenesis is increased, intramitochondrial pregnenolone would inhibit formation of 26-hydroxycholesterol, thus preventing inhibition of de novo sterol synthesis and LDL receptor gene expression. This would ensure availability of substrate for steroidogenesis.

The mechanism by which products of the cholesterol side-chain cleavage enzyme reaction inhibit 26-hydroxylase is not yet known. However, it is worth remembering the previously reported inhibition of cholesterol side-chain cleavage enzyme by pregnenolone (21). This inhibitory action is believed to be exerted through binding of pregnenolone to a site on the protein other than the substrate binding domain.

Although calcium has been shown to stimulate 26-hydroxylation of cholesterol by isolated mitochondria, it is not known whether calcium has a physiologic role in the control of this reaction, and if so, what the mechanism of its action is. It is noteworthy that calcium also increases pregnenolone formation by isolated adrenal mitochondria in the presence of a NADPH-generating system, perhaps by a mechanism similar to that for 26-hydroxylase (22).

It has been postulated that sterol carrier protein$_2$ (SCP$_2$) can modulate the 26-hydroxylation of cholesterol, presumably through the transport and/or distribution of cholesterol to the mitochondrial membranes (23). This 13.2-kDa basic peptide is present in many tissues, and the mRNA encoding it is upregulated in the ovary by gonadotropic hormones (24). The availability of the cloned cDNA for SCP$_2$ will allow a direct test of this concept through misexpression and assessment of the impact on cholesterol 26-hydroxylase activity.

The mRNA for 26-hydroxylase also appears to be regulated. Treatment of immature rats with PMSG/hCG causes a 2- to 3-fold increase in 26-hydroxylase mRNA. This increase in 26-hydroxylase mRNA may be required to provide more regulatory sterol in cells that are more active in making steroid hormones and synthesizing cholesterol de novo. These findings demonstrate gonadotropic regulation of a cholesterol metabolizing P-450 enzyme gene heretofore unexplored in the ovary.

26-Hydroxycholesterol as an Intracrine Regulator of Ovarian Cholesterol Homeostasis

The observations presented above suggest that 26-hydroxycholesterol could function as intracellular regulator of sterol homeostasis. The suggested role for this compound as an intracrine factor is based on the facts that (a) exogenous 26-hydroxycholesterol is a potent suppressor of cellular de novo sterol synthesis, (b) ovarian cells express the 26-hydroxylase gene, and (c) the regulation of 26-hydroxylase activity is consistent with a role of 26-hydroxycholesterol in cellular cholesterol homeostasis. The notion that 26-hydroxycholesterol is the key cellular effector is consonant with (a) ketoconazole sensitivity of lipoprotein control of cholesterol synthesis and LDL receptor gene transcription (12), and (b) aminoglutethimide blockade of gonadotropin-induced stimulation of HMG/CoA reductase activity (25–27). In the presence ketoconazole de novo sterol synthesis and LDL receptors are upregulated. These sequelae can be accounted for by ketoconazole inhibition of 26-hydroxycholesterol synthesis with resultant increases in HMG/CoA reductase and LDL receptor gene transcription. Stimulation of rat ovarian tissue with hCG causes a prompt rise in progestin secretion and HMG/CoA reductase activity and mRNA. The increase in HMG/CoA reductase is almost completely inhibited in the presence of aminoglutethimide. The interpretation of these observations is that hCG increases progestin synthesis, resulting in diminished 26-hydroxycholesterol formation, which in turn leads to derepression of the HMG/CoA reductase gene. In the presence of aminoglutethimide, progestin synthesis is blocked so that 26-hydroxycholesterol synthesis occurs with attendant inhibition of HMG/CoA reductase gene expression.

If 26-hydroxycholesterol is indeed an intracellular regulator, one would predict that its levels would be tightly controlled by both synthesis and catabolism. We believe that 26-hydroxycholesterol, like other side-chain hydroxylated sterols, can be metabolized to steroid hormones by cytochrome P-450$_{SCC}$ and thus inactivated as a regulator of cholesterol homeostasis (28). 26-hydroxycholesterol may also be subject to side-chain oxidation in mito-

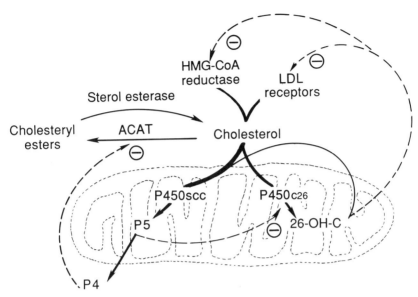

FIGURE 6. Model for regulation of cholesterol metabolism in an ovarian cell. Cholesterol is derived from de novo synthesis in LDL. De novo synthesis and lipoprotein uptake are suppressed by 26-hydroxycholesterol. When steroidogenesis is stimulated, pregnenolone (P5) and progesterone (P4) accumulate, resulting in inhibition of 26-hydroxylase (P-450$_{c26}$) and less production of 26-hydroxycholesterol (26-OH-C), promoting increased de novo cholesterol synthesis and LDL uptake. Progesterone also inhibits acyl CoA: cholesterol acyl transferase (ACAT) with a resultant increase in free cholesterol for utilization for steroid hormone synthesis. (From Rennert H, Fischer RJ, Alvarez JG, Trzaskos JM, Strauss JF, III, Generation of regulatory oxysterols: 26-hydroxylation of cholesterol by ovarian mitochrondria, Endocrinology 1990;127:738–46, with permission.)

chondria or peroxisomes (29) to form 3β-hydroxy-5-cholenoic acid or to esterification. The extent to which these reactions occur in steroidogenic, hepatic, and other cell types may vary considerably and is a topic for further investigation.

The factors that might allow 26-hydroxycholesterol to act on the genome remain to be identified. Although a hepatic oxysterol binding protein has been purified to homogeneity and its cDNA cloned, there is as of yet no evidence that this protein participates in mediating the genomic action of hydroxysterols. This is clearly a subject deserving an intensive investigation.

From our findings that pregnenolone and progesterone inhibit 26-hydroxylase, we would predict that exogenous progestins added in quantities sufficient to inhibit 26-hydroxylase would increase HMG/CoA reductase activity and/or LDL receptor expression. This prediction has been fulfilled in studies by Gal et al. (30) who reported that progesterone treatment stimulates HMG/CoA reductase in several tumour cell lines and Panini et al. (31) who found increased HMG/CoA reductase activity in rat intestinal epithelial cells following treatment with 30-μM progesterone. Since the tumor cells studied by Gal and coworkers did not have progesterone receptors, the increase in HMG/CoA reductase activity needs to be explained by a nonclassical mechanism, consistent with inhibition of 26-hydroxylase activity.

Based on the observations presented above, we propose a model of cholesterol homeostasis in ovarian cells in which 26-hydroxycholesterol is envisioned as the effector that acts to reduce HMG/CoA reductase and LDL receptor gene transcription (Fig. 6). We hypothesize that the formation of 26-hydroxycholesterol is coordinately linked with cholesterol side-chain cleavage activity through inhibition of 26-hydroxylase by pregnenolone and progesterone. This coupled interaction would insure that the cell's ability to acquire cholesterol was directly linked to demand for steroid hormone precursor.

Conclusion

While this chapter has presented arguments in favor of the concept that 26-hydroxycholesterol is a regulator of cholesterol homeostasis, one cannot exclude the possibility that other hydroxysterols derived from metabolism of cholesterol such as 24-hydroxycholesterol or intermediates in cholesterol biosynthesis such as hydroxylanosterols are equally important.

Acknowledgments. Research described in this chapter was supported by UPHS Grant HD-06274 and grants from the Rockefeller and Mellon Foundations. The authors thank Ms. Jeannette Winnick for help on preparation of this manuscript.

References

1. Gwynne JT, Strauss JF, III. The role of lipoproteins in steroidogenesis and cholesterol metabolism in steroidogenic glands. Endocr Res 1982;3:299-329.
2. Strauss JF, III, Schuler LA, Rosenblum MF, Tanaka T. Cholesterol metabolism by ovarian tissue. Adv Lipid Res 1981;19:99-159.
3. Murphy BD, Silavin SL. Luteotrophic agents and steroid substrate utilization. Oxf Rev Reprod Biol 1989;11:179-223.
4. Gwynne JT, Mahafee DD. Lipoproteins and steroid hormone-producing tissues. Methods Enzymol 1986;129:679-90.
5. Goldstein JL, Brown MS. Regulation of the mevalonate pathway. Nature 1990;343:425-30.

6. Golos TG, Strauss JF, III. 8-bromoadenosine cyclic 3', 5'-phosphate rapidly increases 3-hydroxy-3-methylglutaryl coenzyme A reductase mRNA in human granulosa cells: Role of cellular sterol balance in controlling the response to tropic stimulation. Biochemistry 1988;27:3503-6.

7. Kandutsch AA, Chen HW, Heiniger HJ. Biological activity of some oxygenated sterols. Science 1978;201:498-501.

8. Taylor FR, Kandutsch AA. Oxysterol binding protein. Chem Phys Lipids 1985;38:187-94.

9. Dawson PA, Ridgway ND, Slaughter CA, Brown MS, Goldstein JL. cDNA cloning and expression of oxysterol-binding protein, an oligomer with a potential leucine zipper. J Biol Chem 1989;264:16798-803.

10. Rajavashisth TB, Taylor AK, Andalibi A, Svenson KL, Lusis AJ. Identification of a zinc finger protein that binds to the sterol regulatory element. Science 1989; 254:640-3.

11. Feldman D. Ketoconazole and other imidazole derivatives as inhibitors of steroidogenesis. Endocr Res 1986;7:409-20.

12. Takagi K, Alvarez JG, Favata MF, Trzaskos JM, Strauss JF, III. Control of low density lipoprotein receptor gene promoter activity: Ketoconazole inhibits serum lipoprotein but not oxysterol suppression of gene transcription. J Biol Chem 1989;264:12352-7.

13. Gupta A, Sexton RC, Rudney H. Modulation of regulatory oxysterol formation and low density lipoprotein suppression of 3-hydroxy-3-methyl glutaryl coenzyme A (HMG-CoA) reductase activity by ketoconazole. A role for cytochrome P450 in the regulation of HMG-CoA reductase in rat intestinal epithelial cells. J Biol Chem 1986;261:8348-56.

14. Dhar AK, Teng JI, Smith LL. Biosynthesis of cholest-5-ene-3β, 24 diol (cerebrosterol) by bovine cerebral cortical microsomes. J Neurochem 1973; 21:51-60.

15. Wikvall K. Hydroxylations in biosynthesis at bile acids isolation of a cytochrom P450 from rabbit liver mitochondria catalyzing 26-hydroxylation of C27-steroids. J Lipid Res 1976;17:366-72.

16. Oftebro H, Bjorkhem I, Skrede S, Schreiner A, Pedersen JI. Cerebrotendinous xanthomatosis. A defect in mitochondrial 26-hydroxylation required for normal biosynthesis of cholic acid. J Clin Invest 1980;65:1418-30.

17. Schuler LA, Scavo L, Kirsch TM, Flickinger GL, Strauss, JF, III. Regulation of de novo biosynthesis of cholesterol and progestins, and formation of cholesteryl ester in rat corpus luteum by exogenous sterol. J Biol Chem 1979;254:8662-69.

18. Rennert H, Fischer RJ, Alvarez JG, Trzaskos JM, Strauss JF, III. Generation of regulatory oxysterols: 26-hydroxylation of cholesterol by ovarian mitochrondria. Endocrinology 1990;127:738-746.

19. Andersson S, Davis DL, Dahlbeck H, Jornvall H, Russell DW. Cloning, structure, and expression of the mitochondrial cytochrome P450 sterol 26-hydroxylase, a bile acid biosynthetic enzyme. J Biol Chem 1989;264:8222-9.

20. Oonk RB, Krasnow JS, Beattie WG, Richards JS. Cyclic AMP-dependent and -independent regulation of cholesterol side-chain cleavage cytochrome P450 (P-450scc) in rat ovarian granulosa cells and corpora lutea cDNA and deduced amino acid sequence of rat P-450scc. J Biol Chem 1989;264:21934-42.

21. Koritz SB, Hall PF. End-product inhibition of the conversion of cholesterol to pregnenolone in an adrenal extract. Biochemistry 1964;9:1298-1304.
22. Simpson ER, Jefcoate CR, McCarthy JL, Boyd GL. Effect of calcium ions on steroid-binding spectra and pregnenolone formation in rat-adrenal mitochondria. Eur J Biochem 1974;45:181-188.
23. Lidström-Olsson B, Wikvall D. The role of sterol carrier protein$_2$ and other hepatic lipid-binding proteins in bile-acid biosynthesis. Biochem J 1986;238: 870-84.
24. Billheimer JT, Strehl LL, Davis GL, Strauss JF, III, Davis LG. Characterization of a cDNA encoding rat sterol carrier protein$_2$. DNA 1990;9:159-65.
25. Schuler LA, Toaff ME, Strauss JF, III. Control of 3-hydroxy-3-methylglutaryl coenzyme A reductase and acyl coenzyme A: Cholesterol acyl transferase. Endocrinology 1981;108:1476-86.
26. Azhar S, Chen YDI, Reaven GM. Gonadotropin modulation of 3-hydroxy-3-methylglutaryl coenzyme A reductase activity in desensitized luteinized rat ovary. Biochemisty 1984;23:4533-8.
27. Puryear TK, Mclean MP, Khan I, Gibori G. Mechanism for control of hydroxy-methylglutaryl coenzyme A reductase and cytochrome P450 side-chain cleavage message and enzyme in corpus luteum. Endrocrinology 1990;126:2910-8.
28. Toaff ME, Schleyer H, Strauss JF, III. Metabolism of 25-hydroxycholesterol by rat luteal mitochondria and dispersed cells. Endocrinology 1982;111:1785-90.
29. Krisans SK, Thompson SL, Pena LA, Kok E, Javitt NB. Bile acid synthesis in rat liver peroxisomes: Metabolism of 26-hydroxycholesterol to 3β-hydroxy-5-cholenoic acid. J Lipid Res 1985;26:1324-32.
30. Gal D, MacDonald PC, Simpson ER. Cholesterol metabolism in human cancer cells in monolayer, V. The effect of progesterone in the regulation of 3-hydroxy-3-methylglutaryl coenzyme A reductase activity by low density lipoprotein. J Clin Endocrinol Metab 1981;53:29-33.
31. Panini SR, Grupta A, Sexton RC, Parish EJ, Rudney A. Regulation of sterol biosynthesis and 3-hydroxy-3-methylglutaryl coenzyme A reductase activity in cultured cells by progesterone. J Biol Chem 1987;262:14435-40.

Part IV

Relevance of Resident Ovarian White Blood Cells

12

Leukocyte Chemo-Attraction and Periovulatory Follicular Processes

W.J. MURDOCH AND R.J. MCCORMICK

A role for white blood cells in ovarian physiology has been suspected for many years (1). Indeed, these cells have been described within follicles and corpora lutea as associated with the mechanisms of atresia (2), ovulation (3), and luteolysis (4). Very little information is currently available concerning the nature of the signaling processes involved in ovarian leukocyte chemoattraction or the cause-and-effect relationships that could exist between tissue resident leukocytes and the endocrine/exocrine functions of the ovary. In contrast, a plethora of research work has been accomplished with respect to the involvement of the white blood cell in generalized immune/ inflammatory reactions.

The purpose of this brief review is to *(a)* make note of the primary chemical messengers of site-directed leukocyte migration that have been characterized to date, *(b)* outline the basic response of a leukocyte to a chemotactic stimulus, *(c)* discuss what is known regarding leukocytic infiltration of the ovary, and *(d)* describe the kinds of bioactive substances secreted from white blood cells and how they might participate in ovarian phenomena.

Immune/Inflammatory Mediators of Leukocyte Chemotaxis

Chemotaxis is defined as the process by which a cell migrates along a concentration gradient in the direction of origin of a specific chemical signal. It is distinguished from chemokinesis, or random migration.

Leukocytes can be attracted by compounds of widely diverse chemical composition. Some of these are of endogenous derivation (e.g., products of activation of the complement cascade and metabolites of arachidonic acid). Others are produced by foreign invaders (e.g., formylated methionyl peptides released from micro-organisms).

Complement 5a. *Complement* (C) is a term used to describe a group of thermolabile proteins present in serum. Many of these proteins are zymogens, which require enzymatic cleavage to become activated. The complement system constitutes a major effector pathway of host defense (and possibly autoimmune) responses. Complement can kill cells by either the classical or alternative (i.e., antibody-independent) pathways (5).

Complement proteins are assembled sequentially on the surface of target cells. During generation of the so-called lytic membrane attack complex, a by-product of the α-chain of the fifth component of complement, C5a, is liberated. Human C5a is a glycoprotein composed of 74 amino acid residues. It is a powerful chemo-attractant for polymorphonuclear leukocytes and monocytes (6, 7).

Once white blood cells are mobilized into a site of allergic inflammation, they operate to phagocytize cells lysed by complement and/or cytotoxins released as a result of their own activation. Complement serves an important role here as well. It opsonizes cells (via C3b) so that they can be readily recognized by the leukocyte (5).

Whether the complement cascade is of any significance to ovarian physiology is not known. There is sparse experimental data to indicate that complement activity is enhanced in atretic (2) and ovulatory (8), compared to cystic, follicles.

Leukotriene B_4. Lipid-derived molecules also possess chemoattractant qualities. Most notable among these are the metabolites of arachidonate, in particular Leukotriene (LT) B_4. This lipoxygenase product is capable of evoking chemotactic responses equivalent to those induced by C5a or the N-formylated oligopeptides (6).

LTB_4 is produced by ovarian tissues. Accordingly, lipoxygenase catabolites of arachidonic acid have been implicated in the processes of ovulation and luteal regression (9–14).

N-Formyl Peptides. These substances are not synthesized by eukaryotic organisms, but are released from bacteria during an inflammatory reaction. Because N-formylated peptides can be synthesized in the laboratory and made available in large quantities, they have afforded investigators a convenient tool by which to study structure/function relationships of leukocyte locomotion. The most potent of these compounds is N-fMet-Leu-Phe. It does not appear that leukocytes of the farm species contain receptors for the N-formyl peptides (6, 7, 15).

Other Factors. An array of additional compounds have been shown to attract white blood cells. This list includes the neutrophil chemotactic factor, eosinophil chemotactic factor of anaphylaxis, lymphocyte-derived chemotactic factor, crystal-induced chemotactic factor, platelet-activating factor (PAF), platelet-derived growth factor, and platelet factor 4. Other yet ill-defined chemo-attractants are released during blood clotting/fibrinolytic processes (16) and as degradation products from damaged tissues (7).

Leukocyte Responses to a Chemotactic Gradient

Extravascular trafficking of leukocytes involves several steps. Cells adhere to endothelium, change shape by cytoskeletal reorganization, and develop pseudopodia, which seek out gaps between endothelial cells (Fig. 1). The latter process is aided by an increase in vascular permeability brought about by inflammatory mediators, such as histamine.

Receptors for chemotactic agents (which are distinct entities, at least for C5a, LTB_4, and N-formyl peptides) are not distributed uniformly over the cellular membrane at a given point in time, but rather are concentrated within the leading front of a (crawling) podia. Analogous to mechanisms involved in the desensitization of an endocrine organ to a hormone, ligand-receptor complexes undergo endocytosis and are internalized. Downregulation of receptors is followed by retraction of the pseudopodia. Preferential expres-

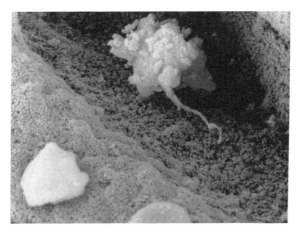

FIGURE 1. Scanning electron micrograph of a white blood cell marginated along a post-capillary venule of a preovulatory ovine follicle. (From Cavender JL, Murdoch WJ, Biol Reprod 1988;39:989–97, reproduced with permission from the Society for the Study of Reproduction.)

sion of receptors at a different surface location presumably takes place as the leukocyte reorients toward the concentration gradient.

Motility of leukocytes is dependent upon calcium. Calcium can be supplied by transmembrane influx and/or by mobilization from intracellular stores. Cyclic nucleotides and products of phosphoinositide metabolism appear to act as second messengers in the mechanics of stimulus-response coupling (16).

Ovarian White Blood Cells

To our knowledge, quantitative information pertaining to the types of leukocytes that infiltrate the follicular wall at various periovulatory times has only been reported for the sheep (17). Neutrophils and eosinophils were observed to accumulate within the extravascular compartment of the theca interna several hours before ovulation. Evidence of vascular injury and formation of microthrombi were observed at ovulation. Extravasated monocytes/macrophages were apparent following ovulation. There were no significant changes in numbers of extravascular lymphocytes throughout the periovulatory period. Nonetheless, lymphocytes were often seen marginated along endothelium in ovulatory and postovulatory follicles. Basophilic cells were found in close proximity to angiogenic sprouts within the formative corpus luteum. These data imply that preovulatory follicles produce a chemo-attractant for granulocytes, while postovulatory follicles secrete a chemotactic agent for monocytes. Granulocytes characteristically arrive into inflamed areas before phagocytic monocytes (18).

In a subsequent study, using a linear under-agarose chemotactic assay, we demonstrated that ovine follicles secreted a low molecular weight chemo-attractant for granulocytes and monocytes (19). A preliminary attempt at purification of this substance indicated that it was a peptide, rich in glycine. Because every third amino acid residue of the main body chain of collagen is glycine (20), thecal collagen is degraded during the process of follicular rupture (21–23), and synthetic collagen-like polypeptides (comprised of the repeating triplet glycine-proline-proline or glycine-hydroxyproline-proline and lacking helical structure) have been shown to possess chemotactic properties (24), we proposed that the chemo-attractant isolated from tissue-conditioned media was a fragment of collagen, liberated during disruption of the connective tissue matrix of the follicular wall. However, our initial amino acid analysis (19) did not include determinations for either proline or hydroxyproline, which, in addition to glycine, are rather uniquely predominate to the structure of collagen (20). Reanalysis of the sample confirmed the presence of these amino acids (unpublished observation). Curiously, C1q, which acts to bind the first component of complement to immune complexes and membranes, contains within its structure a fibril-like moiety that resembles collagen (5). This (N-terminal) region is about 80 amino acid residues in length and contains repeating sequences of glycine-X-Y, where X and Y are often hydroxyproline or proline.

A chemotactic protein for neutrophils was recently isolated from human follicular fluid. This protein was heat labile, trypsin sensitive, and of high (about 100 kDa) molecular weight (25).

Involuting corpora lutea apparently also produce chemo-attractants for leukocytes (15, 26, 27). The nature of such compounds has not yet been elucidated.

Secretory Products of Leukocytes: Possible Implications in Ovarian Function

Mobility is not the only response of a leukocyte to a chemo-attractant agent. Contents of lysosomes and secretory granules are also released after such exposure. The threshold for a secretory event is greater than that necessary to elicit chemotaxis (16).

A broad spectrum of bioactive chemicals are produced by leukocytes. These compounds contribute to the injury of tissue that usually accompanies an inflammatory reaction and, somewhat paradoxically, are probably involved in subsequent extracellular matrix remodeling/wound repair.

Proteolytic Enzymes. Granulocytes represent a crucial element of the cellular host defense mechanism against microbial/parasitic infections. When marshalled into tissue sites of inflammatory or allergic insult, they can cause tissue damage via release of proteases. Neutrophils contain collagenases, elastases, and chymotrypsins (28). These enzymes would presumably be capable of acting on connective tissue targets within the thecal layer of the follicle and thereby be involved in the weakening of the follicular wall that precedes ovulation and/or the reorganization of tissues affiliated with transformation of the ovulated follicle into a corpus luteum.

Toxic Oxidants. Granulocytes also contain peroxidases (28, 29). Reactive oxygen species, released in a burst upon cellular activation, can cause serious injury to tissues (30). Hydrogen peroxide exerted antigonadotropic effects toward rat luteal cells in vitro (31). It was suggested that H_2O_2 produced by leukocytes attracted into the corpus luteum could be of relevance to the luteolytic process. Eosinophil peroxidase augmented the ability of macrophages to lyse tumor cells (32). Macrophages are probably responsible for phagocytosis of dead luteal cells (15, 26).

Arachidonate Metabolites. Products of both the cyclo-oxygenase and lipoxygenase pathways of metabolism of arachidonic acid are liberated by white blood cells (33–35). It is well established that prostaglandins are critical intermediates in the mechanics of ovulation (36), and luteolysis (37), and as already mentioned, lipoxygenase products might likewise be involved. Furthermore, related compounds secreted by leukocytes, such as PAF, appear to play a role in ovarian function (38). Eicosanoids provoke diverse pathophysiological effects generally associated with inflammation and tissue trauma (39, 40), which are processes certainly akin to ovulation and luteolysis.

Cytokines. The cytokines represent a group of leukocyte-derived soluble factors that act as mediators of immune/inflammatory responses. A nonexclusive list of these compounds would encompass the interleukins, tumor necrosis factors, and interferons (41). That cytokines can modify ovarian functions is becoming increasingly evident.

Interleukin-1 is a polypeptide produced by the monocyte/macrophage lineage of white cells in response to acute infection and antigenic challenge. It activates lymphocytes and stimulates metabolism of arachidonate (42). IL-1 was detected in relatively high amounts in follicular fluid (43). Differentiation/luteinization of pig and rat granulosal cells was inhibited by IL-1 (44, 45). Macrophages exerted a seemingly inconsistent (i.e., tropic) influence on human luteal cells (46).

Corpora lutea of rabbits produced a tumor necrosis factor-like material in response to lipopolysaccharide (27). TNF is a cytotoxic agent secreted by activated macrophages. It appears to play a role in the relatively uncommon occurrence of spontaneous regression of some cancers (47). In many respects, the corpus luteum resembles a solid tumor that undergoes cyclic degeneration. A hallmark of tumor regression induced by TNF entails endothelial cell necrosis (47). Vascular damage and tissue ischemia are amongst the earliest morphological signs of luteal regression (48). Thus, a cause-and-effect relationship could exist between luteal accumulation of TNF, blood vessel injury, and luteolysis. The vascular system of the theca interna is likewise compromised during the ovulatory process. Blood vessels become completely disrupted in the area of the ovulatory stigma (49, 50).

Gamma interferon is secreted by T-lymphocytes. One of its actions is to upregulate the expression of cell-surface major histocompatibility complex (MHC) molecules (41, 51). With this background in mind, Fairchild and Pate (52) recently demonstrated that gamma interferon stimulated the appearance of MHC antigens on cultured bovine luteal cells. They suggested that autoimmune recognition of luteal cells could lead to a cell-mediated cytotoxic reaction underlying the mechanism of luteolysis.

Examples of other cytotoxins secreted by white blood cells include the major basic protein of eosinophils (29) and the pore-forming protein (perforin) of cytotoxic T-lymphocytes and natural killer cells (53). Both substances disrupt membranes. Perforin forms transmembrane lesions in a manner similar to that which occurs during polymerization of the ninth component of complement.

Angiogenic and Growth Factors. Neovascularization is a prominent feature of the formative corpus luteum. Several of the putative angiogenic factors (e.g., fibroblast growth factor and heparin) are produced by ovarian tissues (54). Macrophages and mast cells are known sources of angiogenic substances (55). Ovarian growth factors could serve an array of other generalized roles in follicular development and function (56).

Conclusion

There is an evolving interest in the concept that cellular elements of the immune/inflammatory system play a vital role in ovarian physiology. Leukocytes are undoubtedly attracted into the ovary during follicular atresia, ovulation, and luteolysis. We have partially purified a peptide chemo-attractant secreted by periovulatory ovine follicles that would appear to be a by-product of degradation of thecal collagen. Leukocytes produce a wide range of potent biologically active substances.

References

1. Warbritton V. The cytology of the corpora lutea of the ewe. J Morphol 1934; 56:181-220.
2. Farookhi R. Atresia: A hypothesis. In: Schwartz NB, Hunzicker-Dunn M, eds. Dynamics of ovarian function. New York: Raven Press, 1981:13-23.
3. Espey LL. Ovulation as an inflammatory reaction—a hypothesis. Biol Reprod 1980;22:73-106.
4. Murdoch WJ, Steadman LE, Belden EL. Immunoregulation of luteolysis. Med Hypotheses 1988;27:197-9.
5. Ross GD, ed. Immunobiology of the complement system. Orlando, FL: Academic Press, 1986.
6. Snyderman R, Goetzl EJ. Molecular and cellular mechanisms of leukocyte chemotaxis. Science 1981;213:830-7.
7. Becker EL. Chemotactic factors of inflammation. Trends Pharmacol Sci 1983; 4:223-5.
8. Fahmi HA, Hunter AG. Effect of estrual stage on complement activity in bovine follicular fluid. J Dairy Sci 1985;68:3318-22.
9. Reich R, Kohen F, Slager R, Tsafriri A. Ovarian lipoxygenase activity and its regulation by gonadotropin in the rat. Prostaglandins 1985;30:581-90.

10. Heinonen PK, Punnonen R, Ashorn R, Kujansuu E, Morsky P, Seppala E. Prostaglandins, thromboxane and leukotriene in human follicular fluid. Clin Reprod Fertil 1986;4:253-7.
11. Steadman LE, Murdoch WJ. Production of leukotriene B_4 by luteal tissues of sheep treated with prostaglandin $F_{2\alpha}$. Prostaglandins 1988;36:741-5.
12. Carvalho CB, Yeik BS, Murdoch WJ. Significance of follicular cyclooxygenase and lipoxygenase pathways of metabolism of arachidonate in sheep. Prostaglandins 1989;37:553-8.
13. Espey LL, Tanaka N, Okamura H. Increase in ovarian leukotrienes during hormonally induced ovulation in the rat. Am J Physiol 1989;256:E753-9.
14. Milvae RA, Alila HW, Hansel W. Involvement of lipoxygenase products of arachidonic acid metabolism in bovine luteal function. Biol Reprod 1986; 35:1210-5.
15. Murdoch WJ. Treatment of sheep with prostaglandin $F_{2\alpha}$ enhances production of a luteal chemoattractant for eosinophils. Am J Reprod Immunol Microbiol 1987; 15:52-6.
16. Snyderman R, Lane BC. Inflammation and chemotaxis. In: DeGroot LJ, ed. Endocrinology. 2nd ed. Philadelphia: WB Saunders, 1989:2466-79.
17. Cavender JL, Murdoch WJ. Morphological studies of the microcirculatory system of periovulatory ovine follicles. Biol Reprod 1988;39:989-97.
18. Anderson JR. Inflammation. In: Anderson JR, ed. Muir's textbook of pathology. London: Arnold, 1976:33-58.
19. Murdoch WJ, McCormick RJ. Production of low molecular weight chemoattractants for leukocytes by periovulatory ovine follicles. Biol Reprod 1989;40:86-90.
20. Harper E. Collagenases. Annu Rev Biochem 1980;49:1063-78.
21. Espey LL. Ovarian proteolytic enzymes and ovulation. Biol Reprod 1974; 10:216-35.
22. Reich R, Tsafriri A, Mechanic GL. The involvement of collagenolysis in ovulation in the rat. Endocrinology 1985;116:522-7.
23. Murdoch WJ, Peterson TA, Van Kirk EA, Vincent DL, Inskeep EK. Interactive roles of progesterone, prostaglandins, and collagenase in the ovulatory mechanism of the ewe. Biol Reprod 1986;35:1187-94.
24. Laskin DL, Berg RA. Chemotactic properties of synthetic collagen-like peptides. Prog Leukocyte Biol 1986;5:379-84.
25. Seow WK, Thong YH, Waters MJ, Cummins JM. Isolation of a chemotactic protein for neutrophils from human ovarian follicular fluid. Int Arch Allergy Appl Immunol 1988;86:331-6.
26. Paavola LG. Cellular mechanisms involved in luteolysis. Adv Exp Med Biol 1979;112:527-33.
27. Bagavandoss P, Wiggins RC, Kunkel SL, Remick DG, Keyes PL. Tumor necrosis factor production and accumulation of inflammatory cells in the corpus luteum of pseudopregnancy and pregnancy in rabbits. Biol Reprod 1990;42: 367-76.
28. Janoff A. Neutrophil chemotaxis and mediation of tissue damage. In: Kaley G, Altura BM, eds. Microcirculation; vol 3. Baltimore: University Park Press, 1980:165-84.

29. Gleich GJ, Adolphson CR. The eosinophilic leukocyte: Structure and function. Adv Immunol 1986;39:177-253.
30. Schraufstatter IU, Hyslop PA, Jackson J, Cochrane CC. Oxidant injury of cells. Int J Tiss Res 1987;4:317-24.
31. Behrman HR, Preston SL. Luteolytic actions of peroxide in rat ovarian cells. Endocrinology 1989;124:2895-900.
32. Nathan CF, Klebanoff SJ. Augmentation of spontaneous macrophage-mediated cytolysis by eosinophil peroxidase. J Exp Med 1982;155:1291-1308.
33. Janniger CK, Racis SP. The arachidonic acid cascade: An immunologically based review. J Med 1987;18:69-80.
34. Parker CW. Lipid mediators produced through the lipoxygenase pathway. Annu Rev Immunol 1987;5:65-84.
35. Samuelsson B, Dahlen S-E, Lindgren JA, Rouzer CA, Serhan CN. Leukotrienes and lipoxins: Structures, biosynthesis, and biological effects. Science 1987; 237:1171-6.
36. Lipner H. Mechanisms of mammalian ovulation. In: Knobil E, Neill JD, eds. The physiology of reproduction. New York: Raven Press, 1988:447-88.
37. Niswender GD, Nett TM. The corpus luteum and its control. In: Knobil E, Neill JD, eds. The physiology of reproduction. New York: Raven Press, 1988:489-525.
38. Harper MJK. Platelet-activating factor: A paracrine factor in preimplantation stages of reproduction? Biol Reprod 1989;40:907-13.
39. Davies P, Bailey PJ, Goldenberg MM, Ford-Hutchinson AW. The role of arachidonic acid oxygenation products in pain and inflammation. Annu Rev Immunol 1984;2:335-57.
40. Denzlinger C, Rapp S, Hagmann W, Keppler D. Leukotrienes as mediators in tissue trauma. Science 1985;230:330-2.
41. Harrison LC, Campbell IL. Cytokines: An expanding network of immuno-inflammatory hormones. Mol Endocrinol 1988;2:1151-6.
42. Dinarello CA. Biology of interleukin 1. FASEB J 1988;2:108-15.
43. Khan SA, Schmidt K, Hallin P, Di Pauli R, De Geyter CH, Nieschlag E. Human testis cytosol and ovarian follicular fluid contain high amounts of interleukin-1-like factor(s). Mol Cell Endocrinol 1988;58:221-30.
44. Fukuoka M, Mori T, Taii S, Yasuda K. Interleukin-1 inhibits luteinization of porcine granulosa cells in culture. Endocrinology 1988;122:376-9.
45. Gottschall PE, Katsuura G, Dahl RR, Hoffman ST, Arimura A. Discordance in effects of interleukin-1 on rat granulosa cell differentiation induced by follicle-stimulating hormone or activators of adenylate cyclase. Biol Reprod 1988;39:1074-85.
46. Halme J, Hammond MG, Syrop CH, Talbert LM. Peritoneal macrophages modulate human granulosa-luteal cell progesterone production. J Clin Endocrinol Metab 1985;61:912-6.
47. Old LJ. Tumor necrosis factor. Sci Am 1988;258:59-75.
48. Keyes PL, Wiltbank MC. Endocrine regulation of the corpus luteum. Annu Rev Physiol 1988;50:465-82.
49. Kitai H, Yoshimura Y, Wright KH, Santulli R, Wallach EE. Microvasculature of preovulatory follicles: Comparison of in situ and in vitro perfused rabbit ovaries following stimulation of ovulation. Am J Obstet Gynecol 1985;152:889-95.

50. Murdoch WJ, Cavender JL. Effect of indomethacin on the vascular architecture of preovulatory ovine follicles: Possible implication in the luteinized unruptured follicle syndrome. Fertil Steril 1989;51:153-5.
51. Billiau A. Interferons and inflammation. J Interferon Res 1987;7:559-67.
52. Fairchild DL, Pate JL. Interferon-γ induction of major histocompatibility antigens on cultured bovine luteal cells. Biol Reprod 1989;40:453-7.
53. Podack ER, Olsen KJ, Lowrey DM, Lichtenheld M. Structure and function of perforin. Curr Top Microbiol Immunol 1988;140:11-7.
54. Koos RD. Potential relevance of angiogenic factors to ovarian physiology. Semin Reprod Endocrinol 1989;7:29-40.
55. Folkman J. Tumor angiogenesis. Adv Cancer Res 1985;43:175-203.
56. Hammond JM, Hsu CJ, Mondschein JS, Canning SF. Paracrine and autocrine functions of growth factors in the ovarian follicle. J Anim Sci 1988;66 (suppl 2):21-31.

13

The Role of IL-1 in the Ovary

MARY LAKE POLAN, JILL A. LOUKIDES, AND PAMELA NELSON

The relationship of the reproductive system and immune secretory products has become a major focus of investigation (1). Attention has centered on the influence of macrophage products, such as interleukin-1 (IL-1) on ovarian function. IL-1 is found in follicular fluid (2) and influences in vitro granulosa cell differentiation and activity (3, 4, 5, 6). Conversely, the ovarian steroids affect monocyte production of IL-1 (7, 8).

The macrophage has been viewed as a moderator of acute inflammatory response and as a luteal phagocytic agent (9, 10) within the ovary. However, the role of ovarian macrophages has broadened as their influence on steroid production throughout the cycle became apparent (3, 4, 5, 11). In light of this increasing body of evidence, we have examined periovulatory human follicular fluid from IVF-ET cycles for the presence of macrophages and monocytes and their secretory product IL-1.

Materials and Methods

Isolation of Cells from Follicular Fluid

Cells were isolated from follicular aspirates obtained from 20 women undergoing transvaginal oocyte retrieval in the Yale University In Vitro Fertilization (IVF) and Embryo Transfer (ET) Program. Of the 20 women, 14 suffered from tubal disease or male factor infertility, 3 had unexplained infertility, and 3 had moderate or severe endometriosis. The women were treated with hMG (3 ampules/day, Pergonal, Serono Labs, Inc.) from day 3 through day 7 of their menstrual cycle followed by 1 to 4 ampules daily until

TABLE 1. Percent resident follicular monocytes/macrophages in follicular fluid isolated at the time of IVF-ET, as determined by flow cytometry.

Follicular Fluid Condition	% Staining with EBM-11 Antibody	% Staining with Leu-M5 Antibody
Clear, oocyte +	5	1
Bloody, pooled patients	17	5
Clear, pooled patients	12	2
Oocyte +	8	5
Oocyte +	2	2
Oocyte +	4	6
Pooled patients	25	28
Oocyte +	7	12
Bloody, oocyte −	12	51
Clear, oocyte −	42	60
Pooled patients	12	10
Oocyte +	25	19
Oocyte −	32	33
Oocyte +	21	18
Oocyte −	36	63
Oocyte +	19	16
Oocyte −	6	10

Note: Values have been corrected for circulating monocytes/macrophages from peripheral blood.

serum estradiol was ≥600 pg/mL and at least 3 follicles of ≥1.6-cm diameter were visible by ultrasound. hCG (10,000 IU) was then administered intramuscularly 32–34 hours prior to oocyte harvesting.

After each woman's IVF oocyte retrieval, the entire contents of 4–6 follicles were pooled as described in Table 1 to provide sufficient numbers of cells to examine. One mL of the pooled follicular fluid was subjected to a complete blood count (CBC). The remaining fluid was measured, layered over lymphocyte separation medium (LSM, Organon Technika), and centrifuged in a Beckman TJ-6 at 2500 rpm for 15 min to remove red blood cells, tissue debris, and dead cells. The cells at the interface (the "buffy coat") were removed and washed once with 12–14 mL RPMI (Gibco) and collected by centrifugation at 1200 rpm for 6 min. Cells were resuspended in 1–2 mL B-cell medium (1.75-g bovine serum albumin in 250-mL phosphate buffered saline containing 0.01% sodium azide) and counted in a hemacytometer.

All follicular fluids were subjected to CBC analysis, including red blood cell content, white cell content, and differential white cell counts. This was done to determine the relative number of macrophages and monocytes present due to contaminating peripheral blood in the following way. We made the standard assumption that one monocyte/macrophage is present per

10^4 red blood cells in peripheral blood. Monocytes/macrophages due to contaminating blood were then calculated from total RBC counts of the follicular fluids. Since monocytes/macrophages and tissue cells (granulosa/luteal cells) are indistinguishable by light microscopy, their combined percentage present in the differential count was multiplied by the total number of white cells found in the fluid to give the number of monocytes/macrophages plus granulosa/luteal cells present in the follicular fluid. After subtracting the number of contaminating peripheral monocytes, the remaining number of follicular fluid-derived granulosa/luteal cells and monocytes/macrophages were calculated. The percent monocytes/macrophages in this follicular-derived cell population was determined by flow cytometry (see below) after subtracting the number of contaminating peripheral monocytes.

Flow Cytometry

In this phase, 200,000 to 500,000 cells suspended in B-cell medium were placed in each of 3 tubes at a final volume of 20–100 µL. Addition of 5 µL of primary antibody, either EBM-11 DAKO-macrophage (CD68) (DAKOPATTS), diluted 1:5 in B-cell medium, or anti-human Leu-M5 (CD11c) (Becton-Dickinson), diluted 1:5 in B-cell medium, was made to each of 2 tubes, and nothing was added to the control tube. Cells were incubated for 15 min at room temperature (RT) in the dark, washed with 2 mL of B-cell medium, and then collected as above. Supernatants were decanted, and 5 µL of secondary antibody (goat anti-mouse fluoresceine isothiocyanate conjugated, Accurate Chemical Scientific Corp.) were added to all tubes. The tubes were again incubated for 15 min at RT in the dark, followed by washing with B-cell medium as described. After decanting the supernatant, 100 µL of 1% paraformaldehyde was added to each tube. The cells were stored at 4°C until analysis (no longer than 24 h) by flow cytometry (Epics Profile I, Coulter Cytometry).

We also tested the EMB-11 and Leu-M5 antibodies on white cell populations obtained from human peripheral blood. The buffy coat was treated as described for the follicular fluid and incubated with the EBM-11 and Leu-M5 antibodies. When subjected to flow cytometric analysis, the non-lymphocyte cell population (monocytes and macrophages) contained 90% positively staining cells, further validating the technique.

Immunoperoxidase Staining

Combined cells from 3 of the women undergoing IVF were examined by immunoperoxidase staining to visually compare the percentage of stained cells with the percentage determined by flow cytometry. After LSM separation and initial washing, cells were cytocentrifuged onto glass slides. The slides were stored desiccated at −20°C until used for immunoperoxidase staining. The cells were fixed onto the slide by incubation in acetone for 10 min at RT and then rehydrated in PBS for 10 min at RT. The following steps (until addition of diaminobenzidine) were carried out in a moist chamber at RT. Normal horse serum (from a Vectastain kit, Vector Laboratories) was applied onto the slides and incubated for 20 min. The serum was decanted from the slides and the primary antibodies added (DAKO-macrophage, diluted 1:20 in PBS, Leu-M5 undiluted) for 30 min, followed by a PBS rinse. The negative controls received only PBS during the primary antibody incubation. The secondary antibody (biotinylated goat anti-human, Vectastain kit) was added to each slide for 30 min followed by a PBS rinse. Then the ABC reagent (avidin-biotin-peroxidase complex from Vectastain, see above) was added for 30 min and washed with phosphate buffer (PB) (0.01 M, pH 7.4). A 0.01% diaminobenzidine (DAB) solution (in PB) was then added to the slides for 10 min followed by a water rinse.

Total Cellular RNA Preparation

Cells isolated from follicular fluid were pelleted after washing. As a control, peripheral monocytes were isolated from women in the luteal phase as described previously (7) and all cell pellets, containing between 1 to 5×10^6 cells, were lysed in 500 uL of 4M guanidinium thiocyanate (Ultra-pure, Bethesda Research Labs), pH 7.0, containing 25-mM sodium citrate, 0.5% sarkosyl, and 0.1 m β-mercaptoethanol. Total RNA was extracted by the method of Chomczynski and Sacchi (12). Total RNA was also isolated from A431 cells, a human epidermal carcinoma cell line known to produce IL-1β mRNA, and from Jurkat, a human T-cell line that does not produce IL-1β, and were used as positive and negative controls, respectively. Total RNA was denatured, electrophoresed, transferred to nylon membrane, and hybridized with a human IL-1β cDNA probe, as previously described (7).

Results

Total cellular RNA from follicular fluid cells, freshly isolated peripheral monocytes, A431 cells (positive control) and Jurkat cells (negative control) were co-electrophoresed, blotted, and probed with a ^{32}P-labeled IL-1β cDNA (7). The A431 IL-1β mRNA, which migrates slightly ahead of 18S rRNA, is shown in Figure 1. The follicular fluid cells yielded a distinct IL-1β band.

Experiments were undertaken to determine the numbers of resident macrophages and monocytes in the follicular fluid isolated from 20 women. The numbers of macrophages/monocytes in each sample were determined using 2 fluorescent-tagged antibodies (EBM-11 and Leu-M5) and analyzing the

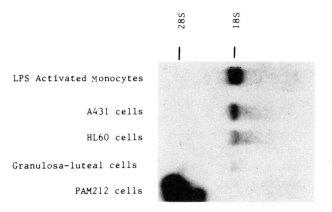

FIGURE 1. Northern blot of RNA of samples loaded at 10 µg per lane: A431 cells (positive control), freshly isolated human peripheral monocytes, Jurkat cells (negative control), and tissue cells from follicular fluids.

samples with a flow cytometer (Table 1). The number of macrophages and monocytes were corrected for contaminating peripheral blood monocytes in each sample (see Materials and Methods section). While the percentages varied from 2–50%, in most cases between 5–15% of the resident nucleated cells in follicular fluid are monocytes or macrophages. In all cases, there was good agreement in the amount of labeling with both antibodies for the same cell population, confirming the reliability of the measurements.

Follicular fluid cells were immunoperoxidase stained using the EMB-11 and Leu-M5 antibodies, respectively, and showed 10% positively staining cells. Similar experiments with both IL-1x and IL-1b antibodies demonstrated that a significant proportion of follicular fluid cells stain positively for the monokine secretory product.

Discussion

Total cellular RNA extracted from the follicular fluid cells isolated from women undergoing IVF/ET was found to contain a small but demonstrable amount of IL-1β mRNA. In the routine handling and counting of cells in follicular fluid, we noted the presence of macrophages, and one purpose of this study was to carefully document the numbers and origin of monocytes and macrophages found in the follicular fluids of women undergoing IVF. Overall, 5–15% of follicular fluid cells were found to be of the macrophage/monocyte lineage originating in the ovary.

An attempt was made to correlate the follicular fluid monocyte/macrophage levels with several parameters, including the presence or absence of an oocyte within the follicle, the degree of peripheral blood contamination, and the principal infertility diagnosis. There was no correlation between the numbers of monocytes/macrophages present (Table 1) and the presence or absence of an oocyte in the follicle nor with the degree of blood contamination of follicular fluid. Only 3 of the women in this study had moderate or severe endometriosis, and in each of these cases, the determinations were done on pooled follicular fluid samples, including fluid from women with tubal occlusion. We found that no pattern emerged to correlate high or low numbers of monocytes with cause of infertility.

Because we consistently found the resident monocyte/macrophage population in follicular fluid to be on the order of 5–15% after subtracting the monocytes and macrophages due to peripheral blood contamination, there appears to be a stable population of these cells within the microenvironment of the ovarian follicle during both follicular and luteal phases. In addition, follicular fluid cells appear to contain the macrophage secretory product IL-1 by immunohistochemical staining. This observation combined with the demonstration of IL-1β message in RNA extracts of total follicular fluid cells suggests active production of monokine. Recent evidence showing the effects of various cytokines on steroid-producing granulosa cells (5, 6) and the steroidal influence on monocyte IL-1 production (7) suggests a possible functional role for the presence of ovarian macrophages beyond that of simple phagocytosis in the corpus luteum. Future studies are needed to define more specifically the function of immune cells and their secretory products during the ovarian cycle.

Acknowledgment. The research reported in this chapter was supported by NIH grant HD-16962 (MLP).

References

1. Adashi EY. Cytokine-mediated regulation of ovarian function: Encounters of a third kind. Endocrinology 1989;124:2043-5.
2. Khan SA, Schmidt K, Hallin P, Pauli R, DeGeyter CH, Nieschlag E. Human testis cytosal and ovarian follicular fluid contain high amounts of interleukin-1-like factor(s). Mol Cell Endocrinol 1988;58:221-30.
3. Fukuoka M, Mori T, Taii S, Yasuda K. Interleukin-1 inhibits luteinization of porcine granulosa cells in culture. Endocrinology 1987;122:367-9.
4. Fukuoka M, Yasuda K, Taii S, Takakura K, Mori T. Interleukin-1 stimulates growth and inhibits progesterone secretion in the cultures of porcine granulosa cells. Endocrinology 1989;124:884-90.
5. Gottschall PE, Uehara A, Hoffman ST, Arimura A. Interleukin-1 inhibits follicle stimulating hormone-induced differentiation in rat granulosa cells in vitro. Biochem Biophys Res Commun 1987;149:502-9.

6. Gottschall PE, Katsura G, Hoffmann ST, Arimura A. Interleukin-1: An inhibitor of luteinizing hormone receptor formation in cultured rat granulosa cells. FASEB J 1988;2:2492-6.

7. Polan ML, Loukides JA, Nelson P, et al. Progesterone and estradiol modulate interleukin-1β messenger ribonucleic acid levels in cultured human peripheral monocytes. J Clin Endocrinol Metab 1989;89:1200-6.

8. Cannon JG, Dinarello CA. Increased plasma interleukin-1 activity in women after ovulation. Science 1985;227:1247-8.

9. Gillim SW, Christenson KA, McLennan CE. Fine structure of the human menstrual corpus luteum at its stage of maximum secretory activity. An J Anat 1969; 126:409-28.

10. Leavitt WW, Basom CR, Bagwell JN, Blaha GC. Structure and function of the hamster corpus luteum during the estrous cycle. Am J Anat 1973;136:235-50.

11. Kirsch TM, Friedman AC, Vogel RL, Flickinger GL. Macrophages in corpora lutea of mice: Characterization and effects on steroid secretion. Biol Reprod 1981;25:629-38.

12. Chomczynski P, Sacchi N. Single-step method of RNA isolation by guanidinium thiocyanate-phenol-chloroform extraction. Anal Biochem 1987;162:156-9.

14

Effects of Bacterial Endotoxin (Lipopolysaccharide) on FSH-Induced Granulosa Cell Activities

PAUL E. GOTTSCHALL AND AKIRA ARIMURA

High amounts of a T-lymphocyte activating factor(s) (interleukin-1-like activity) has been detected in human ovarian follicular fluid (1), and it was suggested that the origin of this activity may have been granulosa cells (GCs). We have been unable to detect IL-1-like activity in conditioned media from GCs obtained from diethylstilbestrol-treated immature rats and cultured under serum-free conditions either in the presence or absence of FSH (unpublished observations). However, our preliminary results have shown that bacterial endotoxin (lipopolysaccharide, LPS) exerted inhibitory effects on FSH-induced formation of LH receptors in rat GCs (2), suggesting the possibility that LPS may act either directly on GCs or may act indirectly by inducing the production of a secondary factor that influences GC function. These experiments were aimed at determining the specific effects of LPS on FSH-induced differentiation of GCs and whether LPS stimulates IL-1-like activity in rat GCs cultured in vitro.

Materials and Methods

Granulosa Cell Culture

CD rats (Charles River Breeding Laboratories, Wilmington, MA), 22 days old, were implanted with a diethylstilbestrol-containing Silastic capsule (10 mm in length) for 5 or 6 days. GCs were harvested by puncturing the follicles with 27-gauge hypodermic needles, and the cells were washed twice and cultured in McCoy's 5A media containing 25-mM HEPES buffer (pH 7.4), 2-mM glutamine (Gibco/Life Technologies, Grand Isle, NY), 0.1-U/mL bovine insulin (Gibco), 0.05% bovine serum albumin (BSA; RIA grade Sigma Chemical Co., St. Louis, MO), and 1% antibiotic/antimycotic solution (Gibco). Cells (3×10^5) were cultured in 1 mL of media in 12×75 polystyrene tubes containing 100-ng/mL FSH (National Pituitary and Hormone Program, oFSH-17) and different concentrations of LPS (055:B5, chromatographically purified, Sigma) and/or human recombinant IL-1β (a gift of Otsuka Pharmaceutical Co. Ltd., Japan; 2×10^7 units/mg protein). After culturing for 72 h, the media was collected for progesterone determination using a commercial radioimmunoassay kit (Diagnostic Products, Los Angeles, CA) and specific [^{125}I]human chorionic gonadotropin (hCG) binding was used to measure LH receptor number on the cells as previously described (3).

In other experiments designed to determine if GCs produce IL-1-like activity, 6×10^6 GCs were cultured in 3 mL of McCoy's 5A media (modified as above) in 60-mm polystyrene dishes, in the presence or absence of LPS (5 μg/mL) and FSH (30 ng/mL) and with or without 2% fetal calf serum (GiBCO). Cells were cultured for 4–48 h, the media was removed and centrifuged to remove any extraneous cellular debris, and the media was concentrated on Centricon-10 microconcentrators (Amicon, Danvers, MA; 10 kDa exclusion). The concentrated media was washed with 3-mL Dulbecco's PBS (GiBCO) and concentrated to a final volume of 300–400 μL. When the samples were assayed for their ability to stimulate thymocyte proliferation, the samples were expressed as μL-equivalent conditioned media without concentration.

Thymocyte Proliferation Assay

The protocol performed for the thymocyte proliferation assay (4) has been modified as previously described (5). Donors of thymocytes were mice of the endotoxin insensitive strain, C3H/HeJ (Jackson Laboratory, Bar Harbor, ME). The animals were sacrificed by excess CO_2 inhalation, and the lobes of the thymus were removed and placed in RPMI 1640 media containing 25-mM HEPES, 10% fetal calf serum, and 1% antibiotic/antimycotic solution (all from Gibco). The cells were dispersed by gently rubbing each tissue between two sterile ground glass slides. The cells were recovered by centrifugation at $200 \times g$ for 10 min, and the cells were washed and resuspended to a dilution of 1×10^7 cells per mL. One hundred microliters of cells, 50 μL of media containing 1-μg phytohaemagglutin (PHA), and 50 μL of sample were added to Titertube micro test tubes (BioRad, Richmond, CA). The tubes were incubated for 72 h in a water-saturated atmosphere of 5% CO_2 and 95% air at 37°C. Twenty h before the end of culture, the cells were pulsed with 0.75 μCi of [methyl-^{3}H]-thymidine (ICN, Cleveland, OH; 2.0 Curies/mM). At the end of culture, the cells were recovered by centrifugation, washed twice with 0.5-mL D-PBS containing 0.1% BSA, and the cell pellets were solubilized in 0.1-N NaOH containing 1% SDS. An aliquot was added to 5-mL Aquasol (Dupont-New England Nuclear, Wilmington, DE), and the vials were counted in a scintillation counter.

Data Analysis

Dose-response curves were evaluated using ALLFIT (6) to estimate an ED_{50} for each curve. Curves from the 4 treatment groups were analyzed by constraining the slopes of the curves to be equal since this did not significantly degrade the fit of the curves. The means of the ED_{50} and all other data were compared by one-way analysis of variance, and individual differences were detected using Tukey's honestly significant difference test. A rejection level of $P < 0.05$ was considered significant.

Results

GCs cultured in the presence of increasing doses of LPS together with FSH for 72 h showed a dose-dependent decline in LH receptor formation and progesterone production (Fig. 1). At the highest dose of LPS (1000 ng/mL), progesterone secretion was suppressed 21%, and LH receptor development was reduced to 28% of that observed in the absence of LPS. To determine if LPS might affect the dose-response curve of IL-1 inhibition of FSH-induced differentiation, GCs were incubated with FSH and LPS in the presence of increasing doses of IL-1 for 72 h. The results of a representative experiment are shown in Figure 2. At low, ineffective doses of IL-1, LPS reduced LH

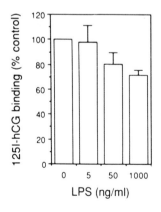
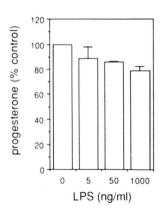

FIGURE 1. Inhibition of FSH (100 ng/mL)-induced LH receptor formation and progesterone production in rat GCs cultured for 72 h by inceasing doses of LPS.

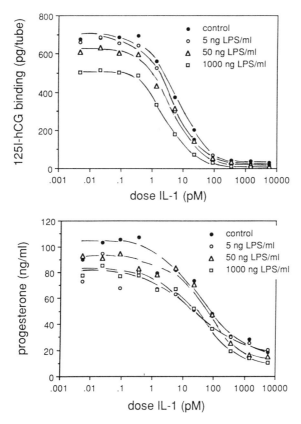

FIGURE 2. Effect of LPS on IL-1 inhibition of FSH (100 ng/mL)-induced LH receptor formation and progesterone production in rat GCs cultured for 72 h.

binding and progesterone secretion similar to that observed in the absence of IL-1. However, at any given effective concentration of IL-1, the reduction in LH receptor development and progesterone secretion was greater in the presence of LPS compared to the absence of LPS. This experiment was repeated twice (n = 3 for each dose), and a mean ED_{50} of the IL-1 dose-response curve calculated for each dose of LPS. In the absence of LPS the ED_{50} for IL-1 inhibition of LH-binding site formation was 5.1 ± 1.3 pM, whereas in the presence of 1000-ng/mL LPS, the ED_{50} was reduced to 1.8 ± 0.5 pM ($P < 0.05$). For the suppression of progesterone secretion, in the absence of LPS, the ED_{50} for IL-1 was 59.0 ± 1.6 pM, but in the presence of 1000-ng/mL LPS, the ED_{50} was 22.2 ± 9.0 pM ($P < 0.05$). There was no significant influence of LPS on the slope of the IL-1 dose-response curves. Therefore, in the presence of the maximal dose of LPS employed, IL-1 was

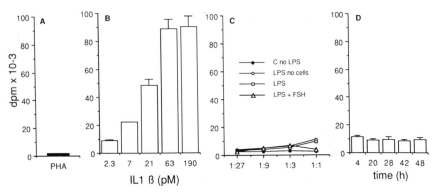

FIGURE 3. Assay of rat GC-condtioned media for IL-1-like bioactivity using [^{3}H]thymidine into thymocytes from C3H/HeJ mice. *A*: A submaximal dose of PHA alone (1 μg/mL, added to all samples) resulted in little incorporation of [^{3}H]thymidine. *B*: In combination with PHA, human recombinant IL-1β caused a dose-related increase in [^{3}H]thymidine incorporation. *C*: Assay of conditioned media from rat GCs, in which 3 mL of media containing 2×10^6 cells/mL were cultured with LPS (5 μg/mL) for 48 h. A control was included that was 3-mL media containing LPS but cultured without cells. The media was concentrated before the assay and the dilution 1:1 was equivalent to 200-μL media. *D*: GC-conditioned media were cultured for various times and assayed for IL-1-like activity. Samples were equivalent to 200-μL conditioned media.

2–3 times more potent in suppressing progesterone secretion and LH receptor development, compared to cells cultured in the absence of LPS.

In an effort to determine if the suppression of LH binding site formation and progesterone secretion by LPS was the result of LPS-stimulated IL-1 production by the GCs themselves, GCs were incubated with LPS and IL-1-like activity measured in the conditioned media using a specific bioassay (i.e., thymocyte proliferation assay). These experiments employed thymocytes from the endotoxin insensitive mouse strain since thymocytes from other strains proliferate in response to LPS. As shown in Figure 3, human recombinant IL-1β produced a dose-dependent stimulation of thymocyte proliferation when cultured in the presence of 1 μg/mL PHA (panel *B*). No IL-1-like activity was observed in conditioned media from unstimulated GCs (panel *C*). In media from GCs stimulated by LPS, there was a dose-dependent stimulation of [^{3}H]thymidine incorporation; however, this was not different from the stimulation observed when media containing identical amounts of LPS (and not cultured with cells) was assayed and used as a control. Media from GCs cultured with LPS and FSH for 48 h showed a reduced activity at the highest dilution, but also was not different from media containing LPS but not cultured with cells. In addition, there was no significant stimulation of [^{3}H]thymidine incorporation when assaying media from LPS and FSH stimulated GCs over a time course (panel *D*). To determine if prostaglandin remaining in the GC media sample might be responsible for inhibiting thymocyte proliferation, concentrated media from FSH-stimulated GCs, either with or without human recombinant IL-1, were assayed for IL-1-like activity. When human recombinant IL-1 was added to the FSH-stimulated sample, there was a significant stimulation of [^{3}H]thymidine incorporation that was not different from the same dose of human recombinant IL-1 assayed without the media sample (data not shown). This suggests that residual prostaglandin in the media sample was not sufficient to inhibit IL-1-stimulated thymocyte proliferation. Also, incubation of GCs in media containing 2% fetal calf serum did not stimulate IL-1-like activity either in the presence or absence of LPS and/or FSH (data not shown).

Discussion

Recently, increasing attention is being directed at studying the possible interactions of the immune and endocrine systems, in large part due to the discovery and isolation of immune regulatory factors, or cytokines, which are produced and elaborated from leukocytes. Cytokines are now known to affect the function of a plethora of cells and tissues, including ovarian function. It is reasonable to assume that cytokines might play a role in the regulation of the ovarian cycle since the appearance and disappearance of resident leukocytes are associated with discrete stages of the estrous cycle (7).

In particular, ovarian macrophages were shown to be absent in developing follicles and abundant in the interstitial tissue. They appear to spread the plane of the follicular surface and may contact with cells resembling steroid-secreting cells (7). Macrophages were also found to be present within atretic follicles (7). Additionally, at least in atretic sheep follicles, macrophage-like cells were observed in the membrana granulosa, and it was suggested that these cells were of GC origin (8).

One of the principal mediators of the acute-phase immune response is a cytokine elaborated from macrophages and monocytes, IL-1, originally detected for its ability to activate T-lymphocytes (9, 10). IL-1 has been shown to exert potent and specific effects on GC function (IL-2 and IL-3 show little or no effect). In GCs obtained from immature rats treated with diethylstilbestrol and cultured in vitro, IL-1 suppressed FSH-induced progesterone and estradiol secretion (11–13) and LH receptor formation (14). Also, IL-1 inhibited androgen production from whole ovarian dispersates (15). A suppression in steroidogenic capacity by IL-1 has also been observed in porcine GCs, and of significant interest is that GCs from small follicles appear to be more responsive to IL-1 than GCs from large antral follicles

(16). Furthermore, the effective concentration of IL-1 that influences GC function in vitro (<10 pM) was similar to the effective concentration of IL-1 that activates T-lymphocytes in vitro (5). Therefore, GCs appear to be a potential target cell for IL-1. However, the source of IL-1 in the ovary that might affect GC function remains in question despite the presence of macrophages in the interstitium.

Several existing sources might be the cellular site of IL-1 biosynthesis in the ovary. One possibility, since IL-1 influences GC function in vitro, is that GCs themselves produce IL-1 and, therefore, may affect GC function in an autocrine/paracrine manner. In support of this possibility, some evidence exists that another macrophage-derived cytokine, tumor necrosis factor (TNF), is present in GCs. GCs immunopositive for TNF were observed in the antral layer of small and large antral follicles and in GCs from atretic follicles (17). In addition, high amounts of IL-1-like bioactivity has been observed in human follicular fluid; although upon partial purification of this activity, several chemical characteristics of this material were different from IL-1α or β (1). We have been unable to detect IL-1-like activity in conditioned media from GCs obtained from immature, diethylstilbestrol-treated rats and cultured under a variety of conditions. Despite the observation that bacterial endotoxin (LPS) influences FSH-stimulated functions in a similar manner to that of IL-1, IL-1-like activity was not detected in the thymocyte proliferation assay, even in response to LPS. Several possiblities exist to explain this result. One, the amount of IL-1 produced by GCs may be below the detectable limit of the assay (1–2 pM). Secondly, cytokines may be produced in GCs in parallel with protease inhibitors that have the ability to bind and inactivate cytokines and growth factors (18). Thirdly, it is possible that the high cell density suppressed the production of IL-1 since several GC functions are dependent on plating density. Lastly, IL-1 may not be produced in GCs.

Finally, significant evidence suggests that granulosa cells are a potential target tissue for IL-1 action. However, further work is required to determine the relevant physiological role that IL-1 might play in follicular development.

References

1. Khan SA, Schmidt K, Hallin P, Di Pauli R, De Geyter C, Nieschlag E. Human testis cytosol and ovarian follicular fluid contain high amounts of interleukin-1-like factor(s). Mol Cell Endocrinol 1988;58:221-30.
2. Gottschall PE, Mori M. Monokines from lipopolysaccaride-stimulated macrophages affect ovarian granulosa cells in vitro. Endocrinology 1989;124 (suppl 1):241.
3. Gottschall PE, Katsuura G, Dahl RR, Hoffmann ST, Arimura A. Discordance in the effects of interleukin-1 on rat granulosa cell differentiation induced by

follicle-stimulating hormone or activators of adenylate cyclase. Biol Reprod 1988;39:1074-85.

4. Symons JA, Dickens EM, Di Giovine F, Duff GW. Measurement of interleukin-1 activity. In: Clemens MJ, Morris AG, Gearing AJH, eds. Lymphokines and interferons: A practical approach. Oxford: IRL Press, 1987:269-89.

5. Gottschall PE, Katsuura G, Arimura A. Interleukin-1 beta is more potent than interleukin-1 alpha in suppressing follicle-stimulating hormone-induced differentiation of ovarian granulosa cells. Biochem Biophys Res Commun 1989; 163:764-70.

6. De Lean A, Munson PJ, Rodbard D. Simultaneous analysis of families of sigmoidal curves: Application to dioassay, radioligand assay, and physiological dose-response curves. Am J Physiol 1978;235:E97-E102.

7. Hume DA, Halpin D, Charlton H, Gordon S. The mononuclear phagocyte system of the mouse defined by immunohistochemical localization of antigen F4/80: Macrophages of endocrine organs. Proc Natl Acad Sci USA 1984;81:4174-7.

8. Hay MF, Cran DG, Moor RM. Structural changes occurring during atresia in sheep ovarian follicles. Cell Tissue Res 1976;169:515-29.

9. Gery I, Gershon RK, Waksman BH. Potentiation of the T-lymphocyte response to mitogens, I. The responding cell. J Exp Med 1972;136:128-42.

10. Gery I, Waksman BH. Potentiation of the T-lymphocyte response to mitogens, II. The cellular source of potentiating mediator(s). J Exp Med 1972;136:143-55.

11. Gottschall PE, Uehara A, Hoffmann ST, Arimura A. Interleukin-1 inhibits follicle-stimulating hormone-induced differentiation in rat granulosa cells in vitro. Biochem Biophys Res Commun 1987;149:502-9.

12. Gottschall PE, Katsuura G, Arimura A. Interleukin-1 suppresses follicle-stimulating hormone-induced estradiol secretion from cultured rat ovarian granulosa cells. J Reprod Immunol 1989;15:281-90.

13. Kasson BG, Gorospe WC. Effects of interleukins 1, 2 and 3 on follicle-stimulating hormone-induced differentiation of rat granulosa cells. Mol Cell Endocrinol 1989;62:103-11.

14. Gottschall PE, Katsuura G, Hoffmann ST, Arimura A. Interleukin-1: An inhibitor of luteinizing hormone receptor formation in cultured granulosa cells. FASEB J 1988;2:2492-6.

15. Hurwitz A, Resnick CE, Hernandez ER, Adashi E. Cytokine-mediated regulation of ovarian function: Interleukin-1 inhibits gonadotropin-induced androgen biosynthesis. Endocrinology 1989;124(suppl 1):244.

16. Fukuoka M, Yasuda K, Taii S, Takakura K, Mori T. Interleukin-1 stimulates growth and inhibits progesterone secretion in cultures of porcine granulosa cells. Endocrinology 1989;124:884-90.

17. Roby KR, Terranova P. Localization of tumor necrosis factor (TNF) in the rat and bovine ovary using immunocytochemistry and cell blot: Evidence for granulosal production. In: Hirshfield AN, ed. Growth factors and the ovary. New York: Plenum Press, 1989:273-8.

18. Gaddy-Kurten D, Hickey GJ, Fey GH, Gauldie J, Richards JS. Hormonal regulation and tissue-specific localization of alpha$_2$-macroglobulin in rat ovarian follicles and corpora lutea. Endocrinology 1989;125:2985-95.

15

TNF α: Altering Thecal and Granulosal Cell Steroidogenesis

P.F. TERRANOVA, K.F. ROBY, M. SANCHO-TELLO,
J. WEED, AND R. LYLES

Tumor necrosis factor α (TNF α) is a 17-kDa protein produced by macrophages in response to lipopolysaccharide (LPS) (1). Recent studies indicate that the ovary contains and produces TNF α (2–6). TNF α has been localized immunohistochemically in the ovary of the rat, cow (3), and human (4), and it has been detected in the human ovary by a bioassay specific for TNF α (5). Granulosa cells are a source of ovarian TNF α based on the presence of immunoreactive TNF α in cultured cells (3, 4) and media (4, 5) and in frozen ovarian sections (3, 4). TNF α also has been shown to alter ovarian steroidogenesis (7–11). Using granulosa cells from the DES-treated immature rat (8, 9, 11, 12) and the adult rat (10), several labs have shown that TNF α inhibits FSH-stimulated progesterone production. In addition, our laboratory has found that TNF α stimulates thecal progestin production in adult rat preovulatory follicles (10). The purpose of this chapter is to review the current literature on TNF α in the ovary and attempt to construct a hypothesis as to the role(s) of TNF α in ovarian function.

Evidence for TNF α in the Ovary

Cow. TNF α has been observed in the corpus luteum (CL) and in antral and atretic follicles of the cow (3). TNF α was observed in the thecal cords that radiate into the central core of the CL from the surrounding thecal capsule. A few TNF α-positive cells were also distributed throughout the remainder of the CL, but were in relatively low numbers compared to the positive cells in the thecal cords. The granulosal cells of antral follicles contained TNF α, which was observed predominantly in the layers of granulosal cells lining the antral cavity. The TNF α also appeared to be in the follicular fluid surrounding the granulosal cells. TNF α has also been found in follicular fluid of the mid-cycle cow (days 8–12) (5). TNF α activity was observed in preovulatory follicles and freshly ovulated follicles, and the TNF α activity was found to be significantly higher than that in the mid-cycle follicles (5).

Rat. In the rat, TNF α has been localized in the CL, throughout the granulosal layer in atretic follicles and in the antral layers of granulosal cells (3). TNF α was observed in fibroblastic-like cells of the central core of the CL. It appeared that the most intense staining for TNF α occurred in the granulosal layer of atretic follicles and in the granulosal cells lining the antral cavity. TNF α appeared to be present in the follicular fluid surrounding the granulosal cells.

Human. TNF α has also been localized in the follicular and luteal compartments of the human ovary (4, 5). Like the rat and cow, healthy antral follicles contained TNF α in the antral layer of granulosa cells, and it also appeared to be secreted by these cells since it was located in the fluid surrounding these cells (4). TNF α was also localized to large lutein-like cells and in theca-derived paraluteal cells of the CL. A recent study using human granulosa cells from an IVF program revealed that TNF α was released from the cells into culture media and that this could be stimulated in vitro by FSH (5). TNF α was detected in the culture media using an L929 mouse fibrosarcoma cell assay. hCG, $PGF_{2\alpha}$, colony stimulating factor, or 8-br-cAMP did not stimulate TNF α production by the granulosa cells. Since the granulosal cell aspirate from the IVF patients contained a small amount of contaminating polymorphonuclear cells (probably monocytes), the effects of FSH on TNF α production was tested directly on monocytes. No effect of FSH was observed on the monocytes. However, is it possible that the FSH could have stimulated the granulosa to produce a factor that induced the monocytes to release TNF α? Additional studies are needed to elucidate conclusively the granulosal cell as the site of TNF α production.

Rabbit. Recent studies using the rabbit have shown that conditioned media from days 5, 17, and 19 luteal tissue contained low or undetectable levels of TNF α (2, 6). Interestingly, lipopolysaccharide (endotoxin) increased TNF α activity in the media from CL on days 17 and 19. Using a cellular bioassay, TNF α activity was not detected in unstimulated and lipopolysaccharide stimulated uterus and nonluteal ovarian tissue in vitro. It was also found that the TNF α activity in the culture medium could be neutralized by an antibody to rabbit TNF α, indicating some specificity to the action of TNF α.

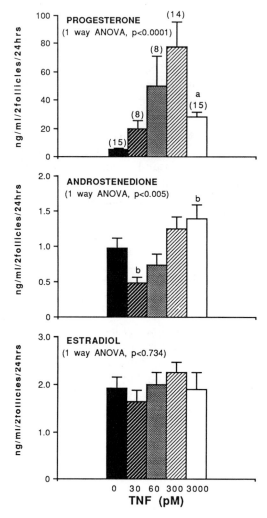

FIGURE 1. Effects of 30 to 3000-pM TNF α on rat follicular progesterone, androstenedione, and estradiol production in vitro. Two preovulatory follicles were incubated in 1-mL M-199 with TNF α for 24 h. (Numbers above bars are the number of replications of each experiment; letters indicate the level of significance as follows: a, P < 0.05 vs. 0 TNF α, P < 0.001 vs. 300-pM TNF α; b, P < 0.05 vs. 0 TNF α.) (Reprinted from Roby KF and Terranova PF, Tumor necrosis factor alpha alters follicular steroidogenesis in vitro, Endocrinology 1988;123:2952–4.)

Effects of TNF α on Ovarian Cells

Adult Cyclic Rats

The first report of the effects of TNF α on ovarian function was from our laboratory in 1988 (7). We observed that TNF α increased progesterone production by proestrous rat follicles. Dose-related increases in progesterone were revealed with TNF α in the physiologic range (30–300 pM) (Fig. 1). The highest dose of TNF α (3000 pM) reduced progesterone production significantly compared to 300-pM TNF α, but progesterone production still remained significantly higher than controls. Androstenedione production by the proestrous follicles was reduced slightly by the lowest dose of TNF α and stimulated by the highest dose in vitro. Estradiol production by the ovarian follicles was unaffected by TNF α during the 24-h incubation, but compared to another study, basal estradiol production was quite low (10). We later reported that these follicles were atretic in vitro due to the low concentration of oxygen (5% CO_2 and air, which is 20% oxygen) in the culture media (10). Nevertheless, a time-course using 300-pM TNF α revealed that progesterone remained low during the first 12 h of incubation and then increased significantly by hour 24 (Fig. 2). Neither androstenedione nor estradiol production by the follicles was altered during the time-course. Interestingly, 160-pM LH increased progesterone and androstenedione at hour 6 of incubation, and it remained elevated throughout hour 24; estradiol was unaffected by LH under these culture conditions (Fig. 1). Thus, it appeared that the time-course effects of TNF α on progesterone were quite different than LH.

In the same study, we showed that TNF α (30 pM), pre-absorbed with 1000-fold excess monoclonal antibody to TNF α, did not increase progesterone production by the follicles in vitro (Fig. 3). Thus, there appeared to be a degree of specificity of the TNF α in stimulating progesterone.

In a later study from our laboratory, we revealed that the culture conditions could drastically affect the responses of the preovulatory follicle to TNF α in vitro (10). This led us to discover that theca was a major target of TNF α in increasing progesterone, that the follicles in low oxygen (5% CO_2 and air) were becoming atretic, and that TNF α could stimulate the estradiol production if the follicle was healthy. The effects of high (95% O_2 and 5% CO_2) and low (5% CO_2 and air) oxygen on the cultured follicles was of interest in order to account for the low estradiol production observed in our previous study (7). Follicles cultured in low oxygen exhibited extensive atresia, whereas after 24 h of culture in high oxygen, the follicles were healthy. TNF α did not appear to alter the histology of the follicle within 24 h of culture.

To determine the site in the follicle at which TNF α was acting to increase production of progesterone, we separated the follicle into thecal and granulosal compartments (15). TNF α increased progesterone production by the theca similar to its effect on the whole preovulatory follicle (Fig. 4).

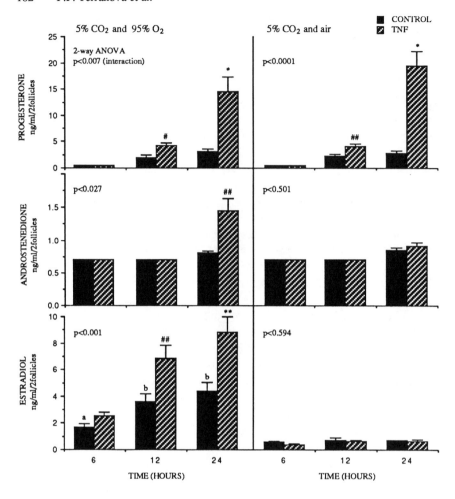

FIGURE 2. The effect of TNF α on follicular progesterone, androstenedione, and estradiol production at 6, 12, and 24 h of culture under the conditions of 5% CO_2 and 95% O_2, or 5% CO_2 and air. Steroids are expressed as ng/mL/2 follicles. The P values of the interactions between time and treatment were determined by 2-way ANOVA. Specific comparisons were performed using Student's t-test. (## P < 0.025; # P < 0.01; ** P < 0.005; * P < 0.001, TNF α vs. control. a, P < 0.025; b, P < 0.005, 5% CO_2 and 95% O_2 vs. 5% CO_2 and air for estradiol controls. (Reprinted from Roby KF and Terranova PF, Effects of tumor necrosis factor alpha in vitro on steroidogenesis of healthy and atretic follicles of the rat: Theca as a target, Endocrinology 1990;126:2711–8.)

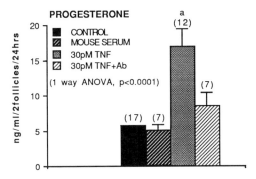

FIGURE 3. Effects of immunoneutralization of TNF α with monoclonal antibody to TNF α on in vitro progesterone production by rat preovulatory follicles. (a, 0 < 0.001 vs. mouse serum.) (Reprinted from Roby KF and Terranova PF, Tumor necrosis factor alpha alters follicular steroidogenesis in vitro, Endocrinology 1988;123: 2952–4.)

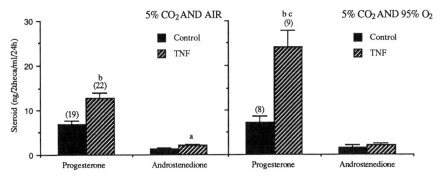

FIGURE 4. The effects of culture condition on thecal steroid production. Theca (2/well) were cultured for 24 h under the condition of 5% CO_2 and air or 5% CO_2 and 95% O_2. Steroid production is expressed as ng/2 theca/24 h/mL. (a, P < 0.05; b, P < 0.001. Students t-test, TNF α-treated vs. control. c, P < 0.001 TNF α-treated, 5% CO_2 and air vs. 5% CO_2 and 95% O_2.)

Interestingly, TNF α had a slight but inhibitory effect on basal granulosal cell production of progesterone, and this was further accentuated when it was observed that TNF α could inhibit FSH stimulated progesterone in vitro (Table 1). Thus, TNF α could stimulate thecal progesterone and inhibit granulosal progesterone, actions which are opposing within the follicle.

Immature Rats

Using granulosal cells from the immature DES-treated rat, Emoto and Baird showed that TNF α inhibited in a concentration dependent fashion, FSH-

TABLE 1. Effect of TNF α and FSH on granulosal progesterone production (100,000 viable granulosa cells [~2 follicle equivalents] from preovulatory rat follicles, cultured for 24 h).

Culture Condition	Progesterone (ng/mL)
Control (media alone)	0.94 ± 0.04 (8)
TNF α (5 ng)	0.78 ± 0.02 (11)[a]
FSH (250 ng)	86.8 ± 3.59 (6)
FSH and TNF α	73.2 ± 4.60 (6)[b]

Source: Roby KF and Terranova PF, Effects of tumor necrosis factor alpha in vitro on steroidogenesis of healthy and atretic follicles of the rat: Theca as a target, Endocrinology 1990;126:2711–8.

[a] $P < 0.001$, control vs. TNF α.

[b] $P < 0.05$, FSH vs. FSH and TNF α.

stimulated aromatase activity (8). A time-course study revealed that TNF α did not reduce aromatase activity per se, but prevented its induction by FSH. Thus, TNF α could inhibit the induction of additional aromatase activity induced by not only FSH but also by TGF β. TNF α also decreased progesterone synthesis that was stimulated by both FSH and TGF β.

Studies by Adashi et al. (9, 12) also revealed that TNF α could inhibit FSH-induced aromatase in cultured granulosal cells of the DES-treated rat. A minimal time requirement of 48-h exposure to TNF α was needed to inhibit the FSH-induced aromatase. Interestingly, cAMP-generating compounds, such as PGE_2, choleragen, and VIP, also stimulated aromatase, and their actions on aromatase were reduced by TNF α. TNF α did not inhibit FSH binding to the granulosa, but was capable of blocking forskolin-induced accumulation of cAMP and reduced adenylate cyclase activity. TNF α was quite potent in inhibiting the ability of FSH to increase extracellular cAMP. TNF α inhibited the production of progesterone and 20α-dihydroprogesterone, while it stimulated an increase in S^{35} incorporation into extracellular proteoglycans, but inhibited FSH increased proteoglycan biosynthesis. The findings of Adashi et al. and Emoto and Baird have recently been confirmed and extended (11). A study by Darbon et al. (11) found that TNF α inhibited in a dose-dependent manner LH receptor formation induced by FSH, cholera toxin, forskolin or 8-br-cAMP; for FSH, this action was observed as early as 24 h after TNF α exposure and was due to a decrease in the number of LH receptors, not a decrease in their affinity. As shown by Adashi et al., TNF α inhibited the cAMP production induced by FSH (9), and it also inhibited FSH-induced progesterone biosynthesis (8, 9).

Human

Recently, we reported that TNF α could increase progesterone and hCG binding in granulosal cells of the human (13). It was reported that hCG stimulated progesterone production by granulosa/luteal cells in a time- and dose-dependent manner. Progesterone production in the absence of hCG increased on days 2 and 4 of culture, then declined to a basal level throughout the remainder of the 10-day culture. Addition of hCG (0.05–1.0 IU/mL) increased progesterone production for the first 4 days, and it plateaued throughout the remaining 10 days. The plateau phase was not maintained with the lowest dose (0.01 IU) of hCG tested, but it was above control levels. Progesterone was maximally stimulated with doses of 0.05- to 1.0-IU hCG during days 6–10 of culture. TNF α alone significantly increased progesterone production above nonstimulated controls by day 10 of culture. Using a maximally stimulating dose of hCG, progesterone increased above controls on days 2–10. With a maximal dose of hCG, progesterone production increased steadily until day 4 of culture, and thereafter it remained unchanged. TNF α and a maximally stimulating dose of hCG closely followed the pattern of progesterone production stimulated by hCG alone for the first 2–4 days. However, progesterone continued to increase for the remainder of the 10-day culture period under the influence of TNF α and hCG. We have repeated this in 5 patients, and the results are consistent. These data are presented by Clinton et al. in this volume (see Chapter 58).

In order to gain insight into the synergism between TNF α and hCG, we assessed hCG binding in the granulosal cells on day 10, a time when progesterone was elevated in the presence of TNF α and hCG. On day 10 of culture, the specific binding of hCG to granulosa cells was significantly higher in cells treated with TNF α alone and hCG alone than in controls. hCG binding in the group treated with TNF α alone was greater than the hCG group. hCG binding in the TNF α group was not statistically different from the combination of TNF α and hCG. However, hCG binding in the hCG plus TNF α group was greater than that stimulated by hCG alone.

In the human granulosa/luteal cell, TNF α has been shown a 3- to 4-fold increase in $PGF_{2\alpha}$ (5). However, in the presence of FSH the effect of TNF α was not apparent. Similar to the results described for the human, TNF α also slightly increased basal progesterone production by the human granulosa/luteal cells in vitro. Interestingly, the level of progesterone production induced by TNF α and $PGF_{2\alpha}$, each alone, were similar, indicating that TNF α may stimulate $PGF_{2\alpha}$, which increases progesterone secretion. The stimulation of both $PGF_{2\alpha}$ and progesterone production by TNF α appeared to be biphasic as higher doses of TNF α reduced in vitro levels of the hormone secretion.

Role of TNF α in Ovarian Function

Based on the current observations given in this review, we have developed several hypotheses as to a role of TNF α in ovarian function. The hypotheses can be divided into two significant areas of ovarian function: luteal and follicular. We will discuss each of these separately since each is an entity on its own and appears to be independent of the other.

Luteal Function

It is evident from several sources in the literature that macrophages are present in the corpus luteum (2, 6, 14–17). The question arises as to what are they doing in the corpus luteum. In our opinion, they are participating in the normal functioning of the corpus luteum as luteotropically active cells and/or participating in the destruction of the corpus luteum (luteal regression). Let's take the luteotropic role first. Original studies of Kirsch et al. (15, 16) proposed a luteotropic role since progesterone secretion increased when macrophages were in contact with luteal cells of the mouse in vitro. Most recently, TNF α, a principal product of activated macrophages, has been shown to increase progesterone secretion (5, 7, 13) and hCG binding in human granulosal luteal cells in vitro (13). Thus, it appears plausible that resident ovarian macrophages may play a role in stimulating luteal progesterone secretion. However, it has been proposed that granulosal cells are a source of ovarian TNF α; this is evidenced by immunohistochemical staining of TNF α in the ovary of 3 species: cow, rat, and human (3, 4). Thus, the question arises as to whether the granulosa cell is a macrophage. This question could be partly answered using immunocytochemistry of corpora lutea (granulosa) with some of the highly specific monoclonal antisera to macrophages during the various stages of the cycle and pregnancy.

In regard to luteal regression, one study indicates that corpora lutea are invaded by macrophages (6). Knowing that macrophages are phagocytic and can contact and ingest follicular cells (15, 18–22), it seems feasible that the cells may initiate luteal regression and/or destroy the luteal cells after they have functionally regressed (stop secreting progesterone). TNF α has been shown to attenuate hCG-stimulated progesterone in luteinized granulosa cells of the rat (12), indicating that it might modulate the responsiveness of the corpus luteum to gonadotropins. Thus, the signal that turns on the luteal regression still remains elusive although another factor, TNF α, has entered the system. It seems to us that factors regulating the responsiveness of the luteal cells to TNF α might be important in determining the mechanism of corpus luteum regression. If the luteal cells cannot respond to TNF α, then it seems that luteal function would be altered. We would like to hypothesize for a moment. Let's assume that TNF α is luteolytic. A study presented by

Sancho-Tello et al. (see Chapter 59) has shown that TNF α action could be reduced by stimulators of the protein kinase C (PKC) pathway and that TNF α itself might work through the PKC pathway in stimulating follicular (thecal) progesterone secretion. It is well known that LH can stimulate luteal secretion of progesterone through both the protein kinase A and C pathways (23–25). If both of these pathways are highly stimulated (by LH and other luteotropins), it is feasible that TNF α would not be able to exert its actions because the PKC would be saturated. In addition, a prior study has shown that stimulation of the PKC pathway leads to a downregulation of TNF α receptors (26). Thus, regulation of TNF α action might occur at the receptor level as well as at the level of the PKC path. As soon as LH loses its stimulation of the PKC path, maximal stimulation would not be accomplished, TNF α receptors would appear, and TNF α would then exert its inhibitory action on the corpus luteum. In our lab, future studies are directed at further understanding the mechanism of action of TNF α and also ascertaining the factors regulating TNF α receptors in the ovary.

In regard to follicular atresia, we have observed immunoreactive TNF α in all antral follicles of the human (4), rat, and cow (3). In addition, it appears that atretic follicles contained more immunoreactive TNF α than healthy follicles (3) although strict quantitative measurements have not been performed. A study by Hirshfield has shown that atresia is rare in follicles without antra (27), and atresia is common in follicles with antra. Thus, some correlation exists between the appearance of TNF α and the increased incidence of atresia. The question arises as to how might TNF α induce atresia of follicles. Studies by Adashi et al. (9, 12), Emoto and Baird (8), Darbon et al. (11), and Roby and Terranova (7, 10) may give some insight into how this occurs. First of all, it must be recognized that all antral follicles exhibit immunoreactive TNF α, but all follicles don't become atretic. Therefore, we return to our luteal hypothesis that states as long as the PKC path is stimulated, TNF α cannot exhibit significant action on follicular steroidogenesis; this is because TNF α receptors are downregulated, and the PKC path is maximally utilized. As soon as FSH/LH no longer maximally stimulate PKC, TNF α receptors appear on the follicle. Since TNF α can inhibit FSH-stimulated aromatase activity of the granulosa, follicular function would be compromised, and atresia would occur. Interestingly, Emoto and Baird elegantly showed that TNF α did not inhibit aromatase per se, but inhibited further induction of aromatase by FSH. In light of atresia, this might be interpreted that TNF α could participate in atresia at various stages of follicular development. One characteristic of atretic follicles is that thecal progesterone secretion increases as well as thecal hypertrophy. The mechanisms by which this occurs are unknown. Interestingly, we have reported that TNF α stimulates thecal progesterone in vitro. Thus, TNF α produced by the granulosal cell may stimulate thecal progesterone secretion, a characteristic of atretic follicles. In our early studies, we observed that low doses of TNF α could stimulate progesterone secretion and inhibit androstenedione synthesis; it is evident this would lead to follicular atresia. Proof that TNF α is causal in atresia is lacking. Our studies are to be directed at whether in vivo correlations exist among follicular atresia, the onset of responsivity to TNF α, and the hormonal regulation of TNF α production by the follicle.

References

1. Carswell EA, Old LJ, Kassel RL, Green S, Fiore N, Williamson B. An endotoxin-induced serum factor that causes necrosis of tumors. PNAS 1975;3666-70.
2. Bagavandoss P, Kunkel SL, Wiggins RC, Keyes PL. Tumor necrosis factor α (TNF α) production and localization of macrophages and T lymphocytes in the rabbit corpus luteum. Endocrinology 1988;122:1185-7.
3. Roby KF, Terranova PF. Localization of tumor necrosis factor (TNF) in rat and bovine ovary using immunocytochemistry and cell blot: Evidence for granulosal production. In: Hirshfield, AN. Growth factors and the ovary. New York: Serono Symposia, USA/Plenum Press, 1989;273-8.
4. Roby KF, Terranova PF. Localization of immunoreactive tumor necrosis factor (I-TNF) in the human ovary. Biol Reprod 1989;40(suppl 1):171.
5. Zolti M, Meirom R, Shemesh M, et al. Granulosa cells as a source and target organ for tumor necrosis factor-α. FEBS Lett 1990;261:253-5.
6. Bagavandoss P, Wiggins RC, Kunkel SL, Remick DG, Keyes PL. Tumor necrosis factor production and accumulation of inflammatory cells in the corpus luteum of pseudopregnancy and pregnancy in rabbits. Biol Reprod 1990;42:367-76.
7. Roby KF, Terranova PF. Tumor necrosis alpha alters follicular steroidogenesis in vitro. Endocrinology 1988;123:2952-4.
8. Emoto N, Baird A. The effect of tumor necrosis factor/cachectin on follicle-stimulating hormone-induced aromatase activity in cultured rat granulosa cells. Biochem Biophys Res Commun 1988;153:792-8.
9. Adashi EY, Resnick CE, Croft CS, Payne DW. Tumor necrosis factor α inhibits gonadotropin hormonal action in nontransformed ovarian granulosa cells. J Biol Chem 1989;264:11591-7.
10. Roby KF, Terranova PF. Effects of tumor necrosis factor-α in vitro on steroidogenesis of healthy and atretic follicles of the rat: Theca as a target. Endocrinology 1990;126:2711-8.
11. Darbon JM, Oury F, Laredo J, Bayard F. Tumor necrosis factor-α inhibits follicle-stimulating hormone-induced differentiation in cultured rat granulosa cells. Biochem Biophys Res Commun 1989;163:1038-46.
12. Adashi EY, Resnick CE, Packman JN, Hurwitz A, Payne DW. Cytokine-mediated regulation of ovarian function: Tumor necrosis factor alpha inhibits gonadotropin-supported progesterone accumulation by differentiating and luteinized murine granulosa cells. Am J Obstet Gynecol 1990;162:889-96.
13. Roby KF, Lyles R, Terranova PF. Tumor necrosis factor-alpha increases progesterone secretion and chorionic gonadotropin binding in human granulosa-lutein cells. 72nd Annual Meeting of the Endocrine Society. Atlanta, 1990.

14. Bulmer D. The histochemistry of ovarian macrophages in the rat. J Anat 1964;98:313-9.
15. Kirsch TM, Friedman AC, Vogel RL, Flickinger GL. Macrophages in corpora lutea of mice: Characterization and effects on steroid secretion. Biol Reprod 1981;25:629-32.
16. Kirsch TM, Vogel RL, Flickinger GL. Macrophages: A source of luteotropic cybernins. Endocrinology 1983;113:1910-2.
17. Halme J, Hammond MG, Syrop CH, Talbert LM. Peritoneal macrophages modulate human granulosa-luteal cell progesterone production. J Clin Endocrinol 1985;61:912-6.
18. Byskov AG. Atresia. In: Midgley AR, Sadler WA, eds. Ovarian follicular development and function. New York: Raven Press, 1979.
19. Hay MF, Cran DG, Moor RM. Structural changes occuring during atresia in sheep ovarian follicles. Cell Tissue Res 1976;169:515-29.
20. Hay MF, Moor RM, Cran DG, Dott HM. Regeneration of atretic sheep ovarian follicles in vitro. J Reprod Fertil 1979;55:195-207.
21. Peluso JJ, England-Charlesworth C, Bolender DL, Steger RW. Ultrastructural alterations with the initiation of follicular atresia. Cell Tissue Res 1980;211: 105-15.
22. Saidapur SK. Follicular atresia in the ovaries of nonmammalian vertebrates. Int Rev Cytol 1978;54:225-44.
23. Marsh JM. The role of cyclic AMP in gonadal steroidogenesis. Biol Reprod 1976;14:30-53.
24. Davis JS, Weakland LL, Farese RV, West LA. Luteinizing hormone increases inositol triphosphate and cytosolic free Ca^{2+} in isolated bovine luteal cells. J Biol Chem 1987;262:8515-21.
25. Shinohara O, Knecht M, Feng P, Catt KJ. Activation of protein kinase C potentiates cyclic AMP production and stimulates steroidogenesis in differentiated ovarian granulosa cells. J Steroid Biochem 1986;24:161-8.
26. Johnson SE, Baglioni C. Tumor necrosis factor receptors and cytocidal activity are down-regulated by activators of protein kinase C. J Biol Chem 1988;263:5686-92.
27. Hirshfield AN. Size-frequency analysis of atresia in cycling rats. Biol Reprod 1988;38:1181-8.

16

TNF α Modulation of Ovarian Steroidogenesis in the Rat

DONNA W. PAYNE, ARYE HURWITZ, JEFFREY N. PACKMAN,
CRISTIANA L. ANDREANI, CAROL E. RESNICK,
AND ELI Y. ADASHI

It has been suggested (1, 2, 3) that resident ovarian macrophages act as in situ regulators of ovarian function since they send out processes to adjacent luteal cells, engage in heterophagy of damaged luteal cells and constitute a major cellular component of the interstitial compartment (1, 4, 5). It is likely that macrophages influence ovarian function via release of regulatory protein(s) called "cytokines" (6). One such macrophage product, tumor necrosis factor α (TNF α) is a 157 amino acid polypeptide originally named for its oncolytic activity in the serum of β-chorionic gonadotropin immunized, endotoxin challenged mice (7). However, it has become clear that TNF α may have pleiotropic regulatory activities as well. In the ovary, these include attenuation of gonadotropin-dependent granulosa cell differentiation (2, 8, 9) and promotion of complex steroidogenic alterations in explanted preovulatory follicles (10, 11).

In this report, we characterize the ability of TNF α to modulate gonadotropin-supported steroidogenesis in serum-free primary cultures of granulosa cells from the immature rat.

Materials and Methods

Materials and animals (intact Sprague-Dawley female rats, 26–28 days old) were as described previously (3). Granulosa cells, obtained by follicular puncture, were cultured (1–5×10^5 viable cells/culture) in tissue culture dishes or polystyrene tubes as described previously (3) for 72 or 96 h using 1 mL McCoy's 5a medium (modified, without serum).

High-Pressure Liquid Chromatography (HPLC), as described previously

(3), consisted of ethyl acetate-extracted media steroids separated on a diol column (Lichrosorb Diol, EM Reagents, Gibbstown, NJ), which had been standardized with 27 steroids. Radiolabeled steroids were detected inline by scintillation counting (Flo-One/Beta Detector, Radiomatic Instruments, Tampa, FL). Δ^4-3-oxosteroids were detected at 240 nm. Identity of steroid peaks were confirmed by three criteria (3).

Progesterone Radioimmunoassay (RIA) was determined as described previously (3).

Enzyme-Based Steroid Assays. 3α- and 20α-hydroxysteroids were determined using nonradioimmune, enzyme-based assays as described previously (3). Briefly, the increase in fluorescence of reduced nicotinamide adenine dinucleotide after oxidation with bacterial hydroxysteroid dehydrogenases (12, 13) was measured in fractions after HPLC separation. 20α-dihydroprogesterone (20α-DHP) was detected as a 20α-hydroxysteroid and by UV at 240 nm. 5α-pregnane-3α, 20α-diol (5α-Pdiol) was detected as both a 3α- and 20α-hydroxysteroid. 5α-pregnane-3α-ol-20-one (pregnanolone) was detected as a 3α-hydroxysteroid.

Cell-Free Enzyme Assays. Media were removed from tubes containing attached granulosa cells in culture and replaced with 0.5 mL of the appropriate enzyme buffer (3). Cells were then sonicated and the sonicates assayed for cholesterol side-chain cleavage activity, 3β-HSD/isomerase or 20α-HSD using radiolabeled steroid substrates as described previously (3). 3α-HSD activity was measured at 37°C in sonicates by the conversion of 250,000 cpm [^{3}H]androsterone (10 μM) to labeled androstanedione in a 100-mM HEPES buffer (pH 8) containing 1-mM EDTA, 1-mM DTT, 0.25-M sucrose, and 0.5-mM NAD. Androstanedione was the only product detected. In all the assays, the reaction was stopped by addition of 100-μL 1N-NaOH. The steroids were extracted, and separated by HPLC. Enzymatic activity was expressed as the rate of conversion of substrate to product per 1×10^5 granulosa cells.

Results

Effect of TNF α on Steroid Production in Cultured Granulosa Cells

In cultured granulosa cells, TNF α inhibits the production of FSH-stimulated, radioimmunoassayable progesterone (Fig. 1). Granulosa cells were cultured for 72 h in the absence or presence of FSH (100 ng/mL) with or without 10 ng/mL TNF α. As expected, treatment with FSH substantially increased progesterone accumulation. Progesterone production was significantly inhibited (84% ± 5%) with the addition of TNF α.

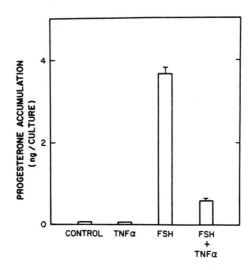

FIGURE 1. Effect of TNF α on basal and FSH-supported progesterone accumulation. Granulosa cells (1×10^5/culture) were cultured for 72 h under serum-free conditions in the absence or presence of FSH (100 ng/mL), with or without TNF α (10 ng/mL). Media progesterone content was determined by RIA (mean ± SE of triplicate determinations). (From Adashi EY, Resnick CE, Packman JN, Hurwitz A, Payne DW, Cytokine-mediated regulation of ovarian function: Tumor necrosis factor α inhibits gonadotropin-supported progesterone accumulation by differentiating and luteinized murine granulosa cells, Am J Obstet Gynecol 1990;162:889–99.)

Similar results were obtained using cultured luteinized granulosa cells (3), i.e., cells that were initially cultured with FSH (30 ng/mL) followed by hCG (10 ng/ML) ± TNF α (10 ng/mL). Under these conditions TNF α inhibited (~60%) the hCG-stimulated progesterone production.

The inhibitory effect of TNF α was reversible. When TNF α was washed from culture, there was a progressive resumption of FSH responsiveness, approximating that of cells never exposed to TNF α by 3 days after its removal (3). The TNF α effect was also dose- and time-dependent (Fig. 2), with a median inhibitory dose of 1.1 ± 0.3 ng/mL and a minimal time requirement of ≥24 h.

Using enzyme-based (nonradiometric) assays, we studied the effect of TNF α on the downstream metabolites of progesterone. In cultured immature granulosa cells, progesterone is metabolized sequentially to 20α-dihydroprogesterone (20α-DHP), 5α-pregnane-3α, 20α-diol (5α-Pdiol), and 5α-pregnane-3α-ol-20-one (pregnanolone) by 20α-hydroxysteroid dehydrogenase (20α-HSD), 5α-reductase, and 3α-HSD (14), as shown in Figure 3.

Granulosa cells were cultured for 72 h in the presence of FSH ± TNF α, and the media progestins determined (Fig. 4). Total FSH-stimulated proges-

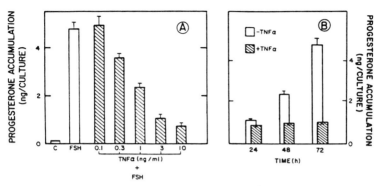

FIGURE 2. TNF α-attenuated progesterone accumulation: Dose and time dependence. Granulosa cells were cultured and media assayed for progesterone as described in Figure 1, except *(A)* cells were cultured with and without increasing concentrations (0.1 to 10 ng/mL) of TNF α or *(B)* for 24 to 72 h with FSH ± TNF α (10 ng/mL). (From Adashi EY, Resnick CE, Packman JN, Hurwitz A, Payne DW, Cytokine-mediated regulation of ovarian function: Tumor necrosis factor α inhibits gonadotropin-supported progesterone accumulation by differentiating and luteinized murine granulosa cells, Am J Obstet Gynecol 1990;162:889-99.)

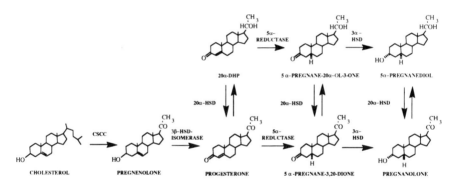

FIGURE 3. Steroidogenic pathway.

tin production was decreased by about 40%. However, the most significant decrease was that of 20α-DHP (60%). Inhibition of 5α-Pdiol and pregnanolone were not as dramatically affected.

Cellular Radiolabeling Studies

To evaluate further the steroidogenic alterations associated with TNF α action, we next explored its overall impact on the steroidogenic pathway (Fig. 3). Granulosa cells were cultured with FSH ± TNF α as described above, followed by addition of [³H]25-hydroxycholesterol (Fig. 5) or [³H]pregnenolone (Fig. 6).

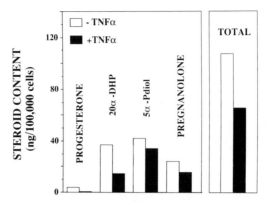

FIGURE 4. Effect of TNF α on FSH-supported total progestin accumulation. Granulosa cells (5×10^5 cells/culture) were cultured for 72 h in the presence of FSH (100 ng/mL) plus androstenedione (10^{-7}M) to enhance overall progestin synthesis ± TNF α (10 ng/mL). Media from 3 dishes per group were pooled, extracted, separated on HPLC, and each fraction assayed for 3α-hydroxysteroid content and 20α-hydroxysteroid content (see text). Progesterone was determined by RIA. Similar results were obtained in a duplicate experiment.

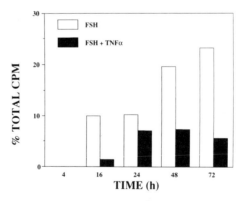

FIGURE 5. Cellular radiolabeling studies with [^{3}H]25-hydroxycholesterol. Granulosa cells were cultured as described in Figure 1, but for 96 h. Thereafter, the media were discarded, the cells washed with fresh media, and media added containing 100,000 cpm of [^{3}H]25-hydroxycholesterol. At the indicated times, media steroids were extracted, fractionated by HPLC, and detected and quantitated by an inline radioactivity detector. (Bars represent the sums of the total metabolic products; results reflect a representative experiment.)

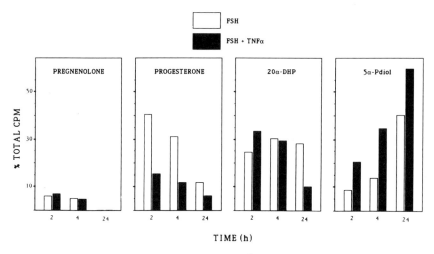

FIGURE 6. Cellular radiolabeling studies with [³H]pregnenolone. Studies were performed as in Figure 5 except that [³H]pregnenolone (250,000 cpm) was used. (From Adashi EY, Resnick CE, Packman JN, Hurwitz A, Payne DW, Cytokine-mediated regulation of ovarian function: Tumor necrosis factor α inhibits gonadotropin-supported progesterone accumulation by differentiating and luteinized murine granulosa cells, Am J Obstet Gynecol 1990;162:889–99.)

When the cultures were labeled with [³H]25-hydroxycholesterol (Fig. 5), metabolism proceeded slowly to pregnenolone, progesterone, 20α-DHP, and 5α-Pdiol. The sum of these total metabolic products was markedly decreased in the presence of TNF α, suggesting that TNF α inhibits cholesterol side-chain cleavage enzyme.

To characterize steroidogenic transformations distal to the cholesterol side-chain cleavage block, granulosa cell cultures were also labeled with [³H]pregnenolone (Fig. 6). Metabolism proceeded rapidly to progesterone and its products. TNF α produced a diminution in the FSH-supported accumulation of progesterone and 20α-DHP (24 h) but an enhancement of 5α-Pdiol. These results suggest that TNF α does not qualitatively alter the steroidogenic pathway, but may have complex quantitative effects wherein progesterone biosynthesis as well as its degradation may be altered.

Effect of TNF α on Steroidogenic Enzymes

In order to determine the effect of TNF α on the enzymes in the steroidogenic pathway, granulosa cells were cultured (as above) with FSH ± TNF α.

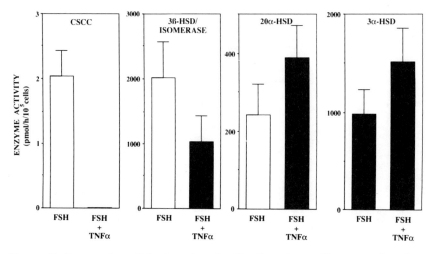

FIGURE 7. Enzymatic activity in cultured cells. Granulosa cells were cultured as described in Figure 1, except that cells were cultured for 96 h in tubes. After culture, the media were discarded and replaced with the appropriate assay buffer and sonicated. The sonicates were assayed for the indicated enzyme activities as described in text. Results represent the mean ± SE of 2–4 different experiments.

Following culture, the media were discarded, and enzyme assays performed on the sonicated cells (Fig. 7).

As shown (Fig. 7), TNF α was a potent inhibitor of cholesterol side-chain cleavage and 3β-HSD/isomerase activity (>90% and 51%, respectively). In contrast, 20α-HSD and 3α-HSD activity were stimulated (1.9- and 1.5-fold respectively). These results suggest that the effect of TNF α to diminish gonadotropin stimulated progesterone accumulation is the result of its action of inhibiting progesterone synthesis and stimulating its degradation.

Summary

In order to evaluate the cellular mechanism(s) underlying TNF α action in the ovarian steroidogenic cascade, granulosa cells were cultured in the absence or presence of gonadotropins, with or without TNF α, and steroidogenesis examined by three approaches. First endogenous media steroids were assayed by RIA and enzyme-based assays. Second, progestin metabolism was monitored by cellular labeling with radioactive precursors. Third, the activities of key steroidogenic enzymes were determined under cell-free conditions.

We have observed that TNF α markedly inhibits the FSH-driven accumulation of progesterone in a dose- and time-dependent and reversible manner. Furthermore, TNF α modulated the production of the downstream metabolites of progesterone. FSH-stimulated 20α-DHP levels were inhibited 60% by the addition of TNF α. In contrast, the distal metabolites, 5α-Pdiol and pregnanolone, were only modestly inhibited. These results are in keeping with the effects of TNF α on enzymatic activities in this system. TNF α inhibited the enzymes leading to progesterone production, but stimulated the enzymes that metabolize progesterone to a 5α-Pdiol. Specifically, cholesterol side-chain cleavage activity and 3β-HSD/isomerase activity were inhibited >90% and 51%, respectively, whereas 20α-HSD and 3α-HSD were stimulated 1.9- and 1.5-fold respectively. These results were confirmed in radiotracer studies using [^{3}H]25-hydroxycholesterol and [^{3}H]pregnenolone as substrates.

The studies described herein involved primary cultures of granulosa cells from immature rats. FSH-primed/hCG-exposed granulosa cells were also studied (with the same result) to better simulate the process of luteinization and thereby provide a crude approximation of granulosa/luteal cell function in the presence of TNF α. In unpublished studies, we have also examined the effect of TNF α on hCG-supported steroidogenesis using cultured whole ovarian dispersates and highly purified theca cells. In these latter systems, TNF α markedly inhibited the hCG-stimulated accumulation of androsterone, apparently via stimulation of 20α-HSD activity and inhibition of 17α-hydroxylase/lyase activity.

Taken together, our findings suggest that TNF α is capable of directly and reversibly attenuating gonadtropin-stimulated steroidogenesis in granulosa, luteal, and thecal compartments via differential modulation of key biosynthetic and degradative enzymes. These observations provide yet another example of the broad range of TNF α actions and underscore its polyfunctional nature. Accordingly, TNF α can now be added to a growing list of regulatory molecules capable of exerting paracrine or autocrine control in the ovary (15).

The known cytotoxic properties of TNF α cannot account for its effect on steroidogenesis in the ovary since the inhibitory effects were reversible, steroidogenesis was robust as determined in radiolabeling studies, and some enzymatic activities were elevated in the presence of TNF α. Furthermore, in these studies, neither cell viability, plating efficiency, number of cells, or their DNA content was changed in the presence of TNF α (2).

In vivo, TNF α may be locally derived from activated resident ovarian macrophages as observed by Keye and coworkers (16) for regressing (but not young) corpora lutea. Alternatively, TNF α may be of granulosa cell origin as suggested by the immunohistochemical studies of Roby and Terranova

(17) wherein antral or atretic granulosa cells have been implicated as possible sites for TNF α gene expression. The association between TNF α elaboration and follicular and luteal decline, as well as our observations that TNF α inhibits gonadotropin-supported synthesis of biologically potent steroids, give further support to the speculation that TNF α may play a role in the still enigmatic processes of atresia and/or luteolysis. Perhaps TNF α of intraovarian origin has a paracrine function in regulating gonadotropin-stimulated hormonal action and plays a role in the processes of follicular and luteal demise.

References

1. Bulmer D. The histochemistry of ovarian macrophages in the rat. J Anat 1964;98:313-9.
2. Adashi EY, Resnick CE, Croft CS, Payne DW. Tumor necrosis factor α inhibits gonadotropin hormonal action in non transformed ovarian granulosa cells. J Biol Chem 1989;264:11591-7.
3. Adashi EY, Resnick CE, Packman JN, Hurwitz A, Payne DW. Cytokine-mediated regulation of ovarian function: Tumor necrosis factor α inhibits gonadotropin-supported progesterone accumulation by differentiating and luteinized murine granulosa cells. Am J Obstet Gynecol 1990;162:889-99.
4. Kirsch TM, Friedman AC, Vogel RL, Flickinger GL. Macrophages in corpora lutea of mice: Characterization and effects on steroid secretion. Biol Reprod 1981;25:629-32.
5. Hume DA, Halpin D, Charlton H, Gordon S. The mononuclear phagocyte system of the mouse defined by immunohistochemical localization of antigen F4/80: Macrophages of endocrine organs. Proc Natl Acad Sci USA 1984;81:174-81.
6. Adashi EY. Do cytokines play a role in the regulation of ovarian function? Prog Neuroendocrinimmunol 1990;3:11-7.
7. Beutler B, Cerami A. Cachectin (tumor necrosis factor): A macrophage hormone governing cellular metabolism and inflammatory response. Endocr Rev 1988;9:57-73.
8. Emoto N, Baird A. The effect of tumor necrosis factor/cachectin on follicle-stimulating hormone-induced aromatase activity in cultured rat granulosa cells. Biochem Biophys Res Commun 1988;153:792-8.
9. Darbon JM, Oury F, Laredo J, Bayard F. Tumor necrosis factor-α inhibits follicle-stimulating hormone induced differentiation in cultured rat granulosa cells. Biochem Biophys Res Commun 1989;163:1038-46.
10. Roby KF, Terranova PF. Tumor necrosis factor alpha alters follicular steroidogenesis in vitro. Endocrinology 1988;123:2952-4.
11. Roby KF, Terranova PF. Effects of tumor necrosis factor-α in vitro on steroidogenesis of healthy and atretic follicles of the rat: Theca as a target. Endocrinology 1990;126:2711-8.
12. Payne DW, Talalay P. Isolation of novel microbial 3α-, 3β, and 17β-hydroxysteroid dehydrogenases. J Biol Chem 1985;260:13648-55.

13. Payne DW, Holtzclaw WD, Adashi EY. The steroidogenic characteristics of primary testicular cell cultures from adult hypophysectomized rats: Enhanced formation of C21 steroids. Biol Reprod 1988;39:581-92.
14. Goldring NB, Orly J. Concerted metabolism of steroid hormones produced by cocultured ovarian cell types. J Biol Chem 1985;260:913-20.
15. Hsueh AJW, Adashi EY, Jones PBC, Welsh TH, Jr. Hormonal regulation of the differentiation of cultured ovarian granulosa cells. Endocr Rev 1984;5:76-127.
16. Bagavandoss P, Wiggins RC, Kunkel SL, Keyes PL. Localization of macrophages and T-lymphocytes and induction of tumor necrosis factor-α (TNF-α) in corpora lutea of pregnant and pseudo-pregnant rabbits. Biol Reprod 1988;38:56.
17. Roby KF, Terranova PF. Localization of tumor necrosis factor (TNF) in the rat and bovine ovary using immunocytochemistry and cell blot: Evidence for granulosal production. In: Hirshfield AN, ed. Growth factors and the ovary. New York: Plenum Press, 1989;273-8.

17

Inflammatory Cells in the Rabbit Corpus Luteum: Relationship to Luteal Involution

P. BAGAVANDOSS, R.C. WIGGINS, S.L. KUNKEL,
D.G. REMICK, AND P.L. KEYES

A remarkable characteristic of the mammalian corpus luteum is its ability to undergo rapid regression following the loss of progesterone synthesis at the end of the luteal phase. The loss of progesterone secretion has been attributed to prostaglandin $F_{2\alpha}$ (1, 2, 3), which has led to the concept of $PGF_{2\alpha}$ as the luteolytic hormone. Associated with or following the termination of progesterone synthesis, the corpus luteum degenerates through mechanisms that are not well understood. Paavola (4) has provided evidence for a potential role of macrophages, and Adashi and coworkers (5) have reported that tumor necrosis factor α can inhibit ovarian cell steroidogenesis. Here we recapitulate recent evidence from our laboratory that macrophages and TNF α activity are associated with end-stage regression of the corpus luteum, and that pregnancy postpones accumulation of macrophages in the corpus luteum (6, 7).

Methods

Pseudopregnant and pregnant rabbits were anesthetized with sodium pentobarbital on designated days (day 0 is day of mating to vasectomized or fertile male), and the corpora lutea was removed and frozen for eventual detection of macrophages and T-lymphocytes by immunofluorescence or mildly fixed for immunocytochemistry (7). Other corpora lutea were incubated with or without lipopolysaccharide (LPS), and the conditioned medium was assayed for TNF α activity by bioassay (7, 8). For enumeration of macrophages and T-lymphocytes, all samples were coded, and the cells were counted in 5 random microscopic fields in each of 1 to 4 corpora lutea per rabbit.

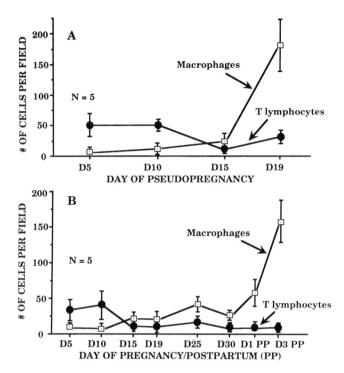

FIGURE 1. Quantification of macrophages and T-lymphocytes in the corpora lutea of pseudopregnancy *(A)* and pregnancy *(B)*. T-lymphocytes were present as early as day 5 of pseudopregnancy and pregnancy, with no detectable significant changes in numbers of these cells at other stages of pseudopregnancy or pregnancy. In contrast, during involution of the corpus luteum, the numbers of macrophages increased dramatically as observed on day-19 pseudopregnancy ($P < 0.01$) and day-3 postpartum. ($P < 0.01$; mean ± SEM; n = 5 rabbits at each stage of pseudopregnancy and pregnancy, total of 60 animals.) (From Biology of Reproduction 1990;42:367, with permission.)

Results and Discussion

T-lymphocytes were observed in corpora lutea at all stages of pregnancy and pseudopregnancy, and the numbers of these cells did not vary significantly among the stages (days). Few macrophages were observed in sections of corpora lutea until the very end of pseudopregnancy (day 19) or until several days after parturition, when the number of macrophages increased dramatically (Fig. 1). The paucity of macrophages in a corpus luteum of day 19 pregnancy is shown in Figure 2A and contrasts with the heavy infiltration of macrophages on day 19 of pseudopregnancy (Fig. 2B).

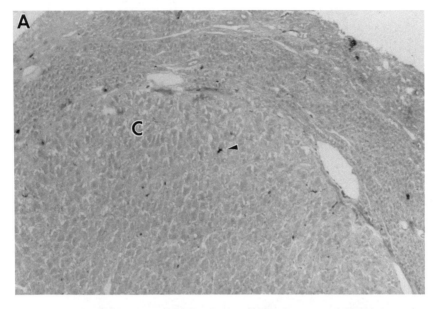

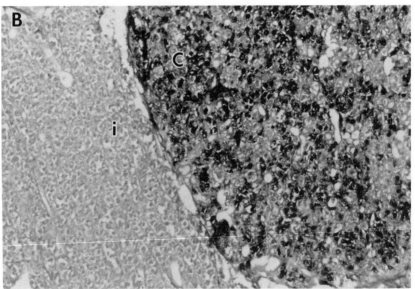

FIGURE 2. *A*: Immunohistochemical localization of macrophages in a section of corpus luteum (C) from a day-19 pregnant rabbit. Only a few scattered macrophages (arrow) were observed. *B*: Macrophages in a section of corpus luteum from a day-19 pseudopregnant rabbit. The corpus luteum is heavily infiltrated with macrophages (black deposits), while the adjacent interstitial tissue (i) is devoid of macrophages (×51). (From Biology of Reproduction 1990;42:367, with permission.)

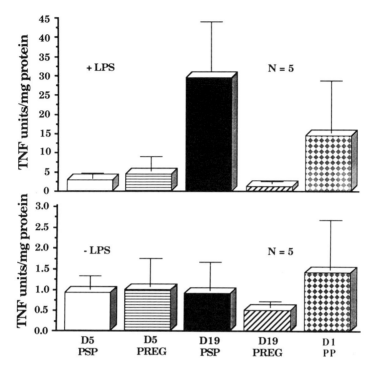

FIGURE 3. TNF α activity in medium of luteal tissue incubated with or without lipopolysaccharide (LPS). Corpora lutea were removed from pseudopregnant (PSP), pregnant (PREG), and postpartum (PP) rabbits. In the absence of LPS, low but detectable TNF α activity was observed (*bottom*). Upon stimulation with LPS (*top*), the nonregressing corpora lutea on day 5 of pseudopregnancy and on days 5 and 19 of pregnancy produced 2- to 4-fold TNF α compared to TNF α values from luteal tissue not stimulated with LPS. However, a 10- to 30-fold increase in activity was observed respectively in the regressing corpora lutea on day-1 postpartum and day-19 pseudopregnancy ($P < 0.05$). (Mean ± SEM; n = 5 rabbits each day; tissues in top (+LPS) and bottom (–LPS) panels are from same animals.) (From Biology of Reproduction 1990;42:367, with permission.)

In response to lipopolysaccharide, TNF α activity in medium was greatest on day 19 of pseudopregnancy, a time when macrophage infiltration was high. However, lipopolysaccharide stimulated TNF α release from luteal tissue at all stages, and in the absence of lipopolysaccharide, low TNF α activity was observed (Fig. 3).

These results indicate that the milieu of pregnancy postpones the accumulation of macrophages until after parturition. Further, the timing of macrophage infiltration suggests that these cells are not instrumental in terminating progesterone secretion by the corpus luteum. The signals that lead to macrophage infiltration and the role of TNF in the corpus luteum are intriguing subjects for future investigation.

Acknowledgment. The research reported in this chapter was supported by NIH grant HD-07127 (PLK) and by 2-P30-HD-18258, Standards and Reagents and Morphology Core Facilities.

References

1. McCracken JA, Schramm W, Barcikowski B, Wilson L, Jr. The identification of prostaglandin F2α as a uterine luteolytic hormone and the endocrine control of its synthesis. Acta Vet Scand [Suppl] 1981;77:71-88.
2. Thatcher WW, Bazer FW, Sharp DC, Roberts RM. Interrelationships between uterus and conceptus to maintain corpus luteum function in early pregnancy: Sheep, cattle, pigs and horses. J Anim Sci 1986;62(suppl 2):25-46.
3. Wiltbank MC, Guthrie PB, Mattson MP, Kater SB, Niswender GD. Hormonal regulation of free intracellular calcium concentrations in small and large ovine luteal cells. Biol Reprod 1989;41:771-8.
4. Paavola LG. Cellular mechanisms involved in luteolysis. Adv Exp Med Biol 1979;112:527-33.
5. Adashi EY, Resnick CE, Packman JN, Hurwitz A, Payne DW. Cytokine-mediated regulation of ovarian function: Tumor necrosis factor α inhibits gonadotropin-supported progesterone accumulation by differentiating and luteinized murine granulosa cells. Am J Obstet Gynecol 1990;162:889-99.
6. Bagavandoss P, Kunkel SL, Wiggins RC, Keyes PL. Tumor necrosis factor-α (TNF-α) production and localization of macrophages and T lymphocytes in the rabbit corpus luteum. Endocrinology 1988;122:1185-7.
7. Bagavandoss P, Wiggins RC, Kunkel SL, Remick DG, Keyes PL. Tumor necrosis factor production and accumulation of inflammatory cells in the corpus luteum of pseudopregnancy and pregnancy in rabbits. Biol Reprod 1990;42: 367-76.
8. Espevik T, Nissen-Meyer J. A highly sensitive cell line, WEHI 164 clone 13, for measuring cytotoxic factor/tumor necrosis factor from human monocytes. J Immunol Methods 1986;95:99-105.

Part V

Submitted Manuscripts

18

Two Populations of Steroidogenic Cells in the Theca Layer of Chicken Ovarian Follicles

HIROAKI NITTA, YOSHIO OSAWA, AND JANICE M. BAHR

The two-cell theory of steroid production in the chicken ovary states that the granulosa layer of the large preovulatory follicle is the primary site of progesterone synthesis whereas the theca layer produces androgens and estrogens (1–3). As the preovulatory follicles approach ovulation, there is a dramatic increase in progesterone production and a significant decrease in androgen and estrogen synthesis. These changes in steroidogenic capabilities of the preovulatory follicles are associated with a concomitant increase in the activity of 3β-hydroxy-Δ^5-steroid dehydrogenase in the granulosa layer and decrease in the activity of the aromatase enzyme in the theca layer (4–5).

Anatomical and histochemical studies suggest that interstitial cells located between theca interna and externa are the only steroidogenic cells in the theca layer (6–7). However, Onagbesan and Peddie (8) reported that both theca interna and externa of the third (F3) and fourth (F4) largest follicles produce estrogens in the presence of oFSH. In contrast, Pedermera et al. (9) measured significant amounts of testosterone in theca interna cells and low amounts of testosterone and high concentrations of estradiol-17β in theca externa cells. As a result, the precise cellular sites of androgen and estrogen production in the theca layer of the chicken ovarian follicle are still controversial.

Therefore, the purposes of this study were (a) to identify the location of steroidogenic cells in the theca layer by immunolocalization of steroidogenic enzymes and (b) to confirm the results of immunocytochemistry by measuring steroids produced by isolated theca interna and theca externa cells.

Materials and Methods

Single-comb white Leghorn hens, 30–60 weeks of age, with regular laying sequences of 6 eggs or more, were used. The lighting schedule was 15 light:

9 dark, and oviposition time was recorded at hourly intervals in the morning and at 1700. On the day of the experiment, preovulatory follicles were obtained from chickens 2 h after oviposition of the first egg in the sequence and were prepared for immunocytochemistry and static cell culture.

Immunocytochemistry. The fifth largest (F5) follicle was processed for paraffin section. Follicles were fixed in 4% paraformaldehyde (PFA) (Sigma Chemical Co., St. Louis, MO) buffered at pH 7.4 for 1 h. Additional fixation was done in PFA overnight at 4°C after yolk was removed. The fixed tissue was embedded in a block of Paraplast (Brunswick Company, St. Louis, MO) after dehydration. Sections were placed on poly-L-lysine (Sigma) coated glass slides. Deparaffinized sections were immunostained for steroidogenic enzymes with a Rabbit ExtrAvidin™ Staining Kit (Sigma). Polyclonal antisera used were anti-P-450$_{SCC}$ (against bovine adrenal P-450$_{SCC}$), anti-P-450$_{c17}$ (against porcine adrenal P-450$_{c17}$), and anti-P-450$_{arom}$ (against human placental aromatase) for immunolocalization of pregnenolone, androstenedione, and estrogen-producing cells, respectively. Control sections were treated with normal rabbit serum at the same concentration as antisera (1:100) or 1% bovine serum albumin (BSA) (Sigma) in PBS instead of the first antisera. The final product was obtained with a treatment of 3,3'-diaminobenzidine (Sigma) solution.

Static Cell Culture. The F3, F4, and F5 follicles were pooled from 4 chickens. Theca layers were separated from follicles, and theca interna and externa cells were isolated by a time-controlled collagenase digestion (10). Theca layers were placed in a solution of 1000-IU collagenase (Sigma) and 0.04% trypsin inhibitor (Sigma) in avian Ringer's buffer containing 0.1% BSA and 10-mM HEPES (Sigma) at 37°C in a shaking water bath for 10 min. Theca interna cells were removed by scraping the inner part of the theca layer with a surgical blade at room temperature. The remaining theca externa layers were then cut into small pieces and further digested in the collagenase solution with mechanical disruption of tissue at 15 min intervals with disposable plastic pipette. Cells were then filtered through a plastic screen and centrifuged at 700 × g for 10 min at 4°C. Cells were resuspended in avian Ringer's buffer after washing cells 3 times. Viable cells were determined by exclusion of trypan blue. Isolated theca interna (2.5×10^5 cells/mL) and externa cells (5×10^5 cells/mL) were pipetted into plastic culture tubes (12 × 75 mm) (Sarstedt Laboratory, Princeton, NJ) in triplicates. Experimental groups of cells were theca interna, theca externa, and a combination of theca interna and externa. Because the cell ratio obtained from theca interna and externa cells by this cell separation method was 1:2 or greater, a 1:2 ratio of theca interna:theca externa cells was used to duplicate a physiological environment in vitro. Final volume of each tube was 2 mL. Cells were treated with or without ovine luteinizing hormone (oLH) (NIADDK-oLH-26, NIH, Bethesda, MD), 25 ng/mL, at 37°C in a shaking water bath for 3 h. Medium was assayed in duplicate for progesterone, testosterone, and estradiol-17β. Amounts of steroids present in 0 time samples were subtracted from amounts of steroids measured in basal and oLH-treated samples to determine net steroid production. Data were analyzed statistically with simple contrasts of two-way analysis of variance.

Results

Immunolocalization

Two distinct populations of cells containing steroidogenic enzymes were localized in the theca layer of F5 follicles (Fig. 1). Theca interstitial cells, located between theca interna and externa, contained P-450$_{SCC}$ (Fig. 1B) and P-450$_{c17}$ (Fig. 1C), whereas a specific cell population in theca externa contained only P-450$_{arom}$ (Fig. 1D) (compare to a control section in Fig. 1A).

Steroid Production

Steroid production by theca interna and externa cells in response to oLH suggested unique steroidogenic capabilities of the two cell types (Fig. 2). Theca interna cells produced progesterone and testosterone. LH stimulated progesterone and testosterone production by theca interna cells significantly compared to basal production (data are not shown) (P < 0.001). Theca externa cells produced only estradiol-17β, whereas no progesterone and testosterone production was detected. In contrast to theca interna cells, the production of estradiol-17β by theca externa cells was not increased by LH. Estradiol-17β production increased significantly (P < 0.001) when theca interna and externa cells were combined, whereas progesterone and testosterone production was not significantly different compared to the amount of steroid produced by theca interna cells alone.

Discussion

We are reporting the first visual evidence of 2 steroidogenic cell populations in the theca layer of the chicken preovulatory follicles. The immunocytochemical study clearly demonstrates the presence of 2 distinct steroidogenic cell populations in the theca layer. One steroidogenic cell population is the interstitial cells located between the theca interna and theca externa. The other steroidogenic cell population is specific cells in the theca externa.

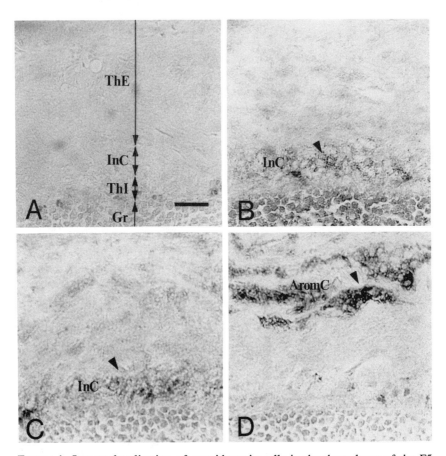

FIGURE 1. Immunolocalization of steroidogenic cells in the theca layer of the F5 follicle. *A*: Control section. Granulosa cells (Gr), theca interna (ThI), interstitial cells (InC), and theca externa (ThE) are shown. *B*: P-450$_{SCC}$ staining. Interstitial cells were stained. *C*: P-450$_{c17}$ staining. Interstitial cells were stained. *D*: P-450$_{arom}$ staining. Specific cells in theca externa, aromatase cells, were only stained. (Arrows indicate immunoreactivity; bar = 25 μm.)

Interstitial cells contain 2 steroidogenic enzymes, P-450$_{SCC}$ and P-450$_{c17}$. These immunoreactivities indicate that interstitial cells produce pregnenolone from cholesterol and can also produce androstenedione from progesterone. It had been reported that interstitial cells are steroidogenic cells and contain 3β-hydroxysteroid dehydrogenase, an enzyme required for progesterone production and androstenedione production (6–7). The cell population in theca externa contained only one steroidogenic enzyme, the P-450$_{arom}$. This evidence indicates that these cells produce estrogens from androgens. We propose to call these cells "aromatase cells."

Data from the short term culture of isolated theca interna and externa cells

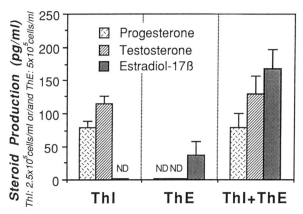

FIGURE 2. Steroid production by theca interna cells (ThI), containing theca interstitial cells, theca externa cells (ThE), and a combination of theca interna and externa cells. Cells were cultured for 3 h at 37°C in the presence of oLH (25 ng/mL). Note that estradiol-17β production by theca externa cells when combined with theca interna cells was significantly increased compared to theca externa cells alone (P < 0.001). (Values represent the mean ± SEM of 4 experiments for progesterone and estradiol-17β production and 3 experiments for testosterone production.)

alone or combined support the results of immunocytochemistry. Theca interna cells secreted progesterone and testosterone and the production of which was stimulated by oLH. In contrast, only estradiol-17β was detected in theca externa cell culture medium. Unlike theca interna cells, theca externa cells were not responsive to oLH. The observation that estradiol-17β production by combined theca interna and externa cells with oLH increased 4.5-fold compared to theca externa cells (P < 0.001) suggests that aromatase cells need androgen as a substrate (e.g., testosterone) to produce estradiol-17β. However, progesterone and testosterone production by combined theca interna and theca externa cells compared to theca interna cells alone was similar even though testosterone was used to produce estradiol-17β. Therefore, the existence of 2 distinct steroidogenic cell populations in the theca layer of the F5 follicles of the chicken was confirmed by our in vitro study.

Findings that indicate estradiol-17β is produced by the theca externa cells of preovulatory follicles in the turkey ovary (10) generally agree with our results in the chicken. However, our observation that estrogen production occurs only in the theca externa disagrees with an earlier publication that reported estrogen production from androstenedione as substrate in the presence of oFSH by both theca interna and externa cells of chicken ovarian follicles (8). This observation may have been caused by contamination of aromatase cells of the theca externa in the theca interna cell culture.

In conclusion, we have demonstrated a unique aspect of steroidogenesis in the theca layer of the smaller preovulatory follicles of the chicken ovary:

(a) The theca layer has two distinct steroidogenic cell populations that are interstitial cells required for progesterone and androgen production and the aromatase cells for estrogen production; (b) the theca layer itself can produce steroids from cholesterol without any substrates from the granulosa layer; and (c) aromatase cells need a substrate, androgen, for estrogen production.

Acknowledgments. We thank Dr. A. Payne, University of Michigan, for her kind donation of P-450$_{SCC}$ and P-450$_{c17}$ antisera. We acknowledge NIDDK and the National Hormone and Pituitary Program for the oLH. This research was supported in part by USDA-Ag-89-37240-4769, the Endocrine Society Student Summer Fellowship, 1989, and the Midwest Society of Electron Microscopists, Inc., Student Grant Program, 1989.

References

1. Huang WY, Kao KJ, Nalbandov AV. Synthesis of sex steroids by cellular components of chicken follicles. Biol Reprod 1979;20:454-61.
2. Bahr JM, Wang SC, Huang WY, Calvo FO. Steroid concentrations in isolated theca and granulosa layers of preovulatory follicles during the ovulatory cycle of the domestic hen. Biol Reprod 1983;29:326-34.
3. Eches RJ, Duke CE. Progesterone, androstenedione and oestradiol content of theca and granulosa tissues of the four largest ovarian follicles during the ovulatory cycle of the hen *(Gallus domesticus)*. J Endocrinol 1984;103:71-6.
4. Armstrong DG. 3β-hydroxy-Δ^5-steroid dehydrogenase activity in the rapidly growing ovarian follicles of the domestic fowl *(Gallus domesticus)*. J Endocr 1982;93:415-21.
5. Armstrong DG. Ovarian aromatase activity in the domestic fowl *(Gallus domesticus)*. J Endocrinol 1984;100:81-6.
6. Gilbert AB, Wells JW. Structure and function of the ovary. In: Cunningham FJ, Lake PE, Hewitt D, eds. Reproductive biology of poultry. Br Poult Sci, 1984: 15-27.
7. Wells JW, Gilbert AB. Steroid hormone production by the ovary. In: BM Freeman, eds. Physiology and biochemistry of domestic fowl. Boca Raton, FL: Academic Press, 1984:323-43.
8. Onagbesan OM, Peddie MJ. Calcium-dependent stimulation of estrogen secretion by FSH from theca cells of the domestic hen *(Gallus domesticus)*. Gen Comp Endocrinol 1989;75:177-86.
9. Pedermera E, Velazquez P, Gomez Y, Gonzalez del Pliego M. Isolation of steroidogenic cell subpopulations in the follicular theca of the ovary in the domestic fowl. In: Hirshfield AN, ed. Growth factors and the ovary. New York: Serono Symposia, USA/Plenum Press, 1989:351-5.
10. Porter TE, Hargis BM, El Halawani ME. Different steroid production between theca interna and theca externa cells: A three-cell model for follicular steroidogenesis in avian species. Endocrinology 1989;125:109-16.

19

Localization of mRNAs That Encode Steroidogenic Enzymes in Bovine Ovaries

R.J. RODGERS AND H.F. RODGERS

Immunocytochemical localization of the steroidogenic enzymes in bovine follicles and corpora lutea (1, 2) allowed the identification of the steroidogenic properties of ovarian cells in situ. To further extend this work, we present here the localization of cholesterol side-chain cleavage cytochrome P-450 (P-450$_{SCC}$) mRNAs and of 17α-hydroxylase (P-450$_{17\alpha}$) mRNAs in bovine ovaries by in situ hybridization (J. Reprod. Fertil., submitted) and compare these results with that of the immunolocalization of the enzymes they encode (1, 2). These enzymes convert cholesterol into pregnenolone and then into androgen, respectively.

Materials and Methods

Bovine follicles (10 follicles, 5 mm in diameter; 6 follicles, 5–10 mm; 2 follicles >10 mm) and corpora lutea (2 of class II, 6 of class III, and 2 of class IV) regressing corpora lutea from cyclic animals as classified by the method of Ireland et al. (3) were collected at an abattoir and embedded in OCT compound (Miles, Inc., Elkhart, IN) and stored at –70°C. Sections (6 μm) were air dried onto gelatin-coated slides and fixed at 4°C for 5 min in 4% glutaraldehyde and 20% dimethylsulphoxide in 0.1-M phosphate buffer (pH 7.3) prior to in situ hybridization. Sections were rinsed in 0.6-M NaCl and 60-mM sodium acetate solution and then prehybridized in 50% formamid, 0.6-M NaCl, 5-mM EDTA, 0.02% Ficoll 400, 0.02% bovine serum albumin, 0.02% polyvinylpyrrolidone, and 10-μg denatured salmon sperm DNA/mL in 50-mM phosphate buffer (pH 7.0). Prehybridization was carried out at 40°C for approximately 5 h and hybridization, for approximately 36 h. The slides were then washed stepwise to the most stringent conditions of 0.15-M NaCl and 15-mM sodium acetate at 40°C.

Hybridizations were performed with ^{32}P-labeled DNA (>10^8cpm/ug DNA) and the concentrations of the 3 DNA probes used in each experimental batch were similar (>10^8cpm/mL). Both the bovine P-450$_{SCC}$ cDNA probe and the bovine P-450$_{17\alpha}$ cDNA probe have been shown to hybridize to single bands of mRNA on Northern blots of bovine ovaries (4), and pBR322 DNA was used as a control. Autoradiography was performed using emulsion K5 or G5 (Ilford, Australia Pty. Ltd., Mt. Waverley, Aust.) and sections were counterstained with hematoxylin and eosin.

Results

The results of the localization of the P-450 mRNAs are presented here (Figs. 2, 4, and 6) and compared with that obtained for the P-450 enzymes (Figs. 1, 3, and 5) previously (1, 2). In the ovarian stroma, only background levels of P-450 mRNAs and enzymes could be detected.

Follicles

In all follicles examined, the positive staining for P-450$_{SCC}$ mRNAs was observed in the theca interna layer (Fig. 2), and weak-to-strong (as in Fig. 2) levels of staining were observed in the membrana granulosa. The theca externa had only background levels, similar to those seen in the ovarian stroma with the P-450$_{SCC}$ cDNA probe and to those observed with pBR322 DNA probe. The localization of the P-450$_{SCC}$ enzyme was similar (Fig. 1), with strong staining observed in the theca interna and weak-to-strong staining in the membrana granulosa.

Strong staining for P-450$_{17\alpha}$ mRNAs was detected in the theca interna layer of follicles, with only background levels present in the theca externa and membrana granulosa (Fig. 4). The pattern of staining did not appear to be

———————————————————————————————▶

PLATE A. *Left Panels:* Light micrographs of immunofluorescence staining of bovine follicle walls (Fig. 1, 6-mm follicle; Fig. 3, 4-mm follicle) and a mature stage III corpus luteum (Fig. 5). Anti-P-450$_{SCC}$ IgG was used in Figures 1 and 5, and anti-P-450$_{17\alpha}$ IgG was used in Figure 3. *Right panels:* Emulsion autoradiograms of tissue sections of a bovine follicle wall (Figs. 2 and 4, the same 5-mm follicle) and a mature stage III corpus luteum (Fig. 6) following in situ hybridization. A P-450$_{SCC}$ cDNA probe was used in Figures 2 and 6, and a P-450$_{17\alpha}$ cDNA probe was used in Figure 4. Sections were stained with hematoxylin and eosin. (TE = theca externa; TI = theca interna; G = granulosa cell layers; bars are 20 μm.) (From J. Reprod. Fertil., with permission.)

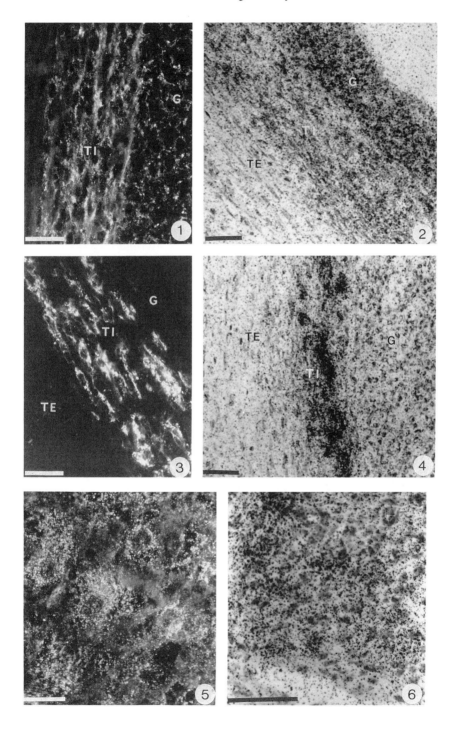

as diffuse as that observed for P-450$_{SCC}$ mRNA, suggesting that some cells had higher levels of P-450$_{17\alpha}$ mRNAs than other cells within the theca interna layer. P-450$_{17\alpha}$ enzyme was also localized to only the theca interna layer of the follicle wall (Fig. 3).

Corpora Lutea

P-450$_{SCC}$ mRNAs were localized to the areas of the corpora lutea containing the steroidogenic luteal cells and not to areas dominated by blood vessels or connective tissue elements (Fig. 6). No positive staining for P-450$_{17\alpha}$ mRNAs was detected in any of the corpora lutea examined, and no positive staining for P-450$_{SCC}$ mRNAs or P-450$_{17\alpha}$ mRNAs was detected in regressing corpora lutea. Similarly P-450$_{SCC}$ enzyme was localized to the steroidogenic luteal cells (Fig. 5), as confirmed by staining enzymatically dissociated cells where cells were readily identified on the basis of their size (2). No positive staining for P-450$_{17\alpha}$ enzyme was observed in corpora lutea (1).

Discussion

The results of localization in bovine ovaries of both the P-450$_{SCC}$ mRNAs and P-450$_{17\alpha}$ mRNAs agree well with those of the localization of the enzymes that these mRNAs encode (1, 2). Similarly, they accord well with the known steroidogenic capacities of the ovarian compartments (see 6) and thus the results support the original suggestion (4) that the amount and type of steroid hormone produced by the ovary and its compartments are dependent upon the amount and type of steroidogenic P-450 enzyme present in those ovarian compartments, which, in turn, are due to the amount and type of P-450 mRNAs that encode them. This suggestion explains the day-to-day changes in ovarian hormone secretion. However, from more recent studies (see 6), it appears that the relationship is more qualitative rather than quantitative, and it appears to hold true only during growth and maturation of follicles and corpora lutea and not necessarily during regression of corpora lutea when, presumably, other steps in the steroidogenic pathway of synthesis and secretion become rate limiting. The mechanisms whereby changes in the expression of P-450 genes occur in concert with ovarian cell differentiation still remain to be determined.

Acknowledgments. We thank Jenny Penschow for helping us establish the in situ hydribization technique, Drs. E.R. Simpson and M.R. Waterman for providing cDNA probes and the National Health and Medical Research Council of Australia for financial support.

References

1. Rodgers RJ, Rodgers HF, Hall PF, Waterman MR, Simpson ER. Immuno-localization of cholesterol side-chain-cleavage cytochrome P-450 and 17α-hydroxylase cytochrome P-450 in bovine ovarian follicles. J Reprod Fertil 1986;78: 627-38.
2. Rodgers RJ, Rodgers HF, Waterman MR, Simpson ER. Immunolocalization of cholesterol side-chain cleavage cytochrome P-450 and ultrastructural studies of bovine corpora lutea. J Reprod Fertil 1986;78:639-52.
3. Ireland JJ, Murphee RL, Coulson PB. Accuracy of predicting stages of bovine estrous cycle by gross appearance of the corpus luteum. J Dairy Sci 1980;63: 155-60.
4. Rodgers RJ, Waterman MR, Simpson ER. Levels of messenger ribonucleic acid encoding cholesterol side-chain cleavage cytochrome P-450, 17-hydroxylase cytochrome P-450, adrenodoxin, and low density lipoprotein receptor in bovine follicles and corpora lutea throughout the ovarian cycle. Mol Endocrinol 1987;1: 274-9.
5. Rodgers RJ, Waterman MR, Simpson ER. Cytochromes P-450$_{SCC}$, P-450$_{17\alpha}$, adrenodoxin and reduced nicotinamide andenine dinucleotide phosphate-cyto-chrome P-450 reductase in bovine follicles and corpora lutea. Changes in specific contents during the ovarian cycle. Endocrinology 1986;118:1366-74.
6. Rodgers RJ. Steroidogenic cytochrome P-450 enzymes and ovarian steroidogen-esis. Reprod Fertil Dev 1990;2:153-63.

20

Fetal Calf Serum: Eliciting Phosphorylation of Ca^{++}/Calmodulin-Dependent Protein Kinase II in Cultured Rat Granulosa Cells

TAKASHI OHBA, YASUTAKA OHTA, KOHJI MIYAZAKI, HITOSHI OKAMURA, AND EISHICHI MIYAMOTO

It is well known that a number of factors affect the proliferation, differentiation, and steroidogenesis of cultured rat granulosa cells. Two multifunctional protein kinases, such as cAMP-dependent protein kinase and protein kinase C, are thought to mediate intracellular signals in granulosa cells. Follicle stimulating hormone (FSH) induces granulosa cell differentiation and the steroidogenesis, which are mediated by the action of cAMP-dependent protein kinase (1–3). In contrast, phorbol ester inhibits FSH actions, such as cAMP formation, LH receptor expression, cholesterol side-chain cleavage enzyme synthesis, and progesterone production (4–7) via the activation of protein kinase C.

Ca^{++} also appears to play an important role as a second messenger in granulosa cells (8, 9). Although it has been suggested that the cAMP and inositol-phospholipid systems are involved in the regulation of granulosa cell functions, little is known about the intracellular Ca^{++} system, namely, the role of Ca^{++}/calmodulin-dependent protein kinases. Ca^{++}/calmodulin-dependent protein kinase II (CaM kinase II) is suggested to be involved in the regulation and coordination of various cellular processes (10–13). A class of the kinases is identified in brain and other tissues and appears to have a relatively broad substrate specificity in vitro (14). Recently, we have identified CaM kinase II in rat embryo fibroblast 3Y1 cells (15). The enzyme has a major 50-kDa subunit and undergoes autophosphorylation in a Ca^{++}/calmodulin-dependent manner in vitro. The addition of fetal calf serum (FCS) and growth factors rapidly elicited the phosphorylation of

CaM kinase II in intact 3Y1 cells. In an effort to examine the occurrence and the role of CaM kinase II in rat granulosa cells, we present evidence that CaM kinase II is phosphorylated by the addition of FCS in cultured rat granulosa cells.

Materials and Methods

CaM kinase II was purified from rat brain, as described previously (14). The affinity-purified anti-CaM kinase II antibodies were prepared, as described previously (15). Granulosa cells were freshly prepared from 26-day-old immature female Wistar rats, as previously reported (6). Rat luteal cells were prepared from immature Wistar rats, treated with PMSG (10 IU)/hCG (5 IU), as previously reported (16).

In Vitro Phosphorylation of CaM Kinase II in Cultured Rat Granulosa Cell or Luteal Cell Extracts. Freshly prepared rat granulosa cells were seeded on plastic tissue culture dishes (10-cm diameter) containing 10 mL of serum-free McCoy's 5A medium (Gibco) at a concentration of 3×10^6 cells/dish and were cultured for 96 h. Cultured granulosa cells or freshly prepared luteal cells (3×10^6 cells) were collected and sedimented by centrifugation at 1500 rpm for 5 min. The pellet was suspended in 0.5 mL of a solution containing 20-mM Tris/HCl (pH 7.4), 0.15-M NaCl, 0.5-mM EGTA, 0.1-mM dithiothreitol, 1-mM PMSF, and 2% aprotinin homogenized in a Dounce homogenizer with 20 strokes. Aliquots of the supernatant were immunoprecipitated with the affinity-purified anti-CaM kinase II antibodies as described previously (15). The antibodies were immobilized on 50% (v/v) protein A-Sepharose. The immunoprecipitates were washed and incubated at 30°C for 20 min with a solution (100 μl) containing 20-mM Tris/HCl (pH 7.4), 015-M NaCl, 5-mM MgCl$_2$, 0.1 mM dithiothreitol, and 40-μM [γ^{32}P]ATP in the presence or absence of 1-mM CaCl$_2$ and 3-μM calmodulin. The reaction was stopped by adding 40 μL of the SDS stop solution. The samples were boiled for 2 min and analyzed by SDS-PAGE followed by autoradiography.

Labeling of Cells with [^{32}P]Orthophosphate and Immunoprecipitation with Anti-CaM Kinase II Antibodies. Granulosa cells were cultured on plastic culture dishes (35-mm diameter) at 37°C for 96 h. Then, the cells were labeled for 18 h in 0.9 mL of phosphate- and serum-free RPMI 1640 medium containing carrier free [^{32}P]orthophosphate (0.2 mCi/mL). Cells were incubated at 37°C for various time periods with or without the indicated concentrations of test agents such as FCS (Flow Lab.), FSH (NIAMDD o-FSH-17), estradiol, progesterone, and epidermal growth factor (EGF) (Sigma). After the incubation medium was aspirated, the cell monolayers were quickly washed by saline and frozen with liquid nitrogen.

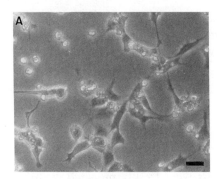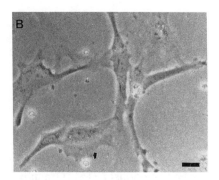

FIGURE 1. Comparison of the shape of rat granulosa cells cultured with or without FCS. Rat granulosa cells were cultured for 48 h in the absence (A) and presence (B) of 10% FCS. (Bars = 20 μm.)

The whole cell extract was immunoprecipitated with anti-CaM kinase II antibodies as previously described (15). Immunoprecipitates were eluted from protein A-Sepharose by adding 60 μL of the SDS sample buffer and boiling for 2 min. The samples were centrifuged at $15,000 \times g$ for 1 min. The supernatants were collected and the eluted phosphoproteins were analyzed by SDS-PAGE. The gels were stained with Coomassie brilliant blue, dried, and exposed to Kodak X-Omat film for autoradiography. The relative ^{32}P incorporation into each band was determined by direct liquid scintillation counting of the excised band.

Results

FCS induced dramatic morphological changes of cultured granulosa cells. When granulosa cells were cultured in McCoy's 5A medium alone, nonspread and round-up cells were mostly observed (Fig. 1A). On the other hand, when the cells were cultured with the medium containing FCS, the cells were well spread and underwent marked hypertrophy within 48 h (Fig. 1B). The findings of the morphological changes of the cells with FCS were in good agreement with those reported previously (17, 18).

When in vitro phosphorylation of CaM kinase II was performed in the cytosolic extract of rat granulosa cells, a 50-kDa protein was phosphorylated in a Ca^{++}/calmodulin-dependent manner. It suggested that the 50-kDa protein may be a major subunit of CaM kinase II in rat granulosa cells (Fig. 2B). Minor bands, around 60 kDa, were also faintly phosphorylated in a Ca^{++}/calmodulin-dependent manner. In contrast, Ca^{++}/calmodulin-dependent

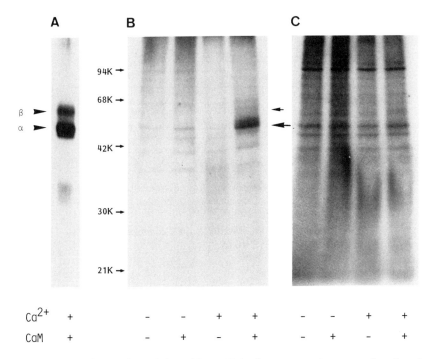

FIGURE 2. Phosphorylation of CaM kinase II in the extract of rat granulosa/luteal cells. Purified rat brain CaM kinase II (*A*) and the immunoprecipitates of granulosa cells (*B*) and luteal cells (*C*) were incubated at 30°C for 20 min with [γ^{32}P]ATP (40 µM) in the presence or absence of Ca^{++}/calmodulin, as described in text. Phosphoproteins were analyzed by SDS-PAGE, followed by autoradiography. (Large and small arrows indicate the positions of the major 50-kDa subunit and the minor 60-kDa subunit, respectively; arrowheads represent the α- and β-subunits of rat brain CaM kinase II.)

phosphorylation was not detected in the cytosolic extract of rat luteal cells (Fig. 2*C*). In the following experiment, we analysed only the major protein of 50 kDa in rat granulosa cells.

We subsequently examined the phosphorylation of CaM kinase II in cultured rat granulosa cells. Cells were labeled with [γ^{32}P]orthophosphate for 18 h, and then freshly dialyzed FCS was added to the cultures at a final concentration of 10% (v/v). The maximal phosphorylation was 1.5-fold in comparison to control at 5 min after the addition of FCS. The phosphorylation subsequently decreased with increasing times of incubation and reached the basal level within 30 min. The phosphorylation reached the lower level than control (0.5-fold) at 60 min after the serum addition. These results suggest that the phosphorylation of CaM kinase II elicited by the addition of serum is relatively

TABLE 1. Effects of various agents on phosphorylation of CaM kinase II in cultured rat granulosa cells, ^{32}P-labeled and treated at 37°C for 5 min for HEPES-buffered saline.

Treatment	^{32}P Incorporation*
FCS (10%)	156 ± 9 (n = 7)
FSH (1 μg/mL)	123 ± 13 (n = 9)
E$_2$ (100 ng/mL)	102 ± 1 (n = 4)
P (1 μg/mL)	109 + 5 (n = 4)
EGF (100 ng/mL)	105 ± 7 (n = 4)

Note: Immunoprecipitation was performed as described in text; the radioactivity of the 50-kDa subunit was determined by liquid scintillation counting.

*Values are expressed as percentage of the control and are represented as means ± SE; $P < 0.05$.

rapid and transient. Serum stimulated the phosphorylation of CaM kinase II in a dose-dependent manner. The maximal effect of FCS on the phosphorylation of CaM kinase II was obtained at a concentration of 10%, and the concentration required to give the half-maximal effect was 1.8%.

The phosphopeptide pattern of the 50-kDa protein phosphorylated in cultured rat granulosa cells in response to 10% FCS was similar to that of the 50-kDa protein phosphorylated in vitro and, moreover, was homologous with that of the autophosphorylated 49-kDa subunit purified from rat brain (data not shown). This verifies that the 50-kDa protein is the subunit of CaM kinase II and suggests that the increase in phosphorylation in response to serum addition may be mainly due to the autophosphorylation of the enzyme.

Table 1 shows the effects of gonadotropin, sex steroid hormones, and EGF on the enhancement of the phosphorylation of CaM kinase II in cultured granulosa cells. Exposure of cells to estradiol, progesterone, and EGF had no significantly stimulative effect on the phosphorylation of CaM kinase II under the conditions used.

Discussion

The present study demonstrates that CaM kinase II occurs in rat granulosa cells and that the addition of serum to intact granulosa cells rapidly elicits the phosphorylation of CaM kinase II. The following lines of evidence suggest that the 50-kDa protein is the major subunit of CaM kinase II in rat granulosa cells: *(a)* The 50-kDa protein is immunoprecipitated with the affinity-purified monospecific antibody to CaM kinase II (Fig. 2B); *(b)* the 50-kDa protein in the immunoprecipitate undergoes in vitro autophosphorylation in a

Ca^{++}/calmodulin-dependent manner; and *(c)* the in vitro phosphorylated 50-kDa protein yielded a similar phosphopeptide pattern to those of the 50-kDa protein phosphorylated in the cultured cells and the autophosphorylated 49-kDa subunit of CaM kinase II purified from rat brain (Fig. 2*A*). In contrast, the Ca^{++}/calmodulin dependently phosphorylated protein(s) was not detected in rat luteal cell extracts immunoprecipitated with affinity-purified CaM kinase II antibody (Fig. 2*C*). These results suggest that the existence of CaM kinase II may correlate with the granulosa/luteal cell differentiation.

In intact granulosa cells, the phosphorylation of CaM kinase II by FCS was rapid and transient. After the addition of FCS, the phosphorylation reached the maximum at 5 min and decreased to the basal level within 30 min. Our previous study showed that serum and growth factors elicited rapid and transient increase in the phosphorylation of CaM kinase II in intact rat fibroblast 3Y1 cells (15). Taken together, CaM kinase II may be involved in the initial phase of the signal transduction pathways and the decrease in the phosphorylation of the enzyme during the time course may be carried out by protein phosphatase(s).

Among various agents tested, FCS is the most potent stimulator of CaM kinase II phosphorylation in intact granulosa cells. FCS has been known to have various effects on the morphology, growth, and steroidogenesis of cultured granulosa cells. Serum also enhanced the growth of the granulosa cells and affected the progesterone production (18; and unpublished data). CaM kinase II may mediate at least some of the biological actions of FCS in intact rat granulosa cells.

References

1. Hunzicker-Dunn M, Birnbaumer L. Adenylyl cyclase activities in ovarian tissues, III. Regulation of responsiveness of LH, FSH, and PGE$_1$ in the prepubertal, cycling pregnant, and pseudopregnant rat. Endocrinology 1976;99:198-210.
2. Knecht M, Amsterdam A, Catt K. The regulatory role of cyclic AMP in hormone-induced of granulosa cell differentiation. J Biol Chem 1981;256:10628-33.
3. Trzeciak WH, Waterman MR, Simpson ER. Synthesis of the cholesterol side-chain cleavage enzymes in cultured rat ovarian granulosa cells: Induction by follicle-stimulating hormone and dibutyryl adenosine 3', 5'-monophosphate. Endocrinology 1986;119:323-30.
4. Kasson BG, Conn PM, Hsueh AJW. Inhibition of granulosa cell differentiation by dioctanoylglycerol—a novel activator of protein kinase C. Mol Cell Endocrinol 1985;42:29-37.
5. Kawai Y, Clark MR. Phorbol ester regulation of rat granulosa cell prostaglandin and progesterone accumulation. Endocrinology 1985;116:2320-6.
6. Shinohara H, Knecht M, Catt KJ. Inhibition of gonadotropin-induced granulosa cell differentiation by activation of protein kinase C. Proc Natl Acad Sci USA 1985;82:8518-22.

7. Trzeciak WK, Duda T, Waterman MR, Simpson ER. Tetradecanoyl phorbol acetate suppresses follicle-stimulating hormone-induced synthesis of the cholesterol side-chain cleavage enzyme complex in rat granulosa cells. J Biol Chem 1987;262:15246-50.

8. Carnegie JA, Tsang BK. Follicle-stimulating hormone-regulated granulosa cell steroidogenesis: Involvement of the calcium-calmodulin system. Am J Obstet Gynecol 1983;145:223-8.

9. Tsang BK, Carnegie JA. Calcium requirement in the gonadotropic regulation of rat granulosa cell progesterone production. Endocrinology 1983;113:763-9.

10. Edelman AM, Blumenthal DK, Krebs EG. Protein serine/threonine kinases. Annu Rev Biochem 1987;56:567-613.

11. Gorelick FS, Wang JKT, Lai Y, Nairn AC, Greengard P. Autophosphorylation and activation of Ca^{2+}/calmodulin-dependent protein kinase II in intact nerve terminals. J Biol Chem 1988;263:17209-12.

12. Miyamoto E. Characterization of a multifunctional Ca^{2+}-calmodulin-dependent protein kinase in the brain. Neuromethods 1986;5:519-50.

13. Nairn AC, Hemmings HC, Greengard P. Protein kinases in the brain. Annu Rev Biochem 1985;54:931-76.

14. Fukunaga K, Yamamoto H, Matsui K, Higashi K, Miyamoto E. Purification and characterization of Ca^{2+}- and calmodulin-dependent protein kinase from rat brain. J Neurochem 1982;39:1607-17.

15. Ohta Y, Ohba T, Fukunaga K, Miyamoto E. Serum and growth factors rapidly elicit phosphorylation of the Ca^{2+}/calmodulin-dependent protein kinase II in intact quiescent rat 3Y1 cells. J Biol Chem 1988;263:11540-7.

16. Thomas JP, Dorflinger LJ, Behrman HR. Mechanism of the rapid antigonadotropic action of prostaglandins in cultured luteal cells. Proc Natl Acad Sci USA 1978;75:1344-8.

17. Lino J, Baranao S, Hammond M. Multihormone regulation of steroidogenesis in cultured porcine granulosa cells: Studies in serum-free medium. Endocrinology 1985;116:2143-51.

18. Orly J, Sato G, Erickson GF. Serum suppresses the expression of hormonally induced functons in cultured rat granulosa cells. Cell 1980;20:817-27.

19. Fukunaga K, Rich DP, Soderling TR. Generation of the Ca^{2+}-independent form of Ca^{2+}/calmodulin-dependent protein kinase II in cerebellar granule cells. J Biol Chem 1989;264:21830-6.

21

Differential Regulation of Cytosolic-Free Calcium in Ovine Small and Large Luteal Cells: Effects on Secretion of Progesterone

P.B. HOYER AND J.A. WEGNER

Two types of morphologically and functionally distinct steroidogenic cells, designated small and large, have been identified in the corpus luteum of many species, including the ewe (1, 2). Unstimulated steroid production by ovine large cells is 5–10 times that of small cells, on a per cell basis (1, 3–5). However, unlike small cells, secretion of progesterone in large cells cannot be stimulated by luteinizing hormone (LH) or by hormone-independent activation of the cAMP-dependent pathway (1, 4, 6–7). Therefore, it appears that steroidogenesis in large cells is independent of LH and cAMP. Luteolysis in many species, including the ewe, is induced by prostaglandin $F_{2\alpha}$ (8–9). However, the exact mechanisms by which luteolysis occurs are not clearly understood. It appears that in the ewe, luteolysis is directly induced in the large cell by $PGF_{2\alpha}$. Large cells contain the majority of high-affinity receptors for $PGF_{2\alpha}$ (10). Recent evidence suggests that the effects of $PGF_{2\alpha}$ are mediated via calcium-induced intracellular events since $PGF_{2\alpha}$ produced a transient peak and sustained increase in cytosolic-free calcium ($[Ca^{++}]_i$) in large but not small cells (11–12; Wegner et al., submitted for publication). Luteolytic effects have been associated with intracellular calcium-mediated pathways in ovine large cells in which basal secretion of progesterone was inhibited ($P < 0.05$) by the phorbol ester TPA, a known activator of the calcium, phospholipid-dependent protein kinase (13–14). Phosphorylation of several endogenous proteins by activation of endogenous calcium-dependent protein kinases was greater in large than in small cells (15).

In addition to the induction of calcium-dependent second messenger pathways, the actions of $PGF_{2\alpha}$ may also be mediated by the maintenance of elevated $[Ca^{++}]_i$ above a level that is optimal for cellular function and progesterone secretion. Studies with myocardial cells (16–17) and hepatocytes (18) have demonstrated that cellular function is disrupted in the presence of sustained high levels of $[Ca^{++}]_i$ and cell death occurs if these levels are not returned to resting. Since the end result of luteal regression is cell death, a $PGF_{2\alpha}$-induced cytotoxicity resulting from sustained increases in $[Ca^{++}]_i$ might facilitate cellular degeneration.

Although the evidence from previous studies indicates that the effect of $PGF_{2\alpha}$ is mediated by alterations in $[Ca^{++}]_i$ in large luteal cells, several aspects of the $PGF_{2\alpha}$-induced calcium response and the role of calcium in luteolysis are still unclear. A better understanding of luteal function with regard to the initiation and mediation of luteolysis may require a greater knowledge of cellular localization and movement of calcium, as well as an appreciation of differences in calcium metabolism between large and small cells. The present study was conducted to compare the ability of ovine large and small luteal cells to regulate $[Ca^{++}]_i$ and to determine whether alterations in $[Ca^{++}]_i$ affect secretion of progesterone in either cell type.

Materials and Methods

Unless otherwise indicated, all chemicals were purchased from Sigma Chemical Co. (St. Louis, MO); and the antibody to progesterone (GDN 337) was provided by Dr. G.D. Niswender.

Tissue Preparation. Ovine large and small luteal cells were prepared by elutriation from corpora lutea surgically collected from day 10 superovulated ewes, as described by Hild-Petito et al. (19).

Intracellular Calcium Measurements. Aliquots of large ($5 \times 10^5/3$ mL) or small ($1 \times 10^6/3$ mL) cells were loaded with 2 µM Fura-2AM (Molecular Probes, Eugene, OR). Fura-2 fluorescence was measured in an SLM8000C spectrofluorometer (SLM, Urbana, IL), as described by Martinez-Zaguilan (20) and converted to $[Ca^{++}]_i$ using the following formula: $[Ca^{++}]_i = kDa [(R - R_{min})/(R_{max} - R)]$, where $kDa = 140.9$ nM; $R_{min} = 0.4783$; $R_{max} = 5.079$; and R = ratio of fluorescence at 340 and 380 nm. The pH-corrected values for kDa, R_{min}, and R_{max} were determined by in situ calibration of small luteal cells loaded with Fura-2 (Wegner et al., submitted for publication).

Calcium Efflux and Uptake. Large ($2 \times 10^4/0.5$ mL) or small ($1 \times 10^5/0.5$ mL) cells were preloaded to isotopic equilibrium with 5-µCi/mL $^{45}Ca^{++}$ (17.2 mCi/mg, New England Nuclear, Boston). Efflux was initiated by transfer to incubation medium (37°C; $\pm LaCl_3$) and was terminated by rapid filtration (4°C) followed by liquid scintillation counting (Wegner et al., submitted for publication). Uptake was initiated by addition of large or small cells to medium containing $^{45}Ca^{++}$ (5 µCi/mL) ± $LaCl_3$ (1 mM). Following incubation (37°C), samples were processed by rapid filtration (4°C).

Cellular Incubations. All incubations were performed on suspended cells in complete Hanks medium (pH 7.15). However, when $LaCl_3$ was used, a modified medium was used in which NaH_2PO_4, $NaHCO_3$, and $MgSO_4$ were omitted (modified Hank's, pH 7.15, buffered with HEPES) to prevent formation of a precipitate. In this medium, basal secretion of progesterone and cellular viability were not affected. Cell viabilities were assessed at the end of 2-h incubation by trypan blue dye exclusion and were not affected by any treatment in either cell type.

Progesterone in Media. Media content of progesterone was determined by radioimmunoassay (19) after 2-h incubation in triplicate (37°C) of large (1 × 10^4/mL) or small (5 × 10^4/mL) cells.

Statistical Analysis. Each experiment (n) represents a different tissue preparation (1–3 animals). Statistical differences between multiple treatments were determined by ANOVA followed, where appropriate, by Student-Newman-Kuels multiple range testing.

Results

Steady state $[Ca^{++}]_i$ concentrations were similar in both cell types (large cells, 62 ± 5 nM, n = 5; small cells, 61 ± 4 nM, n = 3). Cytosolic-free $[Ca^{++}]_i$ was increased (P < 0.05) by the calcium ionophore, A23187, in small and large cells (Fig. 1). However, following 2-h incubation with A23187 (1 µM), which did not significantly reduce cellular viability (13), secretion of progesterone was inhibited (P < 0.05) in large cells but was not affected in small (Fig. 1).

The effect of $PGF_{2\alpha}$ (0.5 µM) on $[Ca^{++}]_i$ and secretion of progesterone was measured (data not shown). Large cells responded to $PGF_{2\alpha}$ with an immediate transient peak (87 ± 2 nM; n = 5) and sustained increase (37 ± 2; n = 5; measured after 10 min) above steady state in $[Ca^{++}]_i$. A small but significant decrease (P < 0.05) in secretion of progesterone (83 ± 4% control; n = 6, following 2-h incubation, pH 7.15, 37°C) was consistently produced by this treatment. Conversely, $PGF_{2\alpha}$ had no effect on $[Ca^{++}]_i$ or secretion of progesterone in small cells (data not shown).

Because A23187 had been shown to increase $[Ca^{++}]_i$ in small as well as large cells, but affected secretion of progesterone only in large, an investigation of the effect of blocking transmembrane calcium flux on the two cell types was made. Cellular uptake and efflux of $^{45}Ca^{++}$ were measured in small

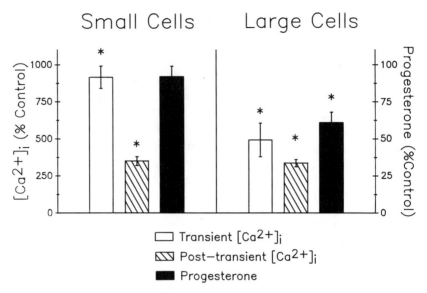

FIGURE 1. The effect of A23187 on $[Ca^{++}]_i$ and secretion of progesterone in small and large cells. Suspensions of small or large cells were incubated $\pm$A23187 (1 μM) as described in text. Measurement of $[Ca^{++}]_i$ was made immediately (open bars) or after 5 min (hatched bars) following addition of A23187. Progesterone content of the media was measured following 2-h incubation. (Values, statistically analyzed as absolute values, represent the mean $\pm$ SE (n = 3); *P < 0.05 different from control.)

and large cells incubated with the calcium antagonist, $LaCl_3$ (Fig. 2). Uptake was inhibited (P < 0.05) by $LaCl_3$ to a similar extent in large and small cells at all time points measured (2–15 min). Efflux of calcium was also inhibited (P < 0.05) by $LaCl_3$ to the same extent in both cell types.

Addition of $LaCl_3$ (1 mM) to suspensions of large cells loaded with Fura-2 caused an increase in flourescence, presumably an increase in $[Ca^{++}]_i$ (Fig. 3). This increase reached a new steady state level within 10 min (the time point shown), which was similar to that observed with $PGF_{2\alpha}$ or $LaCl_3$ + $PGF_{2\alpha}$. Secretion of progesterone in large cells was inhibited (P < 0.05) to a similar extent by $PGF_{2\alpha}$, $LaCl_3$, or $PGF_{2\alpha}$ + $LaCl_3$ (Fig. 3). Preincubation of large cells with $LaCl_3$ (5 min), followed by the addition of $PGF_{2\alpha}$, completely abolished the transient peak of increased $[Ca^{++}]_i$ observed with PGF_{2a} alone (data not shown, Wegner et al., submitted for publication). Although $LaCl_3$ inhibited $^{45}Ca^{++}$ uptake and efflux in small cells (Fig. 2), it did not produce an increase in $[Ca^{++}]_i$ at any time (Fig. 3). In addition, no increase in $[Ca^{++}]_i$ was measured by incubation of small cells with $PGF_{2\alpha}$ or $PGF_{2\alpha}$ + $LaCl_3$. There was also no effect of $PGF_{2\alpha}$, $LaCl_3$, or $PGF_{2\alpha}$ + $LaCl_3$ on secretion of progesterone in small cells.

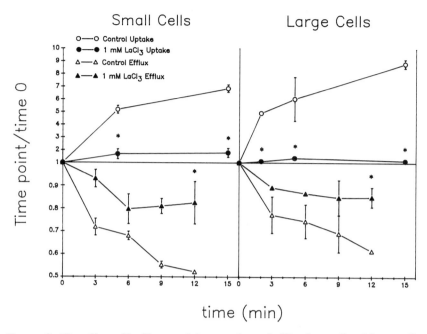

FIGURE 2. The effect of LaCl₃ on calcium uptake and efflux in small and large cells. Small or large cells were incubated (modified Hank's medium) for measurement of cellular uptake or efflux of ^{45}C (as described in text). Incubations were for designated times, ±LaCl₃ (1 mM). (Values, statistically analyzed as absolute values, are mean ± SE ratio relative to time 0 [n = 2, in duplicate]; *P < 0.05 different from control.)

Since La^{+++} antagonizes the action of Ca^{++} by displacement of Ca^{++} from its binding sites (22), there was a possibility that the increase in fluorescence of Fura-2 observed in large cells might be due to La^{+++} binding directly to Fura-2 rather than an actual increase in $[Ca^{++}]_i$. Therefore, a number of control experiments were performed (data not shown). The results of those experiments demonstrated that *(a)* in cell-free incubations, La^{+++} but not Ca^{++} lowered the flourescence of Fura-2 at 360 nm (the isoexcitation wavelength of Fura-2), whereas fluorescence at 360 nm in large cell incubations was not affected by La^{+++}; *(b)* La^{+++} did not produce an increase in flourescence in large cells incubated with BAPTA (5 µM, intracellular chelator of Ca^{++}); *(c)* in large cells co-loaded with Fura-2 and snarf-1 (fluorescent indicator of intracellular pH), La^{+++} produced an increase in $[Ca^{++}]_i$, but no change in intracellular pH; *(d)* the increase in $[Ca^{++}]_i$ stimulated by La^{+++} was observed in large cells pre-incubated with probenecid (2.5 mM, organic anion transport inhibitor), indicating no interaction of La^{+++} with Fura-2 that

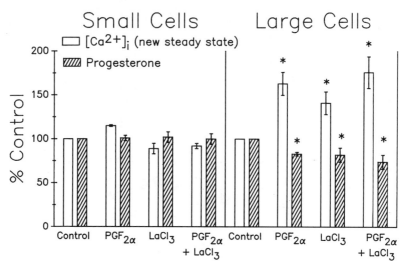

FIGURE 3. The effect of $LaCl_3$ ($\pm PGF_{2\alpha}$) on $[Ca^{++}]_i$ and secretion of progesterone in small and large cells. Suspensions of small or large cells were incubated (modified Hank's medium as described in text) for measurement of $[Ca^{++}]_i$ (open bars) at steady state (control), or 10 min after the addition of $PGF_{2\alpha}$ (0.5 µM), $LaCl_3$ (1 mM), or $PGF_{2\alpha}$ + $LaCl_3$. Measurement of progesterone content of the media was made following 2-h incubation. (Values, statistically analyzed as absolute values, are expressed as mean ± SE; n = 3, $[Ca^{++}]_i$; n = 4, small cells; n = 7, large cells, progesterone; *P < 0.05 different from control.)

had leaked to the extracellular compartment; and *(e)* large cell viability was not affected after 2-h incubation with $LaCl_3$.

Discussion

Several recent studies have presented evidence for the role of calcium and calcium-dependent intracellular pathways in mediating the effects of $PGF_{2\alpha}$ at the level of the luteal cell (11, 13–14, 23–26). However, little information is available regarding luteal cell regulation of $[Ca^{++}]_i$ and the relationship between alterations in $[Ca^{++}]_i$ and secretion of progesterone. The studies performed here demonstrate that ovine large luteal cells respond to various means of increasing $[Ca^{++}]_i$ to a more consistent degree than do small cells, and this increase in $[Ca^{++}]_i$ is related to an inhibition of secretion of progesterone.

The calcium ionophore, A23187, produced an increase in $[Ca^{++}]_i$ in small as well as large cells; however, secretion of progesterone was inhibited (P < 0.05) only in large. Both cell types appear to utilize transmembrane calcium flux (uptake and efflux) in part for maintenance of intracellular $[Ca^{++}]_i$

homeostasis. Furthermore, steady state $[Ca^{++}]_i$ concentrations were the same in resting large and small cells.

Inhibition of transmembrane Ca^{++} flux with $LaCl_3$ in both cell types produced a sustained increase in $[Ca^{++}]_i$ in large but not small cells. These results provide evidence that small cells possess a greater capacity than large to buffer intracellular $[Ca^{++}]_i$. Secretion of progesterone was inhibited in large but not small cells incubated with $LaCl_3$.

Essential to the understanding of the role of calcium in luteal regression is a basic knowledge of the localization and movements of calcium involved in the actions of $PGF_{2\alpha}$. $PGF_{2\alpha}$ induced a transient peak and sustained increase in $[Ca^{++}]_i$ in large but not small cells, and likewise produced an inhibition of secretion of progesterone only in the large. When large cells were pre-incubated with $LaCl_3$, followed by addition of $PGF_{2\alpha}$, the transient peak of increased $[Ca^{++}]_i$ was abolished. These results provide evidence that extra-cellular calcium is involved in producing the transient peak of increased $[Ca^{++}]_i$ induced by $PGF_{2\alpha}$ in large cells. However, nonlinear curve fitting analysis of the recovery phase of the $PGF_{2\alpha}$-induced calcium transient in large cells best fit a two-compartment model consisting of a rapidly and a slowly exchanging compartment (12; Wegner et al., submitted for publication). The transient increase in $[Ca^{++}]_i$ induced in large cells by $PGF_{2\alpha}$ was not abolished in calcium-free medium (Wegner et al., submitted for publication). Therefore, an intracellular as well as an extracellular source of Ca^{++} are likely to both contribute.

The importance of calcium efflux in maintaining calcium homeostasis in large cells has been suggested by two approaches. Cellular efflux was stimu-lated by $PGF_{2\alpha}$ in large cells (12, and Wegner et al., submitted for publica-tion). By kinetic analysis, this appeared to contribute to the decay of $[Ca^{++}]_i$ from the transient peak to the new steady state $[Ca^{++}]_i$ levels. In addition, in the present study, an increase in $[Ca^{++}]_i$ was observed in large but not small cells incubated with $LaCl_3$. If intracellular calcium stores in large cells do not have the ability to adequately buffer calcium and calcium efflux is inhibited, then an increase in $[Ca^{++}]_i$ would be expected. The observation that $LaCl_3$ did not cause an increase in $[Ca^{++}]_i$ in small cells suggests that large and small cells use different strategies to regulate $[Ca^{++}]_i$ and that large cells depend heavily on cellular efflux of Ca^{++} to restore increases in $[Ca^{++}]_i$ to steady state levels. A reduced ability to recover from a calcium load may be involved in large cell susceptibility to cytotoxic effects of increased $[Ca^{++}]_i$ during luteolysis.

There appears to be a relationship between increased $[Ca^{++}]_i$ and inhibi-tion of steroidogenesis in large but not small cells, suggesting a contributory role of $[Ca^{++}]_i$ in mediating functional luteolysis in these cells. Secretion of progesterone was inhibited in large cells by A23187, $PGF_{2\alpha}$, and $LaCl_3$, all agents that produced transient and/or sustained increases in $[Ca^{++}]_i$. It has been observed that reducing the increases in $[Ca^{++}]_i$ induced by $PGF_{2\alpha}$

(under conditions of lower extracellular calcium) prevented the inhibition of secretion of progesterone (Wegner et al., submitted for publication). Whereas, these results suggest that increased $[Ca^{++}]_i$ levels may be directly involved in mediating the inhibition of progesterone secretion, increasing $[Ca^{++}]_i$ for a sustained period of time may also trigger events involved in structural alterations associated with luteolysis.

In summary, the results of these experiments demonstrated a $PGF_{2\alpha}$-induced $[Ca^{++}]_i$ response in ovine large but not small luteal cells. Increases in $[Ca^{++}]_i$ produced by A23187, $PGF_{2\alpha}$, and $LaCl_3$ appear to be linked to inhibition of secretion of progesterone in large cells. In addition, this study provided evidence that large and small cells differ in their ability to regulate cytosolic-free calcium homeostasis. These differences may be critical to the role of $PGF_{2\alpha}$ in producing a direct luteolytic effect on large cells to induce luteal regression.

Acknowledgments. The authors wish to thank Dr. R.J. Gillies and R. Martinez-Zaguilan for contributions to the Fura-2 spectrofluorescence studies, and Dr. M.E. Wise, S. Marion, and W. Englenberg for their assistance. This work was supported in part by NIH grants HD-20613, HL-07249 and BRSG RR-05675.

References

1. Fitz TA, Mayan MH, Sawyer HR, Gamboni F, Niswender GD. Characterization of two steroidogenic cell types in ovine corpus luteum. Biol Reprod 1982; 27:703.
2. Rodgers RJ, O'Shea JD. Purification, morphology and progesterone production and content of three cell types isolated from the corpus luteum of the sheep. Aust J Biol Sci 1982;35:441.
3. Rodgers RJ, O'Shea JD, Findaly JK. Progesterone production in vitro by small and large ovine luteal cells. J Reprod Fertil 1983;69:113.
4. Hoyer PB, Fitz TA, Niswender GD. Hormone-independent activation of adenylate cyclase in large steroidogenic ovine luteal cells does not result in increased progesterone secretion. Endocrinology 1984;114:604.
5. Harrison LM, Kenny N, Niswender GD. Progesterone production, LH receptors, and oxytocin secretion by ovine luteal cell types on days 6, 10 and 15 of the oestrous cycle and day 25 of pregnancy. J Reprod Fertil 1987;79:539.
6. Hoyer PB, Niswender, GD. The regulation of steroidogenesis is different in the two types of ovine luteal cells. Can J Physiol Pharmacol 1985;63:240.
7. Hoyer PB, Niswender GD. Adenosine 3',5'-monophosphate-binding capacity in small and large ovine luteal cells. Endocrinology 1986;119:1822.
8. McCracken JA, Glew ME, Scaramuzzi RJ. Corpus luteum regression induced by prostaglandin $F_{2\alpha}$. J Clin Endocrinol Metab 1970;30:544.
9. Horton EW, Poyser NL. Uterine luteolytic hormone; A physiological role for prostaglandin $F_{2\alpha}$. Physiol Rev 1976;56:595.

10. Balapure AK, Caicedo IC, Kawada K, Watt DS, Rexroad CE, Fitz TA. Multiple classes of PGF$_{2\alpha}$ binding sites in subpopulations of ovine cells. Biol Reprod 1989;41:385.
11. Wiltbank MC, Guthrie PB, Mattson MP, Kater SB, Niswender GD. Hormonal regulation of free intracellular calcium concentrations in small and large ovine luteal cells. Biol Reprod 1989;41:771.
12. Hoyer PB, Wegner JA, Martinez-Zaguilan R, Gillies RJ. Critical levels of cytosolic-free calcium relate to optimal secretion of progesterone in ovine large luteal cells [Abstract]. Endocrine Society, 1990.
13. Hoyer PB, Marion SL. Influence of agents that affect intracellular calcium regulation on progesterone secretion in small and large luteal cells of sheep. J Reprod Fertil 1989;86:445.
14. Wiltbank MC, Knickerbocker JJ, Niswender GD. Regulation of the corpus luteum by protein kinase C, I. Phosphorylation activity and steroidogenic action in large and small ovine luteal cells. Biol Reprod 1989;40:1194.
15. Hoyer PB, Kong W. Protein kinase A and C activities and endogenous substrates in ovine small and large luteal cells. Mol Cell Endocrinol 1989;62:203.
16. Buja LM, Hagler HK, Willerson JT. Altered calcium homeostasis in the pathogenesis of myocardial ischemic and hypoxic injury. Cell Calcium 1988;9:205.
17. Dhalla NS, Panagia V, Singal PK, Makino N, Dixon IMC, Eyolfson DA. Alterations in heart membrane calcium transport during the development of ischemia-reperfusion injury. J Mol Cell Cardiol 1988;20(suppl 2):3.
18. Starke PE, Hoek JB, Farber JL. Calcium-dependent and calcium-independent mechanisms of irreversible cell injury in cultured hepatocytes. J Biol Chem 1986;261:3006.
19. Hild-Petito S, Ottobre AC, Hoyer PB. Comparison of subpopulations of luteal cells obtained from cyclic and superovulated ewes. J Reprod Fertil 1987;80:537.
20. Martinez-Zaguilan R, Martinez GM, Gillies RJ. Simultaneous measurement of intracellular pH and Ca^{2+} using the fluorescence of snarf-1 and fura-2. Am J Physiol (in press).
21. Williams JA, Korc M, Dormer RL. Action of secretagogues on a new preparation of functionally intact, isolated pancreatic acini. Am J Physiol 1987;235:E517.
22. Langer G, Frank J. Lanthanum in heart cell culture. Effect on calcium exchange correlates with its localization. J Cell Biol 1972;54:441.
23. Davis JS, Weakland LL, Weiland DA, Farese RV, West LA. Prostaglandin F$_{2\alpha}$ stimulates phosphatidylinositol 4,5-bisphosphate hydrolysis and mobilizes intracellular Ca^{2+} in bovine luteal cells. Proc Natl Acad Sci USA 1987;84:3728.
24. Conley AJ, Ford SP. TPA and PGF$_{2\alpha}$ inhibition of basal progesterone secretion by ovine luteal cells in different oxygen environments. Biol Reprod 1988; 38(suppl 1):398.
25. Alila HW, Corradino RA, Hansel W. Differential effects of luteinizing hormone on intracellular free Ca^{2+} in small and large bovine luteal cells. Endocrinology 1989;124:2314.
26. Pepperell JR, Preston SL, Behrman HR. The antigonadotropic action of prostaglandin F$_{2\alpha}$ is not mediated by elevated cytosolic calcium levels in rat luteal cells. Endocrinology 1989;125:144.

22

Presence of an Endogenous Inhibitor of Protein Kinase C Throughout Pseudopregnancy in the Rat Ovary

KATHLEEN M. EYSTER

The calcium- and lipid-dependent protein kinase (protein kinase C) is an intracellular messenger for the phospholipase C/polyphosphoinositide pathway. This pathway has been shown to be an important transduction system in hormone action (1) and plays a role in many other cell activities (2–4). It has been proposed that the hormonal control of ovarian function utilizes the phospholipase C/protein kinase C transduction pathway (5). We recently reported that an endogenous inhibitor of protein kinase C was present in the rat ovary on day 7 of pseudopregnancy (6). The presence of an endogenous inhibitor of protein kinase C presents a potential mechanism for regulation of the enzyme in addition to the well-characterized diacylglycerol, phospholipid, and calcium activators. These studies were undertaken to determine whether the activity of the endogenous inhibitor of protein kinase C varied throughout pseudopregnancy in the rat ovary.

Methods

Immature female Sprague-Dawley rats, 27 days old, were injected sc with 20-IU pregnant mares' serum gonadotropin (PMSG) followed 48 h later by a sc injection of 20-IU human chorionic gonadotropin (hCG) to induce pseudopregnancy. Ovaries were obtained throughout pseudopregnancy from 4 sets of rats. In each set of rats, the ovaries were removed on day 0 (immediately after hCG injection) and on days 3, 7, 10, and 13 of pseudopregnancy and the tissues were pooled. Each pool contained tissues from 2–4 rats. The tissues were stored at −70° until use. At that time, the ovaries were homogenized in a Tris-HCl homogenization buffer (pH 7.4) at a dilution of 1:5

(w/v), and cytosol was prepared as previously described (7). All experiments were performed in duplicate on each pool of tissue.

The assay for protein kinase C measured the transfer of the terminal phosphate from [γ^{32}P]ATP to histone III-S as described (7). Enzyme activity was measured in the absence and presence of calcium (0.1 mM) and lipids (0.8-μg/mL 1,2-dioleoyl rac-glycerol and 20-μg/mL phosphatidylserine). Protein phosphorylation in the absence of calcium and lipid was subtracted from phosphorylation in their presence, and the resulting value represented specific calcium- and lipid-dependent protein kinase activity. The limit of detection was 0.1 pM/min; that is, phosphorylation values that did not exceed 0.1 pM/min after subtracting noncalcium- and lipid-dependent phosphorylation were considered to be nondetectable. Protein content was determined by the BioRad Bradford protein assay (8). Data are expressed as picomoles of ^{32}P transferred from [γ^{32}P]ATP to histone III-S per minute times milligrams of sample protein (pM/min × mg). Mixing experiments were performed as described (6). The partial purification of protein kinase C on DEAE ion exchange media utilized a batch technique in a test tube (6). Data were analyzed by analysis of variance. The sources of all chemicals, reagents and other materials have been reported elsewhere (6).

Results

The specific activity of protein kinase C in the cytosols of rat ovaries obtained on days 0, 3, 7, 10, and 13 of pseudopregnancy was minimal and was below the limits of detection in many cytosol samples (Fig. 1). There were no significant differences in protein kinase C activity in ovarian cytosols between days of pseudopregnancy. Protein kinase C activity was significantly increased ($P < 0.05$) after partial purification of the cytosols on DEAE ion exchange matrix (Fig. 1). That is, samples in which protein kinase C activity was undetectable in cytosol contained readily measurable enzyme activity after DEAE purification. Protein kinase C activity in the DEAE eluent did not differ significantly among the test days throughout pseudopregnancy. It was not possible to accurately calculate the percent recovery from the DEAE because of the minimal activity in the cytosol. However, recovery was clearly greater than 100% in all cases.

Ovarian cytosols from days 0, 3, 7, 10, and 13 of pseudopregnancy were mixed with a control source of protein kinase C consisting of rat brain cytosol, which had been partially purified on DEAE. When ovarian cytosols from the test days throughout pseudopregnancy were mixed with control protein kinase C, there was a significant inhibition of control enzyme activity ($P < 0.05$, Table 1). The inhibition by ovarian cytosols did not vary significantly throughout pseudopregnancy.

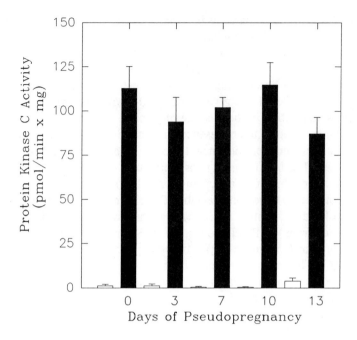

FIGURE 1. Specific activity of protein kinase C in ovarian cytosol (open bars) and after partial purification on DEAE (closed bars) on days 0, 3, 7, 10, and 13 of pseudopregnancy. (Values are the mean ± SEM; n = 8.)

TABLE 1. Rat ovarian cytosol from test days during pseudopregnancy mixed with rat brain DEAE eluent.

	Protein Kinase C Activity (pM/min × mg)	Percent of Control
Control, brain eluent	1409.3 ± 320	100
Control, plus ovarian cytosol		
Day 0	92.6 ± 14*	7
Day 3	84.2 ± 17*	7
Day 7	97.7 ± 20*	8
Day 10	102.9 ± 20*	8
Day 13	86.8 ± 17*	7

Note: Values are the mean ± SEM, n = 8.
*Significantly different from control (P < 0.05).

Discussion

The data indicate that the endogenous inhibitor of protein kinase C is present in the rat ovary throughout pseudopregnancy. The domination of protein kinase C activity in ovarian cytosols by the endogenous inhibitor does not vary over the course of pseudopregnancy nor is there variation in the inhibition of control protein kinase C activity by the addition of ovarian cytosols from the test days throughout pseudopregnancy.

The phospholipase C/polyphosphoinositide system plays a critical role in many cell functions, including hormone action (1), cell growth and differentiation (2), and oncogene action (3). Thus, there are important physiological implications to the identification of an endogenous inhibitor of protein kinase C. The inhibitor adds another site through which regulation of protein kinase C could occur. The role of the endogenous inhibitor of protein kinase C in the pseudopregnant ovary may involve modulation of the action of one or more of the multiple hormones that affect ovarian function, or its role may be related to other aspects of cell function.

There are multiple levels at which regulation of the endogenous inhibitor could occur. For example, the quantity of the inhibitor could be regulated relative to the changing physiology of the rat ovary during pseudopregnancy. However, the data presented herein indicate that the inhibitor activity does not vary significantly throughout pseudopregnancy, which further suggests that regulation of the endogenous inhibitor of protein kinase C in the rat ovary does not occur through regulation of the quantity of the inhibitor.

It may be that the endogenous inhibitor is regulated by phosphorylation (9). For example, hormonal activation of another second messenger pathway such as the adenylate cyclase system could result in phosphorylation of the endogenous inhibitor and cause activation (or inactivation) of the inhibitor. There are interactions between the adenylate cyclase and phospholipase C/polyphosphoinositide pathways (10, 11); perhaps the endogenous inhibitor of protein kinase C is the site of some of these interactions. Hormonal regulation via phosphorylation would not require that the amount of the endogenous inhibitor vary.

Alternatively, the endogenous inhibitor may not be specifically regulated. It may be that the role of the endogenous inhibitor of protein kinase C in the pseudopregnant rat ovary is to hold the enzyme in an inactive state in the cytosol until specific physiologic activation occurs. The inhibition of protein kinase C is not overcome by the presence of calcium, diacylglycerol, and phosphatidylserine; however, the inhibitor does appear to be water soluble. Thus, the translocation of protein kinase C from cytosol to the membrane in vivo might release the inhibition by physically removing the enzyme from its inhibitor. Both cAMP- and cGMP-dependent protein kinases are activated by release of inhibition (12), although by different mechanisms. Release of inhibition through translocation would be a logical method for activation of protein kinase C. However, if this were the case one might expect to find endogenous inhibitors of protein kinase C in all tissues. Endogenous inhibitors of protein kinase C in other tissues have been reported (6, 9, 13–15). However, the endogenous inhibitor has not been shown to dominate the activity of protein kinase C in all of these tissues. If the role of the endogenous inhibitor of protein kinase C is to hold the enzyme in an inactive state until physiological stimulation occurs, then the question remains as to why the activity of protein kinase C of the pseudopregnant rat is dominated by the inhibitor whereas that of many other tissues is not.

On the other hand, translocation of protein kinase C from cytosol to membranes may not remove the enzyme from its inhibitor. If this is the case, then protein kinase C might remain completely inhibited throughout pseudopregnancy in the rat. If protein kinase C is inhibited, then all activation of phosphoinositol turnover would be shunted to the inositol trisphosphate/calcium arm of the phospholipase C/phosphoinositol pathway.

Conclusion

The endogenous inhibitor of protein kinase C appears to maintain a constant level of activity in the rat ovary throughout pseudopregnancy. The physiological role of the endogenous inhibitor in the pseudopregnant rat ovary is unknown. However, studies of the function of the inhibitor show promise both for the elucidation of ovarian function and at the level of the biochemical interactions of protein kinase C and its inhibitor.

Acknowledgments. The author expresses appreciation to Mary S. Waller for her excellent technical assistance. The research reported in this chapter was supported in part by NIH grant HD-26640 and USDSM Parson's Fund.

References

1. Nishizuka N. Studies and perspectives of protein kinase C. Science 1986;233: 305-12.
2. Macara IG. Oncogenes, ions, and phospholipids. Am J Physiol 1985;248:C3-C11.
3. Berridge MJ, Heslop JP, Irvine RF, Brown KD. Inositol lipids and cell proliferation. Biochem Soc Trans 1985;13:67-71.
4. David JD, Faser CR, Perrot GP. Role of protein kinase C in chick embryo skeletal myoblast fusion. Dev Biol 1990;139:89-99.
5. Clark MR, Kawai Y, Davis JS, LeMaire WJ. Ovarian protein kinases. In: Toft DO, Ryan RJ, eds. 5th Ovarian Workshop. Champaign, IL: Ovarian Workshops, 1985:383-401.

6. Eyster KM. An endogenous inhibitor of protein kinase C in the pseudopregnant rat ovary. Biochem Biophys Res Commun 1990;168:609-15.
7. Eyster KM, Clark MR. Nonsteroidal antiestrogen inhibition of protein kinase C in human corpus luteum and placenta. Biochem Pharmacol 1989;38:3497-3503.
8. Bradford MM. A rapid and sensitive method for the quantitation of microgram quantities of protein utilizing the principle of protein-dye binding. Anal Biochem 1976;72:248-54.
9. Pearson JD, DeWald DB, Mathews WR, et al. Amino acid sequence and characterization of a protein inhibitor or protein kinase C. J Biol Chem 1990;265: 4583-91.
10. Beckner SK, Farrar WL. Interleukin 2 modulation of adenylate cyclase. Potential role of protein kinase C. J Biol Chem 1986;261:3043-7.
11. Naghshineh S, Noguchi M, Huang K-P, Londos C. Activation of adipocyte adenylate cyclase by protein kinase C. J Biol Chem 1986;261:14534-8.
12. Roach PJ. Protein kinases. Methods Enzymol 1984;107:81-101.
13. Huang C-K, Oshana SC. Partial characterization of protein kinase C and inhibitor activity of protein kinase C in rabbit peritoneal neutrophils. J Leukocyte Biol 1986;39:671-8.
14. Schwantke N, LePeuch CJ. A protein kinase C inhibitory activity is present in rat brain homogenate. FEBS Lett 1984;177:36-40.
15. Anderson WB, Salomon DS. Calcium, phospholipid-dependent protein kinase C as a cellular receptor for phorbol ester tumor promoters: Possible role in modulating cell growth and tumor promotion. In: Kuo JF, ed. Phospholipids and cellular regulation; vol. 2. Boca Raton, FL: CRC Press, 1985:127-70.

23

Effects of Gonadotropins and PGE$_2$ on Ovarian Adenylate Cyclase in Cellular Membrane from Mature Cyclic Cows

SERGE-ALAIN WANDJI, M.A. FORTIER, AND M.-A. SIRARD

It is well accepted that gonadotropins play a major role in the processes of growth and differentiation of ovarian follicles (1). Although this observation was derived mainly from studies done in the rat (2, for a review), gonadotropins are used today to induce superovulation in domestic animals. However, in cattle, superovulation treatments induce variable responses, which reflect the poor knowledge of folliculogenesis in this species (3, 4). It is widely acknowledged that in many mammalian species, FSH stimulates ovarian adenylate cyclase (AC) activity (5) leading to the accumulation of cAMP in granulosa cells (6). In addition, the role of cAMP as a second messenger in the mechanism of action of FSH has been well demonstrated. This includes stimulation of steroidogenesis and induction of LH receptors— effects that could be mimicked by cAMP analogs (7). Furthermore, prostaglandin E$_2$ (PGE$_2$) also stimulates cAMP production and has been proposed to mimic some of the FSH effects even in granulosa cells that have not already gained full sensitivity to FSH (8). FSH receptors have been demonstrated in granulosa membranes as early as the pre-antral stage in the rat ovary (9).

In this study, we elected to characterize adenylate cyclase response to FSH as a preliminary effort to study the relation between follicular stage, animal age, and FSH responsiveness in cattle. We have found a higher and more consistent effect of PGE$_2$ compared to FSH on bovine ovarian adenylate cyclase in preliminary studies (10). Therefore, the effect of PGE$_2$ was also evaluated in this study.

Materials and Methods

Membrane Preparation. Cow ovaries contralateral to ovulation were obtained at a slaughter house and immediately immersed in a Hank's solution at 4°C until arrival at the laboratory. Ovaries were dissected longitudinally in Hank's solution, and the hile and ligaments were removed. The pieces of gonads were immersed in 5 volumes of cyclase homogenization buffer (CHB, pH 7.6) composed of 0.05-M Na$^+$-N-2-hydroxyethylpiperarazine-N'-2-ethane sulfonic acid (HEPES), 0.001-M ethyleneglycol-bis (β-aminoethylether)-N,N'-tetraacetic acid (EGTA), and 10% dimethyl sulfoxide (DMSO) at 4°C and then minced in pieces smaller than 4 mm. Ovarian minces were further homogenized twice for 15 sec with an interval of 20 sec, using a polytron tissue disintegrator (Brinkman PT-10) at 40% of maximum velocity. The resulting homogenate was then filtered through glass wool and centrifuged at 600 × g for 10 min at 4°C. The supernatant was resuspended in 5 volumes of CHB and centrifuged at 40,000 × g for 20 min at 4°C. The pellet was washed twice, resuspended in CHB to obtain a protein concentration between 1.0 and 1.5 mg/mL, and used fresh.

Adenylate Cyclase Assay. Adenylate cyclase activity was defined as the enzymatic conversion of α-[^{32}P]ATP to [^{32}P]cAMP after 5 min (unless specified otherwise). The method was as used previously for cow endometrium (11) and described in detail elsewhere (12).

In the first round of experiments, 40-μL homogenates of 6 contralateral cow ovaries were incubated for 5 min at 37°C (pH 7.5) in an incubation medium containing 150-mM HEPES, 3-mM IBMX (Sigma Chemical Co., St. Louis, MO), 75-mM MgCl$_2$, 30-mM KCl, 0.2-mg/mL creatin phosphokinase, 2-mM creatin phosphate, 0.25-mM ATP (Boerhringer), 1-mM DTT (Sigma), and approximately 5 × 10^5 CPM [^{32}P]ATP. The final volume of incubation was 150 μL. 5-μg/mL FSH (NIADDK-oFSH-17, a gift from Dr. Raiti, National Hormone and Pituitary program, Maryland) and 10^{-4}M PGE$_2$ (Sigma) were used for hormonal stimulations. FSH and PGE$_2$ treatments were used in the presence of 75-μM GTP. While 300-μM GPP (Boehringer Mannhein, Canada), 10^{-2}M forskolin (Sigma), and 10^{-2}M sodium fluoride were used as positive controls for the stimulation of adenylate cyclase, 10^{-4}M Ca^{++} was used as a negative control of cAMP production. In addition, 3 contralateral ovaries were digested with trypsin (0.030%, Sigma), collagenase (0.020%, Sigma), and DNAse (0.010%, Sigma) as a different method of homogenization, and the resulting 40,000 × g pellet was incubated as described above for adenylate cyclase assay. The reaction was stopped by the addition of 100 μL of a solution containing 40-mM ATP, 10-mM cAMP, 30-mM SDS, and 3 × 10^{4}cpm [^{3}H]cAMP, followed by boiling at 90°C during 3 min. The [^{32}P]cAMP formed was isolated by chromatography using Dowex (AG 50W-X4) and alumina columns as described before (11). The imidazole (Sigma) eluates from alumina column were collected in scintillation vials and counted in a beta counter.

In the second experiment, 2 contralateral ovaries were homogenized as described for the first group in the first experiment. The effect of different concentrations of magnesium (1, 2, 5, 7.5, 10, and 75 mM) on adenylate cyclase activity was evaluated in the presence or absence of 75-µM GTP and 10^{-8}-M FSH. In the third experiment, the effect of different concentrations of GTP (7.5, 25, 50, and 75-µM) on the capacity of FSH to stimulate adenylate cyclase activity was evaluated using 3 ovaries. The incubation medium this time contained only 7.5-mM MgCl$_2$, the second experiment having suggested this Mg^{++} concentration as optimal. Experiment 4 was designed to compare FSH and PGE$_2$ effects on AC activity in optimal assay conditions obtained from the previous experiments. Twelve ovaries were directly homogenized as described above, and AC activity was measured after 15 min incubation at 32.5°C with MgCl$_2$ at 7.5 mM and GTP at 7.5 µM. In all experiments, protein concentration was determined by the method of Lowry et al. (13). Statistical analysis of the data was performed using a paired Student t-test, except for the data of experiment 4, which was analyzed according to the Split plot design (14).

Results

In the first experiment (Fig. 1, A and B) GTP caused 65% and 105% increases in adenylate cyclase activity over basal level (P < 0.001) in the total and the digested homogenate, respectively. FSH did not stimulate AC activity over

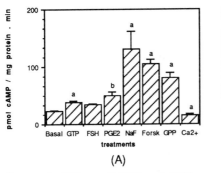
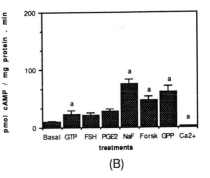

(A)   (B)

FIGURE 1. Effects of FSH and PGE$_2$ on AC activity. A: Whole bovine ovarian homogenate. (a, relative to basal, P < 0.01; DNAse; b, relative to GTP, P < 0.01.) B: Digested bovine ovarian homogenate. (Trypsin, 0.03%; collagenase, 0.02% and 0.01% in 15 mL of solution for 1 h at 37°C.)

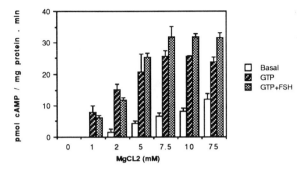

FIGURE 2. Effects of Mg^{++} concentration on the capacity of FSH to stimulate AC activity in bovine ovarian homogenate in the presence of 75-μM GTP. The incubation was for 5 min at 37°C. (Values are mean ± SE of triplicate determination of cAMP production in 2 separate experiments.)

GTP level either in total ovarian homogenate or in the enzymatic prepared membranes. PGE$_2$ induced 32% and 22% increases in cAMP production over GTP (P < 0.001) in total ovarian homogenate and digested cell membranes.

The lack of FSH effect could not be attributed to a disfunction of the AC system since GPP, a potent stimulator of the regulatory component of the enzyme induced a 3.5-fold increase in cAMP production (P < 0.001). Furthermore, forskolin, which stimulates the catalytic moiety of AC, induced a 4.5-fold increase in cAMP production (P < 0.001). The total activity of AC as assessed by fluoride was about 7 times the basal level (P < 0.001). On the other hand, Ca^{++} caused 30% and 74% reductions in AC activity in the total ovarian and in the granulosa membranes, respectively (P < 0.01 and 0.001). These results suggest that the lack of FSH effect could be related to the receptor coupling to the G-protein. Therefore, a second experiment was conducted to evaluate the effect of various concentrations of Mg and GTP on the capacity of FSH to stimulate AC activity.

In the absence of Mg^{++}, AC activity was undetectable and could not be stimulated by GTP, nor could FSH, NaF, GPP, and Forskolin (results not shown). There was an increase in basal production of cAMP in response to Mg^{++} up to 75-mM MgCl$_2$ (Fig. 2). The effect of GTP on cAMP production when expressed as percentage over the basal level averaged 600% between 1 and 7.5 mM and decreased at higher Mg^{++} concentrations. A weak effect of FSH (22% over that of GTP) required at least 5-mM Mg^{++}. Therefore, in the subsequent experiments, Mg^{++} concentration in the incubation medium was fixed at 7.5 mM.

When GTP concentration was increased from 0 to 25 μM, there was a linear increase in cAMP production (P < 0.05) with no further increase up to 75 μM as shown in Figure 3. It is of interest to note that a significant additive effect of FSH over GTP (30%; P < 0.05) was detectable only at 7.5-μM GTP.

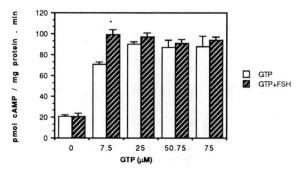

FIGURE 3. Effects of GTP concentration on the capacity of FSH to stimulate AC activity in bovine ovarian homogenate for 5 min at 37°C in the presence of 7.5-mM $MgCl_2$ and various concentrations of GTP. (Values are mean ± SE of triplicate determination of cAMP production in 3 separate experiments; *P < 0.05.)

In a separate experiment performed on bovine follicular homogenates, the effect of FSH on AC activity was optimal after either 15 min at 32.5°C or after 10 min at 37°C (unpublished data). Therefore, in the subsequent experiment, the incubations were carried out at 32.5°C for 15 min.

FSH (10^{-7}M) caused a 1.58-fold increase (P < 0.001) in AC activity compared to GTP after 15 min at 32.5°C in the whole ovarian homogenate (Fig. 4). PGE_2-induced cAMP production was 2.0-folds (P < 0.0001) that of GTP in the whole ovarian homogenate, and the sodium fluoride-induced stimulation of cAMP production was 15.4 times (P < 0.0001) that of the basal level (Fig. 4).

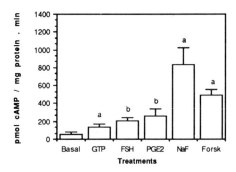

FIGURE 4. Effects of FSH and PGE_2 on AC activity in whole homogenates of 12 bovine ovaries. The homogenates were incubated for 15 min at 32.5°C in the presence of 7.5-mM Mg^{++}. Treatments were basal, 7.5-μM GTP, 5-μg/mL FSH, 10^{-4}M PGE_2, sodium fluoride (NaF), and forskolin. (Values are mean ± SE of triplicate determination of cAMP production in four separate experiments; a, relative to basal, P < 0.0001; b, relative to GTP, P < 0.001.)

Discussion

The results of the first experiment suggested that the AC system was functional since sodium fluoride, GPP, and forskolin all induced significant stimulation of the enzyme activity. On the other hand, Ca^{++} inhibited AC activity in both the whole ovarian homogenate and the enzymatic prepared membranes. Previous studies indicated that Ca^{++} also inhibited FSH-stimulated cAMP production in porcine ovarian cells and in cell-free membranes (15). The lack of FSH effect could then be located prior to the AC system, namely, at the hormone/receptor level. Moreover, PGE$_2$ significantly stimulated cAMP production in total ovarian homogenate, an indication that PGE$_2$ but not FSH receptors might be functionally coupled to the AC system. Therefore, the lack of FSH effect in this first experiment could suggest a weak couplage of FSH with its receptor in our assay conditions. Alternatively, the lack of FSH effect on AC activity could be due to the weak linkage between the FSH/receptor complex and the G-protein, i.e., the regulatory moeity of AC. This hypothesis is supported by results of the third experiment in which high levels of GTP interfere with the FSH effect on adenylate cyclase. It is of interest to note that previous reports on FSH receptors in calf's testis have suggested that GTP might increase the dissociation of the FSH/receptor complex from the regulatory component of AC (16). It is apparent from our results that Mg^{++} is important for basal as well as hormonal stimulation of AC activity. The effect of FSH required at least 5-mM Mg^{++}, which is in accordance with previous reports (15) that Mg^{++} regulates positively FSH receptors.

Granulosa cells of essentially all follicles have been found to possess receptors for FSH (9). The relatively low response of ovarian homogenate in terms of cAMP production in the presence of FSH can be explained using different hypothesis. First, the FSH receptors in small follicles, at least those in the pre-antral stage, may not be coupled to the AC system. The coupling of FSH receptors with AC could be effective only in larger antral follicles. Alternatively, FSH receptors in pre-antral follicles may represent a different population of receptors with lower affinity to the hormone. Therefore, it can be suggested that a threshold concentration of FSH is required to stimulate granulosa cell AC in pre-antral follicles. This is in agreement with the hypothesis that the preovulatory discharge of FSH is the stimulus for the recruitment of pre-antral follicles (17). Finally and more probably, the dilution effect due to protein from the interstitial tissue has to be considered to explain the lower response of the ovarian homogenate. Our results suggest a stimulation of cAMP accumulation by PGE$_2$ in ovarian granulosa cells. This prostaglandin has been found to be produced by ovarian follicles under LH stimulation (18). PGE$_2$ has also been shown to mimic some of the FSH effects on granulosa cells even at early stages of development when follicles do not respond to FSH (8). FSH has been shown to stimulate PGE_2 production in granulosa cells (19). The higher potency of PGE_2 than FSH required to stimulate cAMP production in whole ovarian homogenates may suggest that the action of this prostaglandin upon AC activity is less specific than that of FSH in the different compartments of the ovary.

In summary, our results suggest that PGE_2 together with FSH play an important role in the stimulation of bovine granulosa cells. A detailed study of the effects of FSH on different classes of follicles will probably be useful to assess a coupling index of FSH to its receptor in relation with follicle diameter.

References

1. Hisaw FL. Development of graafian follicle and ovulation. Physiol Rev 1947;27:97-119.
2. Richards JS. Protein hormone action a key to understanding ovarian follicular development. Biol Reprod 1976;14:82-94.
3. Anderson GB. Methods of producing twins in cattle.Therio 1978;9:3-16.
4. Monniaux D, Chapin D, Saumande J. Superovulation response in cattle. Therio 1983;19:55-81.
5. Knecht M, Manta T, Katz MS, Catt KJ. Regulation of adenylate cyclase activity by FSH and GnRH in cultured granulosa cells. Endocrinology1983;112:1247-55.
6. Kolena J, Channing CP. Stimulatory effect of LH, FSH and prostaglandins upon cAMP levels in porcine granulosa cells . Endocrinology 1972;90:1543-62.
7. Knecht M, Amsterdam A, Catt KJ. The regulatory role of cAMP in hormone-induced differentiation of granulosa cells. J Biol Chem 1981;256:10628-33.
8. Lamprecht SA, Zor U, Tsafriri A, Lindner HR. Action of prostaglandine E2 and of LH on ovarian adenylate cyclase, protein kinase and ornthine decarboxylase activity during postnatal development and maturity in the rat. J Endocrinol 1973;57:217-33.
9. Richards JS, Midgley AR, Jr. Protein hormone action: A key to understanding ovarian and luteal follicular development. Biol Reprod 1976;14:82-94.
10. Sirard MA, Fortier MA. Monolayer culture of claf ovaries as a model to study follicular development in the bovine. Biol Reprod 1986;34(suppl):225.
11. Fortier MA, Guilbault LA, Grasso F. Specific properties of epithelial and stromal cells from the endometrium of cows. J Reprod Fertil 1988;83:239-48.
12. Krall JF, Korenman SG. Regulation of uterine smooth muscle cell beta-adrenergic catecholamine-sensitive adenylate cyclase by Mg++ and guanylyl nucleotide. Biochem Pharmacol 1979;28:2771-5.
13. Lowry OH, Rosebrough NY, Farr AL, Randall RJ. J Biol Chem;193:265-75.
14. Snedecor WJ, Cochran WG. In: Cox DF, ed. Statistical methods. Iowa State Press, 1980:325-33.
15. Ford KA, Hunzicker-Dunn M, LaBarbera AR. Dissociated effects of cations on FSH receptors and FSH sensitive adenylyl cyclase in granulosa cells. 5th NIH Ovarian Workshop,1985.

16. Reichert LE, Jr, and Bosukonda D. FSH receptor in testis: Interaction with FSH, mechanism of signal transduction and properties of the purified receptor. Biol Reprod 1989;40:13-26.
17. Schwartz NB. The role of FSH and LH and their antibodies on follicle growth and on ovulation. Biol Reprod 1974;10:236-72.
18. Clark MR, Marsh JM, Lemaire WJ. Mechanism of LH regulation of prostaglandin synthesis in rat granulosa cells. J Biol Chem 1978;253:7757-61.
19. Bauminger S, Lindner RH. Effects of gonadotropin on prostaglandin production in the rat ovary. J Steroid Biochem 1974;5:402-13.
20. Erickson GF, Wang CR, Casper Mattson G, Hofeditz C. Studies on the mechanism of LH receptor control by FSH. Mol Cell Endocrinol 1982;27:17-30.

24

Sphingosine Derivatives, Calmodulin Inhibitors, and TMB-8: Inhibitors of Adenylate Cyclase Activity in Rat Luteal Membranes

M. Lahav, D. Barzilai, and O. Topaz

Prostaglandin $F_{2\alpha}$ (PGF) plays a major role in the initiation of luteal regression in many mammalian species (1). In luteal preparations incubated in vitro, PGF inhibited cAMP accumulation (2, 3). When adenylate cyclase activity was measured in luteal membranes, PGF added directly to the reaction mixture had no effect; however, exposure to PGF of intact corpora lutea in vitro or in vivo resulted in impaired adenylate cyclase activity in subsequently prepared luteal membranes (4).

The mechanism of action of PGF in luteal cells is at present still controversial and may vary among species. For the rat, an increase in calcium concentration and activation of protein kinase C apparently mimicked the effect of PGF (3, 5), but such a mechanism was not compatible with other findings (6–9). Although PGF has been found to stimulate phospholipase C activity in rat luteal tissue (7, 10), this activation did not always correlate with the effectiveness of PGF in suppressing cAMP production in the various preparations (7).

Recently, Sender-Baum and Ahren (5) reported that sphingosine and psychosine inhibited cAMP and progesterone production in rat luteal cell suspensions. Lysosphingolipids are known to inhibit protein kinase C (11); in the present study, we tested their ability to inhibit the activity of adenylate cyclase in luteal membranes.

Phenothiazines and W-7 are drugs known to inhibit calmodulin and protein kinase C, and 8-(N,N-diethylamino)-octyl-3,4,5-methoxybenzoate (TMB-8) has been shown to interfere with several calcium-related processes (references cited in 6, 8, 12). In experiments done in isolated corpora lutea, we observed that at higher concentrations, W-7 and TMB-8 inhibited LH-dependent cAMP accumulation (6, 8). Thus, we examined the effect of these and other drugs on luteal adenylate cyclase activity.

Materials and Methods

Pregnant mare serum gonadotropin (PMSG, 50 IU, sc) was administered to 29-day-old Sprague-Dawley rats; 72 h later, they received human chorionic gonadotropin (hCG, 25 IU, sc). The rats were sacrificed 96 h after hCG administration. Ovarian membranes were prepared essentially as previously described (4). Ovaries were minced and homogenized in sucrose buffer, using a Polytron. The homogenate was centrifuged ($160 \times g$, 5 min), and the supernatant was spun ($10,000 \times g$, 50 min). The sedimented membranes were resuspended in sucrose buffer (35- to 50-μg protein/20 μL).

Adenylate cyclase was assayed according to Torjesen and Aakvaag (13). Total volume of the incubation mixture was 60 μL. Incubation (20 min at 30°C) was usually started by the addition of membranes; when sphingolipids and phosphatidic acid were tested, the enzymatic reaction was started by adding ATP plus regenerating system after 30 min preincubation of all other components at 4°C. The reaction was terminated by boiling the test tubes; the samples were cooled, treated with alumina for 15 min, and centrifuged. The supernatant was then assayed for cAMP by modifications (6, 13) of the Gilman method.

In each individual experiment, 4 incubation tubes were used per treatment. Usually, results from several experiments were combined after normalization within each experiment to the mean value obtained for one treatment.

The sources of most materials have been described previously (6, 8). Chlorpromazine was donated by Dr. Jon Finberg, Department of Pharmacology, Technion Faculty of Medicine. Lipids, forskolin, and all components of the enzymatic reaction mixture were obtained from Sigma (St. Louis, MO). Stock solutions of sphingosine, psychosine, phosphatidic acid, and forskolin in DMSO, and aqueous stock solutions of sphingosylphosphorylcholine and GTPτS, were stored at –20°C.

Results

In the membrane fraction used in our study, adenylate cyclase activity could be stimulated by hCG, LH, and isoproterenol. LH was routinely used at 10 μg/mL. Sphingosine (up to 80 μM) had no significant effect on cAMP production; however, its solubility in the PIPES buffer was visibly inadequate. Since bovine serum albumin inhibited the LH-stimulated enzyme activity, we could not use it as a lipid carrier. Thus, we examined the effect of

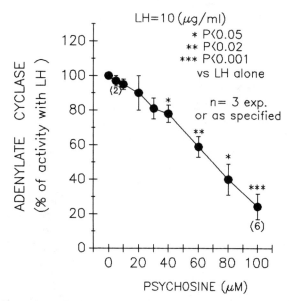

FIGURE 1. Effect of psychosine on adenylate cyclase activity in LH-treated luteal membranes. Presented are averaged results from several (generally 3) experiments, each with 4 incubations per treatment.

psychosine and sphingosylphosphorylcholine, lysosphingolipids with higher water solubility. Figure 1 presents a dose-response curve for psychosine in LH-treated membranes. A quantitatively similar curve was observed with sphingosylphosphorylcholine.

We then examined the effect of W-7 and TMB-8 on adenylate cyclase activity, in the presence of LH, at concentrations previously used in the incubation medium of intact corpora lutea. The inhibition observed was statistically significant, but partial (40%), and higher drug concentration did not increase it. With two phenothiazines, chlorpromazine (Fig. 2) and trifluoperazine, complete inhibition was achieved with similar dose dependence. Phosphatidic acid (0.01–10 μg/mL) did not inhibit the LH-dependent adenylate cyclase activity.

The next series of experiments was designed to locate more precisely the site at which the inhibitors interfered with the activity of adenylate cyclase. Thus, the effect of the inhibitors was examined in the presence of 3 stimulants: LH, GTPτS (a nonhydrolyzable guanine nucleotide, 1 μM), and forskolin (50 μM). The results are summarized in Figure 3.

With forskolin as stimulant, none of the inhibitors reduced adenylate cyclase activity in a statistically significant manner; however, values were more variable than those observed with the other stimulants. In membranes stimulated with GTPτS, all 5 inhibitors significantly suppressed adenylate

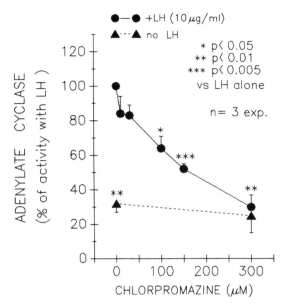

FIGURE 2. Effect of chlorpromazine on adenylate cyclase activity in luteal membranes. Presented are averaged results from 3 experiments.

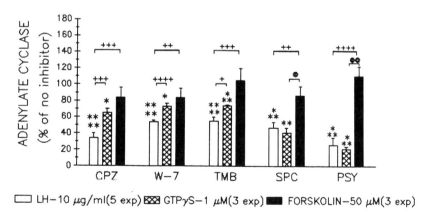

FIGURE 3. Effect of chlorpromazine (CPZ, 300 µM), W-7 (75 µM), TMB-8 (180 µM), sphingosylphosphorylcholine (SPC, 70 µM), and psychosine (PSY, 100 µM) on adenylate cyclase activity in the presence of LH, GTPτS, or forskolin. Presented are averaged results from 5 (LH) or 3 (GTPτS and forskolin) experiments. (*P < 0.025; **P < 0.01; ***P < 0.005; ****P < 0.001 vs. same stimulant but no inhibitor; +P < 0.05; ++P < 0.02; +++P < 0.01; ++++P < 0.005 vs. LH + same inhibitor; @P < 0.02; @@P < 0.005 vs. GTPτS + same inhibitor.)

cyclase activity, compared to the activity with GTPτS alone. In samples exposed to sphingosine derivatives, GTPτS-dependent and LH-dependent activities were both greatly—and similarly—inhibited. In contrast, the effect of the synthetic drugs was significantly smaller in the presence of GTPτS than in the presence of LH.

Discussion

In the present study, we showed that two lysosphingolipids, psychosine and sphingosylphosphorylcholine, inhibit luteal adenylate cyclase activity. Since inhibition occurred with LH and GTPτS as stimulants, but not with forskolin, the compounds probably act at the level of the G_s-protein. Alternatively, the lysophospholipids may act on the catalytic protein, but the mode of interference is such that forskolin abrogates it.

Inhibition of cAMP accumulation in rat luteal cell suspensions was previously reported by Sender-Baum and Ahren (5). However, in intact cells, sphingosine inhibited forskolin-induced cAMP accumulation as well. It is noteworthy that the inhibitory effect of PGF on cAMP in luteal cell suspensions was negligible with forskolin as stimulant (14). Furthermore, when rats were pretreated with a PGF analogue, luteal adenylate cyclase activity was impaired when stimulated with hCG or with a stable guanine nucleotide, but not with forskolin (13).

Presented originally as inhibitors of protein kinase C (13), sphingosine derivatives were later shown to inhibit some calmodulin-dependent enzymes (15) and Na,K-ATPase (14). Suppression of Na,K-ATPase followed a steep dose-response curve, very similar to that observed for adenylate cyclase.

It is intriguing that phenothiazines, and other calmodulin-inhibiting drugs, also demonstrate a similarly broad specificity: they have been reported to inhibit calmodulin, protein kinase C, Na,K-ATPase (12, and references in 8, 10), and now also adenylate cyclase. Interestingly, these drugs as well as sphingosine derivatives possess a positively charged nitrogen and a hydrophobic moiety. The significance of these findings awaits clarification.

Acknowledgments. This study was supported by the Chief Scientist's Office of the Israel Ministry of Health and by the Dario and Mathilde Beraha Fund for Hormones, Cancer, and Aging Research.

References

1. Rothchild I. The regulation of the mammalian corpus luteum. Recent Prog Horm Res 1981;37:183-298.

2. Lahav M, Freud A, Lindner HR. Abrogation by prostaglandin $F_{2\alpha}$ of LH- stimulated cyclic AMP accumulation in isolated rat corpora lutea of pregnancy. Biochem Biophys Res Commun 1976;68:1294-300.

3. Dorflinger LJ, Albert PJ, Williams AT, Behrman HR. Calcium is an inhibitor of luteinizing hormone-sensitive adenylate cyclase in the luteal cell. Endocrinology 1984;114:1208-15.

4. Khan MI, Rosberg S. Acute suppression by $PGF_{2\alpha}$ on LH, epinephrine, and fluoride stimulation of adenylate cyclase in rat luteal tissue. J Cyclic Nucleotide Protein Phosphor Res 1979;5:55-63.

5. Sender-Baum MG, Ahren KEB. Sphingosine and psychosine, suggested inhibitors of protein kinase C, inhibit LH effects in rat luteal cells. Mol Cell Endocrinol 1988;60:127-35.

6. Lahav M, Rennert H, Sabag K, Barzilai D. Calmodulin inhibitors and 8-(N,N-diethylamino)-octyl-3,4,5-trimethoxybenzoate (TMB-8) do not prevent the inhibitory effect of prostaglandin $F_{2\alpha}$ on cyclic AMP production in rat corpora lutea. J Endocrinol 1987;113:205-12.

7. Lahav M, West LA, Davis JS. Effect of prostaglandin $F_{2\alpha}$ and a gonadotropin-releasing hormone agonist on inositol phospholipid metabolism in isolated rat corpora lutea of various ages. Endocrinology 1988;123:1044-52.

8. Lahav M, Davis JS, Rennert H. Mechanism of the luteolytic action of prostaglandin F-2α in the rat. J Reprod Fertil 1989;37(suppl):233-40.

9. Musicki B, Aten RF, Behrman HR. The antigonadotropic actions of prostaglandin $F_{2\alpha}$ and phorbol ester are mediated by separate processes in rat luteal cells. Endocrinology 1990;126:1388-95.

10. Leung PCK, Minegishi T, Ma F, Zhou F, Ho-Yuen B. Induction of polyphosphoinositide breakdown in rat corpus luteum by prostaglandin $F_{2\alpha}$. Endocrinology 1986;119:12-8.

11. Hannun YA, Bell RM. Lysosphingolipids inhibit protein kinase C: implications for the sphingolipidoses. Science 1987;235:670-4.

12. Oishi K, Zheng B, Kuo JF. Inhibition of Na,K-ATPase and sodium pump by the protein kinase C regulators sphingosine, lysophosphatidylcholine, and oleic acid. J Biol Chem 1990;265:70-5.

13. Torjesen PJ, Aakvaag A. Characterization of the adenylate cyclase of the rat corpus luteum during luteolysis induced by a prostaglandin $F_{2\alpha}$ analogue. Mol Cell Endocrinol 1986;44:237-42.

14. Kenny N, Robinson J. Prostaglandin $F_{2\alpha}$-induced functional luteolysis: Interactions of LH, prostaglandin $F_{2\alpha}$, and forskolin in cyclic AMP and progesterone synthesis in isolated rat luteal cells. J Endocrinol 1986;111:415-23.

15. Jefferson AB, Schulman H. Sphingosine inhibits calmodulin-dependent enzymes. J Biol Chem 1988;263:15241-4.

25

Cadherins and Ovarian Follicular Development

RIAZ FAROOKHI AND OREST W. BLASCHUK

The cadherins are a family of integral membrane glycoproteins that mediate calcium-dependent cell adhesion (1). We have shown that granulosa cells from diethylstilbesterol (DES)-primed immature rats adhere to one another in a calcium-dependent manner and express a cadherin that is related to murine E-cadherin (2, 3). Disaggregated rat granulosa cells do not express cadherin (2) and are incapable of FSH-stimulated LH receptor induction in vitro (4). The inclusion of estradiol with FSH in cultures of disaggregated rat granulosa cells restores cadherin expression (3), promotes cell aggregation (3, 4), and re-establishes FSH-stimulated LH receptor induction (2, 4). These observations suggest that cadherin-mediated cell aggregation may be necessary for FSH-stimulated LH-receptor induction in granulosa cells. We have tested this possibility in two ways.

First, we examined the dose effects of estradiol on cadherin expression in disaggregated granulosa cells and related this to the dose effects of estradiol on LH receptor induction in disaggregated granulosa cells cultured with FSH. We have shown previously (4) that high concentrations of steroids are inhibitory for FSH-mediated LH receptor induction in vitro. Second, we examined the effects of including cadherin antibodies in cultures of disaggregated rat granulosa cells containing FSH and estradiol. Specifically, we examined the effects of the antibodies on granulosa cell aggregation and LH receptor induction. Our results support the hypothesis that cadherin-mediated aggregation is necessary for granulosa cell differentiation.

Methods

Preparation and Tissue Culture of Disaggregated Granulosa Cells. Disaggregated granulosa cells were obtained from the ovaries of DES-primed immature rats, as described previously (4). An essential feature of the disaggregation procedure is the trypsin treatment of the cells in the absence of calcium. The disaggregated cells thus obtained are devoid of cell surface cadherin (2, 3). The disaggregated granulosa cells were cultured in 35-mm tissue culture dishes (Falcon, Lincoln Park, NJ) in 2 mL of a 1:1 mixture of Ham's F-12 and Delbecco's Modified Eagle's Medium (H-D media; GiBCO, Burlington, Ont.). Cells were cultured at a density of 2×10^6 viable cells per dish. FSH (15 ng/mL) and/or estradiol (0–200 nM) were included in the H-D media. Penicillin (100 IU/mL) and streptomycin (100 ug/mL) were also included. HEPES (10 mM) was included as buffer. LH receptor induction in cultures of granulosa cells was assessed as described previously (4).

Preparation of Cadherin-Specific Antisera. The following peptides were purchased from Multiple Peptide Systems (San Diego, CA): (1) DWVIPPINLPENSR, (2) RYSVTGPGADQPP, (3) AHAVDVNGNQVEN, (4) DKDQPHTPAWNARY, and (5) DYLNEWGNRFKKLAD. These peptides are derived from the avian N-cadherin sequence (5). Peptides 1–4 correspond to portions of the extracellular domain of cadherin. Peptide 5 corresponds to a portion of the cytoplasmic tail of the molecule. The underlined residues are conserved perfectly among all avian and mammalian cadherins. One of us (OWB) has identified the tripeptide HAV sequence (present in peptide 3) as an important recognition sequence for cell adhesion (6). The peptides were conjugated to keyhole limpet haemocyanin and rabbits were immunized with either a mixture of conjugated peptides 1–4 or conjugated peptide 5. The titre and specificity of the antisera produced were determined by immunoblot procedures (3). Both antisera recognize the same 124-kDa cadherin in granulosa cells cultured with estradiol (Fig. 1). Antibodies were isolated from the antisera by affinity chromatography on a column of protein A (Biorad, Richmond, CA) according to the manufacturer's instructions. The antiserum produced against peptides 1–4 was termed L2 and the antiserum prepared against peptide 5 was designated L4.

Electrophoresis and Immunoblot Procedures. The procedures for SDS-polyacrylamide gel electrophoresis (SDS-PAGE) and immunoblotting have been described previously (2, 3).

Results

Effects of Estradiol on LH Receptor Induction and Cadherin Expression

The effects of increasing concentrations of estradiol on LH receptor induction in disaggregated granulosa cells cultured in the presence of FSH are shown in Figure 2. A maximal induction of LH receptor occurs at an estradiol

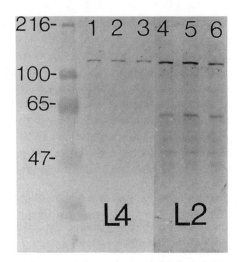

FIGURE 1. Immunoblots of freshly prepared granulosa cell extracts probed with either L4 (lanes 1–3) or L2 (lanes 4–6). Molecular weight markers (in kDa) are indicated in the left-most lane.

concentration of 30 nM. Higher concentrations of estradiol ($\geq$100 nM) are inhibitory for receptor induction. In fact, no LH receptors could be detected at estradiol concentrations greater than 200 nM (not shown).

The immunoblot depicted in Figure 3 indicates that estradiol, but not FSH, regulates cadherin expression in granulosa cell cultures. A maximal expression of cadherin is apparent between 10- to 30-nM estradiol. As was the case

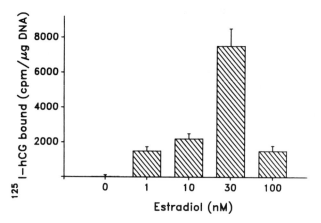

FIGURE 2. LH/hCG receptor content of disaggregated granulosa cells cultured for 72 h with 30 ng FSH and the indicated concentrations of estradiol. Receptor content was assessed by measurement of specific [^{125}I]hCG binding to the cells.

1 2 3 4 5 6 7 8

FIGURE 3. Immunoblot of granulosa cell extracts from 24 h cultures of disaggregated cells. Cells were cultured with either FSH alone (lane 1: 30 ng/mL; lane 2: 100 ng/ mL; lane 3: 200 ng/mL) or estradiol alone (lane 4: 1 nM; lane 5: 10 nM; lane 6: 30 nM; lane 7: 100 nM; lane 8: 200 nM). The blot was probed with L2.

for receptor induction, higher concentrations of estradiol attenuated cadherin expression by these cells. FSH alone did not affect cadherin levels in the granulosa cells.

Effects of Cadherin Antibodies on Culture Morphology

Morphology of the disaggregated granulosa cells cultured for 48 h in either L2 or antibodies from preimmune serum is shown in Figure 4. No significant changes in culture morphology from that depicted at 48 h were seen at 72 h (not shown). Disaggregated cells cultured with L4 or with BSA (not shown) were similar to those maintained with the preimmune antibodies. The inclu-

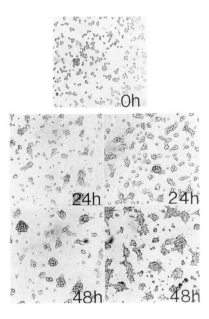

FIGURE 4. Morphology of disaggregated granulosa cells cultured with either L2 (*left panels*) or preimmune antibodies (*right panels*) for 24 or 48 h in the presence of FSH (30 ng) and estradiol (10 nM). Antibodies were added at a concentration of 0.1 mg/mL.

sion of the L2 antibodies attenuated the aggregation of the granulosa cells. Although some aggregates were formed in the cultures that included L2, both the size and the compactness of these aggregates were diminished (compare left to right panel of Fig. 4 at 48 h). Cell attachment and spreading were also decreased in the L2 containing cultures.

Effects of Cadherin Antibodies on LH Receptor Induction

The L2 antibodies were also capable of attenuating LH receptor induction in cultures of disaggregated granulosa cells (Fig. 5). Neither L4 nor antibodies from the preimmune sera blocked LH receptor induction (Fig. 5).

Discussion

The results from the present study further substantiate our contention that direct cell interactions within the membrana granulosa are necessary for cell differentiation. These interactions are mediated by the cell adhesion molecule (CAM), cadherin. The expression of cadherin by granulosa cells is regulated by estradiol. This regulation is biphasic: Low concentrations of estradiol stimulate expression of cadherin; high concentrations are inhibitory.

Takeichi (1) has shown that cadherins play an important role in animal morphogenesis. Little is known, however, about factors that control cadherin

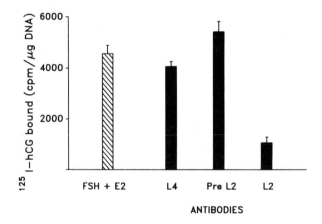

FIGURE 5. LH/hCG receptor induction at 72 h in disaggregated granulosa cells cultured with FSH and estradiol. The hatched bar indicates the receptor induction when no antibodies were added to the culture; the solid bars indicate the effects of adding the various antibody preparations. Antibody was added at the initiation of the culture at a final concentration of 0.1 mg/mL.

expression in developing and differentiating tissues. Our studies have shown that steroid hormones, specifically estrogens, regulate cadherin expression in the developing ovarian follicle (2, 3). Recently, Svalander et al. (7) have shown that ovarian steroids control the expression of a rat uterine epithelium CAM, termed "cellCAM-105." Estrogen stimulates cellCAM-105 expression in the luminal epithelium; progesterone stimulates this CAM in the glandular epithelium. Interestingly, progesterone downregulates cellCAM-105 expression in the luminal epithelium. Choi et al. (8) have also shown that progesterone can enhance cadherin levels in amphibian oocytes.

Cadherins are important in the formation of intercellular junctional complexes. Gumbiner et al. (9) have shown that antibodies to E-cadherin block junctional complex formation in canine kidney cells. Increases in adherens and gap junction formation occur in mouse sarcoma cells after transfection with cDNAs for the avian form of E-cadherin (10, 11). Estrogens have been shown to promote gap junction formation within the membrana granulosa of the rat ovarian follicle (12). Our observation that estrogens regulate cadherin expression in these cells would be compatible with the notion that cell adhesion is a prerequisite for the formation of specialized intercellular junctions and direct cell communication (13, 14).

The physiological implications and molecular mechanisms for the biphasic effects of estradiol on cadherin expression in granulosa cells is unclear. This observation may, however, offer an explanation for why treatment with high concentrations of estrogen can lead to follicular atresia (15, 16). Furthermore, the increases in estrogen biosynthetic activity in the mural granulosa cells of preovulatory follicles may provide a mechanism for dissociation or segregation of these cells from the remaining mass of granulosa cells that will be expelled at ovulation with the oocyte.

Conclusion

In summary, we have demonstrated that cadherins mediate the hormonal responsiveness of granulosa cells. Furthermore, our results suggest that this CAM plays a pivotal role in the program of granulosa cell differentiation. Finally, cadherin expression by granulosa cells may provide a specific marker for estrogenic action in these cells. We are presently attempting to elucidate the mechanisms by which estradiol regulates cadherin expression in granulosa cells.

References

1. Takeichi M. The cadherins: Cell-cell adhesion molecules controlling animal morphogenesis. Development 1988;102:639-55.

2. Farookhi R, Blaschuk OW. E-cadherin may be involved in mediating FSH-stimulated responses in rat granulosa cells. In: Hirshfield AN, ed. Growth factors and the ovary. New York: Serono Symposia, USA/Plenum Press, 1989:257-65.
3. Blaschuk OW, Farookhi R. Estradiol stimulates cadherin expression in rat granulosa cells. Dev Biol 1989;136:564-67.
4. Farookhi R, Desjardins J. Luteinizing hormone receptors in dispersed granulosa cells requires estrogen. Mol Cell Endocrinol 1986;47:13-24.
5. Hatta K, Nose A, Nagafuchi A, Takeichi M. Cloning and expression of cDNA encoding a neural calcium-dependent cell adhesion molecule: Its identity in the cadherin gene family. J Cell Biol 1988;106:873-81.
6. Blaschuk OW, Sullivan R, David S, Pouliot Y. Identification of a cadherin cell adhesion recognition sequence. Dev Biol 1990;139:227-9.
7. Svalander PC, Odin P, Nilsson BO, Obrink B. Expression of cellCAM-105 in the apical surface of rat uterine epithelium is controlled by ovarian steroid hormones. J Reprod Fertil 1990;88:213-21.
8. Choi YS, Sehgal R, McCrea P, Gumbiner B. A cadherin-like protein in eggs and cleaving embryos of xenopus laevis is expressed in oocytes in response to progesterone. J Cell Biol 1990;110:1575-82.
9. Gumbiner B, Stevenson B, Grimaldi A. The role of the cell adhesion molecule uvomorulin in the formation and maintenance of the epithelial junctional complex. J Cell Biol 1988;107:1575-87.
10. Mege R-M, Matsuzaki F, Gallin WJ, Goldberg JI, Cunningham BA, Edelman GM. Construction of epithelioid sheets by transfection of mouse sarcoma cells with cDNAs for chicken adhesion molecules. Proc Natl Acad Sci USA 1988;85:7274-8.
11. Matsuzaki F, Mege R-M, Jaffe SH, et al. cDNAs of cell adhesion molecules of different specificity induce changes in cell shape and border formation in cultured S180 cells. J Cell Biol 1990;110:1239-52.
12. Amsterdam A, Rotmensch S. Structure-function relationships during granulosa cell differentiation. Endocr Rev 1987;8:309-37.
13. Edelman GM. Modulation of cell adhesion during induction, histogenesis, and prenatal development of the nervous system. Annu Rev Neurosci 1984;7:339-77.
14. Takeichi M. Cadherins: A molecular family essential for selective cell-cell adhesion and animal morphogenesis. Trends Genet 1987;3:213-7.
15. Dierschke DJ, Hutz RJ, Wolf RC. Induced follicular atresia in rhesus monkeys: Strength-duration relationship of the estrogen stimulus. Endocrinology 1985;117:1397-403.
16. Sadrkhanloo R, Hofeditz C, Erickson GF. Evidence for widespread atresia in the hypophysectomized estrogen-treated rat. Endocrinology 1987;120:146-55.

26

Differential Regulation of 3β-HSD and 17β-HSD Expression in Granulosa Cells

Y. TREMBLAY, B. MARCOTTE, AND J.F. STRAUSS, III

The enzyme 3β-hydroxysteroid dehydrogenase/Δ^5-Δ^4 isomerase (3β-HSD) catalyzes the transformation of Δ^5-ene, 3β-hydroxy to Δ^4-3-keto steroids and is therefore an essential enzyme in the biosynthesis of all steroid hormones. 3β-HSD deficiency results in decreased formation of cortisol, aldosterone, and sex steroids (1). Clinically, 3β-HSD deficiency causes ambiguous genitalia and lethal adrenal insufficiency in newborns (2). On the other hand, the reversible interconversion of Δ^5-androstenediol to DHEA, testosterone to Δ^4-androstenedione, and estrone to estradiol is mediated by 17β-hydroxysteroid dehydrogenase (17β-HSD), also termed 17-oxidoreductase or 17-ketosteroid reductase. Deficient activity of ovarian 17β-HSD can cause hirsutism and polycystic ovarian disease (3). 3β-HSD and 17β-HSD are both non-cytochrome P-450 enzymes using NAD and NADPH as cofactors, respectively.

Recently, human placental 3β-HSD (4) and 17β-HSD (5) cDNAs clones were isolated and sequenced, providing new tools for studies on the regulation of these enzymes. We have used these cDNAs as probes to study these steroidogenic enzymes in primary cultures of human and porcine granulosa cells. Northern blot analysis of human and porcine granulosa cells shows two 17β-HSD mRNA species of 1.3 kb and 2.2 kb and a single 1.8-kb 3β-HSD mRNA, respectively. Our studies show that treatment of primary cultures of human granulosa cells with cAMP increases the abundance of 3β-HSD mRNA as well as mRNAs for other steroidogenic enzymes. In contrast, cAMP decreases 17β-HSD mRNA accumulation in luteinized human granulosa cells. To evaluate the potential influence of luteinization of granulosa cells in the cAMP response, we performed studies in primary cultures of preovulatory porcine granulosa cells. Both 3β-HSD and 17β-HSD mRNA levels were increased by cAMP in these cells as well as mRNA for cytochrome P-450$_{SCC}$. Treatment of human granulosa cells with the phorbol ester PMA and of porcine granulosa cells with hCG or FSH increased the relative abundance of both 3β-HSD and 17β-HSD mRNAs whereas PRL alone had no significant effect. PRL, on the other hand, caused a decrease in cAMP stimulation of 3β-HSD mRNA levels without a significant effect on the level of 17β-HSD mRNA.

Materials and Methods

Human ovarian luteinized granulosa cells were prepared, separated, and cultured as previously described (6). After 2 days in culture, 8-br-cAMP or phorbol,12-myristate,13-acetate (PMA) was added. Preovulatory porcine granulosa cells were mechanically separated from follicles and cultured in MEM containing 10% (v/v) FCS as described elsewhere (7). After 72 h in culture, porcine granulosa cells were treated with 8-br-cAMP, follicule stimulating hormone (FSH), human chorionic gonadotropin (hCG), or prolactin (PRL). RNA was prepared and equal amounts (10 μg) were electrophoresed (8). All Northern blots were probed with either the nearly full-length (1.5 kb) 3β-HSD clone (4) or with the EcoRI/SacI fragment of the 17β-HSD cDNA (5), labeled using the random primer method (9). Hybridization conditions were as described (10), except for porcine cells which were hybridized with 17β-HSD cDNA in 40% formamide at 37°C.

Results and Discussion

Ovarian granulosa cells synthesize estradiol principally from androgenic precursors provided by theca cells (11). Primary cultures of luteinized human granulosa cells are known to respond to tropic hormones and their cAMP second messenger by secreting progesterone (prog) and accumulating mRNAs for some steroidogenic enzymes (6, 12). Consistent with their important steroidogenic capacity, luteinized granulosa cells contain high levels of 17β-HSD and 3β-HSD mRNA. Figure 1 shows representative autoradiograms of granulosa cell RNA from 3 different individuals hybridized with ^{32}P-labeled cDNA for 17β-HSD and γ-actin (Fig. 1A), and 3β-HSD and adrenodoxin (Fig. 1B). Consistent with our previous results, the 17β-HSD probe hybridized under high stringency conditions with 2 mRNA species of 1.3 kb and 2.2 kb (5, 10), whereas the 3β-HSD probe hybridized with a single 1.8-kb mRNA (4). Treatment of cultured cells with 8-br-cAMP significantly reduced the abundance of the 1.3-kb 17β-HSD mRNA to 14 ± 3% (n = 3) of control (value arbitrarily fixed at 100%), but did not significantly affect the relative abundance of the 2.2-kb 17β-HSD mRNA (100 ± 10%, n = 3). This

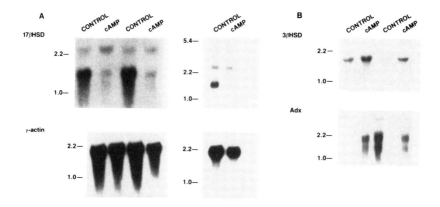

FIGURE 1. Northern blot analysis of total RNA from primary cultures of luteinized human granulosa cells incubated for 24 h with or without 1.5 mM 8-br-cAMP. Panel A shows Northern blots probed with the placental 17β-HSD cDNA, while panel B represents blots probed with 3β-HSD cDNA. The lower part of each panel represents the same blot probed with γ-actin and adrenodoxin cDNAs, respectively. Molecular size markers are HindIII-cleaved bacteriophage PM-2.

dramatic reduction of 17β-HSD mRNA level caused by the cAMP analogue was also observed following long-term treatment (3 days) of granulosa cells (10) and in primary cultures of human cytotrophoblast cells (10). The inhibition observed is highly specific and is not due to toxicity, as probing the same blot for adrenodoxin mRNA showed a 4.3 ± 0.2-fold increase (n = 3) above control levels. Washing and reprobing these blots with ^{32}P-labeled 3β-HSD cDNA showed that cAMP treatment increased 7 ± 1-fold 3β-HSD mRNA (n = 3) as already shown for other steroidogenic enzymes (6, 12). Moreover, this result is in agreement with the capacity of these cells to increase progesterone secretion in response to cAMP.

Human granulosa cells were also incubated with the phorbol ester PMA, which stimulates protein kinase C (Fig. 2). In contrast with the absence of effect of TPA on the accumulation of 17β-HSD mRNA in the trophoblastic tumor cells JEG-3 (10), PMA increased by 4-fold 17β-HSD (panel A) and 3β-HSD (panel B) mRNA levels whereas P-450$_{SCC}$ mRNA was increased 30-fold (panel C).

Since the inhibition of 17β-HSD mRNA levels by cAMP was a somewhat expected finding, we next evaluated the potential role of luteinization in the cAMP response of ovarian cells. Preovulatory porcine granulosa cells were thus used for this study. The same Northern blots were hybridized with 3β-HSD, 17β-HSD (Fig. 3) and γ-actin (not shown) cDNAs. After a 24-h incubation, hCG and FSH and in particular 8-br-cAMP, increased the abun-

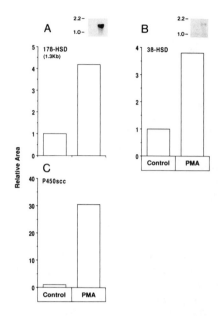

FIGURE 2. Northern blot analysis from primary cultures of human luteinized granu-losa cells (6 individuals) treated for 24 h with 40-nM PMA. Autoradiograms were densitometrically scanned, and the areas under the tracings were expressed relative to control, which were arbitrarily fixed at 1.0.

dance of 3β-HSD mRNA. hCG, FSH, and 8-br-cAMP produce similar in-creases in 17β-HSD mRNA levels. Taken together, these results (Figs. 1 and 3) suggest that inhibition of the estrogen-synthesizing machinery by cAMP may be restricted to the post-luteinization period. Alternatively, there may be species difference in the regulation of the expression of 17β-HSD by cAMP. These findings also reveal clear differences in the responses of 3β-HSD and 17β-HSD mRNAs to different stimuli. Estrogen secretion after the LH surge falls dramatically and the diminution in estradiol secretion may be due, at least in part, to cAMP-mediated suppression of 17β-HSD gene expression.

Fevold (13) and Greep et al. (14) first demonstrated that FSH and LH were required for ovarian steroid biosynthesis. Since then, numerous studies (15) have shown that both 3β-HSD and 17β-HSD activities in granulosa cells are modulated by gonadotropins as well as by other factors, including PRL. In FSH-primed rat granulosa cells in vitro, PRL stimulates progesterone pro-duction in a dose-dependent manner (16) in association with an increase in 3β-HSD activity (17). In contrast, estrogen secretion does not seem to be affected. However, treatment of porcine granulosa cells (18) with PRL de-creases progesterone secretion from small but not large follicles. These studies suggest that the action of PRL may vary between species as well as

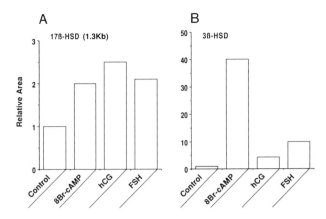

FIGURE 3. Effect of 3-mM 8-br-cAMP, 4-IU/mL hCG, and 50-ng/mL FSH on 17β-HSD (*A*) and 3β-HSD (*B*) mRNAs in porcine granulosa cells. After a 24-h incubation, cells (2.5 × 10⁶ cells/mL) were scraped, pooled (n = 6), and RNA extracted as described in reference 7. The data are shown as histogram bars where the control mRNA level was fixed at 1.0.

according to the stage of granulosa cell differentiation. Based on these data, experiments were designed to assess the effect of PRL on the level of 3β-HSD and 17β-HSD mRNAs in porcine granulosa cells. As shown in Figure 4, PRL caused a partial dose-dependent decrease in the cAMP-stimulation of 3β-HSD mRNA levels, while 17β-HSD levels are not significantly affected.

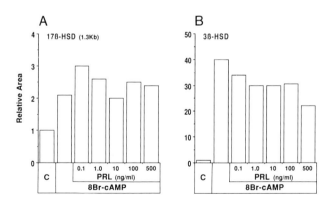

FIGURE 4. Effect of increasing concentrations of PRL (24-h incubation) on 8-br-cAMP-stimulated preovulatory porcine granulosa cells. Each bar represents a pool (n = 6). The filter was probed with 3β-HSD cDNA and reprobed with 17β-HSD cDNA. The areas of the densitometric scans were calculated and compared to the control fixed at 1.0.

Conclusion

The present data show that cAMP can suppress or stimulate ovarian levels of mRNAs encoding steroidogenic enzymes. In fact, the response may be dependent upon the state of differentiation of the cell as well as upon the extent and the duration of stimulation. We have also found that the mRNAs encoding 3β-HSD and 17β-HSD are regulated by the phorbol ester PMA, thus suggesting that pathways using protein kinase A and C are active in human granulosa cells. Moreover, the present results show that PRL treatment has a differential effect on 3β-HSD and 17β-HSD mRNA levels in cAMP-stimulated cells.

References

1. Bongiovani AM. Congenital adrenal hyperplasia due to 3β-HSD deficiency. In: New MI, Levine LS, eds.; vol 13. Basel: Karger, 1984:72-82.
2. White PC, New MI, Dupont B. Congenital adrenal hyperplasia. N Engl J Med 1987;316:1519-24.
3. Pang S, Softness B, Sweeney WJ, New MI. N Engl J Med 1987;316:1295-1301.
4. Luu-The V, Lachance Y, Labrie C, et al. Full length cDNA structure and deduced amino acid sequence of human 3β-hydroxy-5-ene steroid dehydrogenase. Mol Endocrinol 1989;3:1310-2.
5. Luu-The V, Labrie C, Zhao HF, et al. Characterization of cDNAs for human estradiol 17β-dehydrogenase and assignment of the gene to chromosome 17. Mol Endocrinol 1989;3:1301-9.
6. Golos TG, Miller ML, Strauss JF, III. Human chorionic gonadotropin and 8 BrcAMP promote an acute increase in cytochrome P450scc and adrenodoxin mRNAs in cultured human granulosa cells by a cycloheximide-insensitive mechanism. J Clin Invest 1987;80:896-9.
7. Chedrese PJ, Rajkumar K, Murphy BD. Dose response of luteinized porcine granulosa cells in vitro to prolactin: Dependency on exposure to human chorionic gonadotrophin. Can J Physiol Pharmacol 1988;66:1337-40.
8. Cathala G, Savouret JF, Mendez B, et al. A method for isolation of intact translationally active RNA. DNA 1983;2:329-33.
9. Feinberg AP, Vogelstein B. A technique for radiolabelling DNA restriction endonuclease fragments. Anal Biochem 1983:132:6-13.
10. Tremblay Y, Ringler GE, Morel Y, et al. Regulation of the gene for estrogenic 17-Ketosteroid reductase lying on chromosome 17. J Biol Chem 1989;264:20459-62.
11. Erickson GF, Magoffin DA, Dyer CA, Hofeditz C. The ovarian androgen producing cells: A review of structure and function. Endocr Rev 1985;6:371-99.
12. Voutilainen R, Tapanainen J, Chung BC, Matteson KJ, Miller WL. Hormonal regulation of P450scc and P450c17 in cultured human granulosa cells. J Clin Endocrinol Metab 1986;63:202-6.

13. Fevold HL. Synergism of follicle stimulating and luteinising hormone in producing estrogen secretion. Endocrinology 1941;28:33-9.
14. Greep RO, Van Dyke HB, Ghow BF. Gonadotropins of the swine pituitary. Endocrinology 1942;30:63-9.
15. Hsueh AJW, Adashi EY, Jones PBC, Welsh TH. Hormonal regulation of differentiation of cultured ovarian granulosa cells. Endocr Rev 1984;5:76-127.
16. Wang C, Hsueh AJW, Erickson GF. Induction of functional PRL receptors by FSH in rat granulosa cells in vivo and in vitro. J Biol Chem 1979;254:11330-5.
17. Jones PBC, Valk CA, Hsueh AJW. Regulation of progestin biosynthetic enzymes in culture rat granulosa cells. Biol Reprod 1981;29:572-8.
18. Veldhuis JD, Klase P, Hammond JM. Divergent effects of prolactin upon steroidogenesis by porcine granulosa cells in vitro. Endocrinology 1981;107:42-9.

27

Pituitary Hormone Regulation of Ovarian 3β-HSD Gene Expression and Activity in the Rat

CLAUDE LABRIE, CÉLINE MARTEL, JACQUES COUËT,
CLAUDE TRUDEL, VAN LUU-THE, AND FERNAND LABRIE

The enzyme 3β-hydroxysteroid dehydrogenase (EC 1.1.1.145)/Δ^5-Δ^4 isomerase (EC 5.3.3.1), hereafter referred to as 3β-HSD, catalyzes the obligatory oxidation/isomerization of 3β-hydroxy-5-ene steroids into 3-keto-4-ene steroids, thus permitting the formation of progesterone from pregnenolone as well as synthesis of the precursors of ovarian androgens and estrogens. In order to obtain a better understanding of the molecular mechanisms controlling ovarian 3β-HSD activity, we have studied the effects of the gonadotropin hCG/LH, as well as those of prolactin (PRL), on rat ovarian 3β-HSD mRNA levels using a recently isolated rat ovary 3β-HSD cDNA (1). In addition to describing in detail the effects of hCG/LH, the present data demonstrate a potent inhibitory effect of PRL on 3β-HSD gene expression and activity, which could well provide an explanation for at least part of the well-known antifertility effects of hyperprolactinemia in women.

Materials and Methods

Experimental Procedure. Human CG (10 IU; Profasi HP) and ovine PRL (1 mg; NIDDK-o-PRL-19; bio-potency, 31 IU/mg) were administered subcutaneously twice daily, alone or in combination, for 10 days to adult female Sprague-Dawley [CrL:CD(SD)Br] rats hypophysectomized 15 days previously. Truncal blood was collected for measurement of serum progesterone by RIA as described (2). All results are expressed as means ± SEM. Statistical significance was determined according to the multiple-range test of Duncan-Kramer (3).

Quantification of 3β-HSD mRNA. Ovarian 3β-HSD mRNA levels were measured by dot blot hybridization, as previously described (4), using the ^{32}P-labeled full-length rat ovary 3β-HSD cDNA clone 56 (1) as probe. The intensities of the resulting autoradiographic spots were quantified using an Amersham RAS Image Analyzer System. The slopes of the dot intensities of each dilution series were calculated by linear regression, and 3β-HSD mRNA levels are expressed as means ± SEM of 5–7 hypophysectomized rats relative to 3β-HSD mRNA levels in control hypophysectomized rat ovaries. Total RNA from intact adult rat ovaries was used as internal control.

Ovarian 3β-HSD Protein Immunoblotting. Ovarian proteins were size separated on a 5–15% polyacrylamide gel (1.5-mm thick) and transferred to nitrocellulose filters. Purified human placental 3β-HSD and BRL protein weight markers were used as control and for estimation of molecular size, respectively. Rat 3β-HSD was revealed by sequential incubations with rabbit antiserum raised against purified human placental 3β-HSD and ^{125}I-labeled goat anti-rabbit immunoglobulin G (5).

Enzymatic Assay of Ovarian 3β-HSD. Freshly excised whole rat ovaries were homogenized with a Polytron in phosphate buffer (50-mM KH_2PO_4, 20% glycerol, 1-mM EDTA, pH 7.5) containing 1-mM phenyl-methylsulphuryl-fluoride and 5-μg/mL each of pepstatin A, antipain, and leupeptin, and centrifuged for 30 min at 1000 g. Aliquots of the supernatant were incubated for 20 min at 37 °C in 0.5-mL phosphate buffer containing 10-μM unlabeled DHEA, 1-μM TLC-purified [4-^{14}C]DHEA (51-mCi/mM) and 0.8-mM NAD$^+$. [^{14}C]Δ^4-dione was quantified as described after TLC (1).

Results

As illustrated in Figure 1*A*, while hCG alone exerted no effect on the steady state levels of whole ovarian 3β-HSD mRNA, oPRL exerted a potent inhibitory effect (P < 0.01) on the same parameter as compared to the values found in control hypophysectomized animals. Simultaneous treatment with hCG partially (P < 0.01) reversed the inhibitory effect of oPRL, increasing 3β-HSD mRNA levels from 19% (oPRL alone) to 47% of the value found in control hypophysectomized animals. Since hCG and oPRL exerted significant stimulatory (20%) and inhibitory (46%) effects, respectively, on ovarian weight (Fig. 1*B*), it is of interest to express 3β-HSD mRNA content following correction for relative changes in total ovarian weight. Such a measure provides an assessment of the whole ovarian content in 3β-HSD mRNA and, subsequently, of the ovary's capacity for expression of 3β-HSD. It can be seen in Figure 1*C* that hCG caused a 45% (P < 0.05) increase in total 3β-HSD mRNA content while oPRL exerted an 88% inhibition of total ovarian 3β-

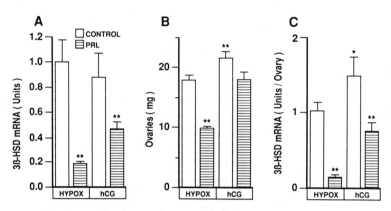

FIGURE 1. Effect of treatment with hCG (10 IU) and oPRL (1 mg), alone or in combination, on ovarian 3β-HSD mRNA (*A*; in units), ovarian weight (*B*), and total ovarian 3β-HSD mRNA content (*C*; in units per ovary) in hypophysectomized rats.

HSD mRNA content (P < 0.01) as compared to the values found in control hypophysectomized rat ovaries.

The potent inhibitory effect of oPRL on ovarian 3β-HSD mRNA content was also observed on the levels of 3β-HSD protein (Fig. 2*A*) and 3β-HSD activity (Fig. 2*B*). In fact, ovarian 3β-HSD protein content and enzymatic activity varied in a manner almost superimposable to 3β-HSD mRNA content (Fig. 1). Thus, oPRL caused decreases of 86% in immunoreactive 3β-HSD protein and 83% in 3β-HSD activity, which were completely reversed by concomitant treatment with hCG. The hCG also reversed the inhibitory effect of oPRL on ovarian 3β-HSD activity. As illustrated in Figures 2*A* and 2*B*, the administration of hCG alone to hypophysectomized animals caused 79% and 46% increases (P < 0.01) in 3β-HSD protein and enzyme activity, respectively.

As can be seen in Figure 2*C*, the effects of treatment with hCG and/or PRL on ovarian weight and 3β-HSD expression and activity translated into qualitatively comparable effects on serum progesterone levels. In fact, oPRL decreased circulating progesterone levels below the limit of detection of the radioimmunoassay (LD = 0.2 nM/L) from a pretreatment value of 1.9 ± 0.4 nM/L. Treatment with hCG completely reversed the inhibitory effect of oPRL on serum progesterone levels (P < 0.01). An additional marker of ovarian steroidogenic function, uterine weight, was measured as an index of ovarian estradiol production (data not shown). hCG treatment markedly increased uterine weight in hypophysectomized females to 302.9 ± 20 from a pretreatment value of 96.0 ± 10 mg (P < 0.01). While oPRL alone did not affect uterine weight, the addition of oPRL to hCG caused a marked reduc-

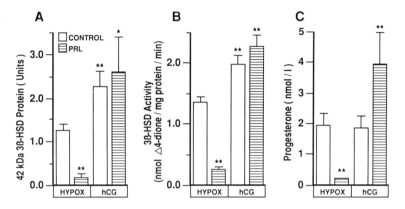

FIGURE 2. Effect of treatment with hCG and oPRL, alone or in combination, on ovarian 3β-HSD protein content (*A*), 3β-HSD enzymatic activity (*B*), and serum progesterone levels (*C*) in hypophysectomized rats.

tion in hCG-induced uterine weight gain, further illustrating the inhibitory effect of oPRL on ovarian steroidogenesis.

Discussion

The present demonstration that PRL exerts a potent inhibitory effect on 3β-HSD expression and activity in the ovaries of hypophysectomized rats confirms and extends previous data concerning the luteolytic effect of PRL under these circumstances. The PRL-induced decrease in 3β-HSD activity translates into a marked inhibition of circulating progesterone levels as well as decreased uterine weight, which reflects reduced estrogen secretion. On the other hand, hCG reverses the inhibitory effect of PRL on 3β-HSD mRNA levels as well as on 3β-HSD protein level and activity. The apparent lack of variation in 3β-HSD mRNA concentration in response to hCG suggests that 3β-HSD could be constitutively expressed in corpora lutea. This phenomenon has been observed for the cholesterol side-chain cleavage P-450 (6) and aromatase cytochrome P-450 mRNAs (7).

The interval between corpus luteum formation and the administration of PRL is critical in determining whether PRL will exert a luteolytic or a luteotrophic effect in the absence of hCG. In mature hypophysectomized rats, delayed (>2 days) PRL treatment dramatically accelerated the normal post-hypophysectomy decline in ovarian weight (8). On the other hand, precocious (<2 days) administration of PRL to hypophysectomized rats in which ovulation had been induced by pretreatment with FSH and LH maintained functional corpora lutea (9).

The present data indicate that PRL, in addition to its inhibitory effect at the hypothalamo/pituitary level (10), can also act directly on ovarian cells to suppress steroidogenic enzyme gene expression, thus providing an additional explanation for the antifertility effects of hyperprolactinemia in women (11, 12). While the present data show a marked reduction in circulating progesterone levels following PRL treatment, the findings of a PRL-induced reduction in uterine weight also suggests decreased estrogen secretion. Recent data have shown that PRL can inhibit the expression of aromatase mRNA in rat granulosa cells prior to and during the early stages of luteinization both in vivo and in cells in culture (13). Such data suggest that decreased aromatase activity could also contribute to the overall reduction in estrogen secretion and uterine weight.

The molecular mechanisms whereby PRL induces luteolysis and inhibits corpora lutea 3β-HSD expression are unknown. Interestingly, hCG and PRL exert opposite effects on 3β-HSD expression, indicating that the 3β-HSD gene(s) probably contain(s) elements responsive to the intracellular mediators of both hormones. The close correlation observed between 3β-HSD mRNA, protein content, and activity levels under a wide range of hormonal conditions—namely, inhibition by PRL and stimulation by hCG—indicates that the modulation of 3β-HSD activity by both hCG and PRL is, at least up to a large extent, related to parallel changes in 3β-HSD gene expression and/or 3β-HSD mRNA stability.

References

1. Zhao H-F, Simard J, Labrie C, et al. Characterization of rat 3β-hydroxysteroid dehydrogenase/Δ^5-Δ^4 isomerase cDNAs and differential tissue-specific expression of the corresponding mRNAs in steroidogenic and peripheral tissues. Submitted.
2. Bélanger A, Caron S, Picard V. Simultaneous radioimmunoassay of progestins, androgens and estrogens in rat testis. J Steroid Biochem 1980;13:185-90.
3. Kramer CY. Extension of multiple-range tests to group means with unequal numbers of replications. Biometrics 1956;12:307-10.
4. Simard J, Hatton AC, Labrie C, et al. Inhibitory effect of estrogens on GCDFP-15 mRNA levels and secretion in ZR-75-1 human breast cancer cells. Mol Endocrinol 1989;3:694-702.
5. Luu-The V, Lachance Y, Labrie C, et al. Full length cDNA structure and deduced amino acid sequence of human 3β-hydroxy-5-ene steroid dehydrogenase. Mol Endocrinol 1989;3:1310-2.
6. Goldring NB, Durica JM, Lifka J, et al. Cholesterol side-chain cleavage P450 messenger ribonucleic acid: Evidence for hormonal regulation in rat ovarian follicles and constitutive expression in corpora lutea. Endocrinology 1987;120:1942.
7. Hickey GJ, Chen S, Besman MJ, et al. Hormonal regulation, tissue distribution,

and content of aromatase cytochrome P450 messenger ribonucleic acid and enzyme in rat ovarian follicles and corpora lutea: Relationship to estradiol biosynthesis. Endocrinology 1988;122:1426-36.

8. Malven PV, Sawyer CH. A luteolytic action of prolactin in hypophysectomized rats. Endocrinology 1966;79:268-74.

9. Malven PV, Sawyer CH. Formation of new corpora lutea in mature hypophysectomized rats. Endocrinology 1966;78:1259-63.

10. Marchetti B, Labrie F. Prolactin inhibits pituitary luteinizing hormone-releasing hormone receptors in the rat. Endocrinology 1982;111:1209-16.

11. Schultz KD, Geiger W, Del Pozo E, Lose KH, Kunzig HJ, Lancranjan I. The influence of the prolactin inhibitor bromocriptine (CB154) on human luteal function in vivo. Arch Gynecol 1976;221:93.

12. Micic S, Svenstoup B, Neilsen J. Treatment of hyperprolactinemic luteal insufficiency with bromocriptine. Acta Obstet Gynecol Scand 1979;58:379.

13. Krasnow JL, Hickey GJ, Richards JS. Regulation of aromatase mRNA and estradiol biosynthesis in rat ovarian granulosa and luteal cells by prolactin. Mol Endocrinol 1990;4:13-21.

28

Molecular Cloning of Rat 3β-HSD: Structure of Two Types of cDNAs and Differential Expression of Corresponding mRNAs in the Ovary

Jacques Simard, Hui Fen Zhao, Claude Labrie, Claude Trudel, Eric Rhéaume, Eric Dupont, Nathalie Breton, Van Luu-The, Georges Pelletier, and Fernand Labrie

Following cleavage of the aliphatic side-chain of cholesterol, thus leading to the formation of pregnenolone and related Δ^5-3β-hydroxysteroids, the next obligatory step in the formation of all classes of steroid hormones—namely, progesterone, mineralocorticoids, glucocorticoids, androgens and estrogens—requires the oxidation and isomerization of these Δ^5-3β-hydroxysteroid precursors into Δ^4-3-ketosteroids. This irreversible oxidative conversion is catalyzed by the enzymatic complex Δ^5-3β-hydroxysteroid dehydrogenase/Δ^5-Δ^4 isomerase (3β-HSD). This membrane-bound enzymatic system is found in steroidogenic tissues such as the placenta, adrenal cortex, testis, and ovary (1–5), as well as in several peripheral tissues including the prostate, breast, brain, and liver (6–10).

The human 3β-HSD cDNA recently isolated by our group using polyclonal antibodies raised against purified human placental 3β-HSD (1, 2) encodes a 42,126-Da protein of 372 amino acids, having a predicted NH_2-terminal amino acid sequence identical to the unique 29 NH_2-terminal amino acids determined by Edman degradation of the purified enzyme. The human 3β-HSD gene was assigned by in situ hybridization to the p11-p13 region of the short arm of chromosome 1 (11). Furthermore, we have recently characterized bovine 3β-HSD cDNA encoding a 42,093-Da protein also containing 372 amino acid residues (4).

Results

In order to identify cDNAs encoding rat 3β-HSD, the ^{32}P-labeled human hp3β-HSD63 cDNA insert (1) was used to screen 4 × 10[5] plaques from a rat ovary λgt11 library. Putative positive clones showing a strong hybridization signal were detected at a frequency of approximately 30/10[4] plaques. Of these, 66 clones were identified on duplicate filters to give positive signals with the ^{32}P-labeled EcoRI/AvaII restriction fragment corresponding to the first 121 nucleotides of the 5' end of the hp3β-HSD63 cDNA clone. These 66 presumably full-length putative 3β-HSD clones were isolated, purified, and characterized by restriction enzyme and Southern analysis using the full-length human 3β-HSD as probe (1, 2). Using this approach, it was possible to discriminate between two types of cDNA clones based on the absence (type I) or presence (type II) of an internal XbaI site. Based on this finding, the 3 longest type I clones (ro3β-HSD56, 63, and 95) as well as the 3 longest type II clones (ro3β-HSD48, 66, and 112) were subcloned into the BS-KS vector. All six clones were then sequenced in both orientations by the dideoxy-chain termination method.

This first in-frame ATG codon in the cDNA sequence of both types is designated as position 1 and is preceded by an in-frame terminator codon TGA 120 nucleotides upstream. The sequences of type I and type II cDNAs have an open reading frame of 1119 nucleotides showing 33 differences between the two types. The longest type I (ro3β-HSD56) and type II (ro3β-HSD112) cDNA inserts contain 5'-untranslated 171 and 152 bp, respectively, with only 2 differences in their overlapping region. The type I and type II inserts include 355 bp and 369 bp 3'-untranslated regions, respectively. There are 8 different nucleotides in these 3'-untranslated regions, while there is an insertion of 14 additional nucleotides at position 1140 of type II cDNA. The polyadenylation consensus signal AATAAA is located 14 nucleotides upstream from the poly(A) tail in both cDNA types. The overall nucleotide sequence similarity between the two types of rat 3β-HSD cDNAs is 96.5%. Moreover, the nucleotide sequences of the expected coding regions of type I and type II cDNAs share 77.7% and 77.3% similarity, respectively, with that of bovine 3β-HSD (4), while the percentage of similarity with the corresponding human 3β-HSD sequence (1) is 78.3% for both types of rat cDNAs.

Type I 3β-HSD cDNA thus encodes a 41,911-Da protein, while a 42,150-Da protein is deduced from type II 3β-HSD cDNA, both having 372 amino acid residues (excluding the first methionine) as previously demonstrated for the human (1) and bovine (4) 3β-HSD proteins (Fig. 1). The deduced amino acid sequences of types I and II 3β-HSD share 93.8% similarity with only 23 nonidentical residues. The similarities of rat type I and type II 3β-HSD amino acid sequences with that of the predicted human protein are 72.3% and

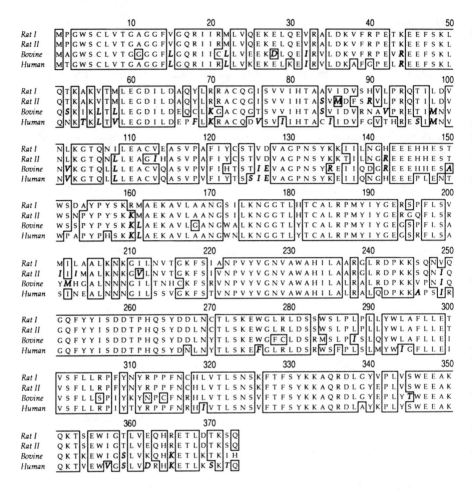

FIGURE 1. Comparison of the deduced amino acid sequences of rat type I, rat type II, bovine, and human 3β-HSD proteins. Amino acid sequences are designated by the universal single-letter code. Amino acid residues are numbered relative to the first NH₂-terminal methionine. Residues common to at least 3 of the 4 deduced sequences are boxed. Residues that are functionally conserved in comparison to rat 3β-HSD type I are indicated by bold italic characters.

71.5%, respectively, while both rat sequences share 74.2% similarity with that of the bovine enzyme.

As illustrated in Figure 2, two major protected fragments are seen following S_1 nuclease digestion of ovarian RNA using 3β-HSD type I (lane 2) or 3β-HSD (lane 5) while no signal is detected using, as control, the same amount of spleen RNA hybridized to type I (lane 3) or type II (lane 4) 3β-HSD probes. The longest protected fragment in the respective reactions was

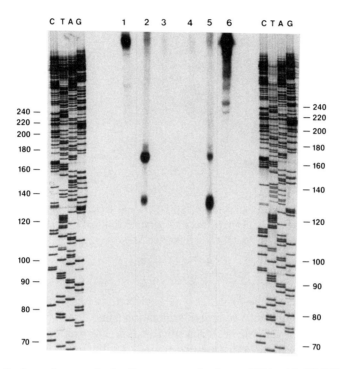

FIGURE 2. S₁ nuclease analysis of rat ovary and spleen mRNA with 3β-HSD type I and type II cDNA probes. Total RNA (70 μg) extracted from rat ovaries or spleens were hybridized with 5'-end-labeled single-stranded probes synthesized using, as primer, the oligonucleotide corresponding to the noncoding strand extending from nucleotides 713 to 742 of both 3β-HSD type I (ro3β-HSD56) and type II (ro3β-HSD112) cDNA clones. Lanes 1 and 6 correspond to untreated 3β-HSD type I and type II probes, respectively.

of the expected length of 177 nucleotides, thus corresponding to the region 565 to 742 of type I (lane 2) or type II (lane 5) 3β-HSD cDNA sequence with the respective probes. This result is also confirmed by analysis of parallel sequencing reactions of each corresponding template using the same primer used to synthesize the probes.

The shortest protected fragment of about 131 nucleotides results from an efficient cleavage by S₁ nuclease in the region 598 to 611 containing 7 expected mismatches in the DNA/RNA heteroduplexes formed following annealing of type I probe with the type II mRNA species (lane 2) or type II probe with the type I mRNA species (lane 5), respectively. These findings strongly suggest the predominance of the type I 3β-HSD mRNA species in the rat ovary. This observation has also been confirmed by ribonuclease protection assay (data not shown).

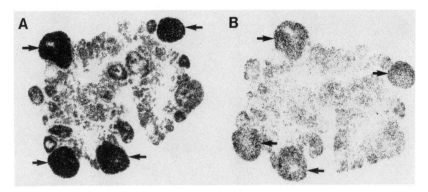

FIGURE 3. Subtissular localization of 3β-HSD type I (A) and type II (B) mRNA species in the rat ovary. Typical autoradiographs following in situ hybridization performed as previously described in reference 5.

Predominance of the 3β-HSD type I mRNA species in the rat ovary is also clearly suggested by in situ hybridization using 5'-end-labeled 24-mer oligonucleotides specific for each mRNA type corresponding to nucleotides 596 to 619 in the antisense orientation. As illustrated in Figure 3, the ovarian subtissular localization of type I 3β-HSD (panel A) is superimposable to that of the type II 3β-HSD mRNA population (panel B), the highest levels being found in the corpora lutea, which are well recognized as the active sites of progesterone biosynthesis. Weaker but significant labeling of 3β-HSD mRNA was also observed in interstitial and thecal cells as ascertained by light microscopy examination (5).

Discussion

The proteins encoded by the two rat mRNAs may be isoenzymes that display subtle differences in their affinities for Δ^5-3β-hydroxysteroids, or they may be localized in different subcellular organelles as suggested by the differences in their predicted transmembrane segments. The presence of multiple genes encoding 3β-HSD certainly offers additional sites of control of expression of this enzyme in various tissues during development and under various physiological conditions in developed tissues. The multiple 3β-HSD mRNAs present in the rat may thus be expressed in a tissue-specific manner. Already, the present data show the predominance of type I 3β-HSD mRNA in the ovary. Moreover, both type I and type II rat 3β-HSD mRNAs are present in classical steroidogenic tissues, such as the adrenals and gonads, as well as in adipose tissue.

References

1. Luu-The V, Lachance Y, Labrie C, et al. Full length cDNA structure and deduced amino acid sequence of human 3β-hydroxy-5-ene steroid dehydrogenase. Mol Endocrinol 1989;3:1310-9.

2. Luu-The V, Takahashi M, Labrie F. Purification of microsomal and mitochondrial 3β-hydroxysteroid dehydrogenase/Δ^5-Δ^4 isomerase from human placenta. Ann NY Acad Sci 1990;595:386-8.

3. Dupont E, Luu-The V, Labrie F, Pelletier G. Light microscopic immunocytochemical localization of 3β-hydroxy-5-ene-steroid dehydrogenase/Δ^5-Δ^4 isomerase (3β-HSD) in the gonads and adrenal glands of the guinea pig. Endocrinology 1990;126:2906-9.

4. Zhao HF, Simard J, Labrie C, et al. Molecular cloning, cDNA structure and predicted amino acid sequence of bovine 3β-hydroxy-5-ene steroid dehydrogenase/Δ^5-Δ^4 isomerase. FEBS Lett 1989;259:153-7.

5. Dupont E, Zhao HF, Rheaume E, et al. Localization of 3β-hydroxysteroid dehydrogenase/Δ^5-Δ^4 isomerase in the rat gonads and adrenal glands by immunocytochemistry and in situ hybridization. Endocrinology 1990;127 (in press).

6. Lacoste D, Bélanger A, Labrie F. Biosynthesis and degradation of androgens in human prostatic cancer cell lines. Ann NY Acad Sci 1990;595:389-91.

7. Abalain JH, Quemener E, Carre JL, et al. Metabolism of androgens in human hyperplastic prostate. Evidence for a differential localization of the enzymes involved in the metabolism. J Steroid Biochem 1989;34: 467-71.

8. Abul-Hajj YJ. Metabolism of dehydroepiandrosterone by hormone dependent and hormone independent human breast carcinoma. Steroids 1975;26:488-501.

9. Jung-Testas I, Hu ZY, Baulieu EE, Robel P. Neurosteroids: Biosynthesis of pregnenolone and progesterone in primary cultures of rat glial cells. Endocrinology 1989;125:2083-91.

10. Lax ER, Schriefers H. Sex specific action of antiandrogens on androgen induced changes in hepatic microsomal 3β-hydroxysteroid dehydrogenase and 5a-reductase activity in the rat. Acta Endocrinol (Copenh) 1981;98:261-6.

11. Bérubé D, Luu-The V, Lachance Y, Gagné R, Labrie F. Assignment of the human 3β-hydroxysteroid dehydrogenase gene (HSDB3) to the p13 band of chromosome 1. Cytogenet Cell Genet 1989;52:199-200.

29

The Signal Transduction System in Luteotrophic Stimulation of Expression of the 3β-HSD Gene in Porcine Granulosa Cells in Culture

P. JORGE CHEDRESE, DANIEL SCHOTT, DAVID ZHANG, AND BRUCE D. MURPHY

The enzyme 3β-hydroxy-Δ^5-steroid dehydrogenase (3β-HSD) catalyses the formation of Δ^4-3ketosteroids from Δ^5-ene, 3β-hydroxysteroids (1). Because it converts pregnenolone to progesterone, it is central to the production of steroid hormones. In rat granulosa cells, follicle stimulating hormone (FSH) and human chorionic gonadotrophin (hCG), which stimulate steroidogenesis, increase the velocity of 3β-HSD, while gonadotrophin releasing hormone, which inhibits steroidogenesis, reduces the velocity, but the K_m is unaffected by these hormones (2, 3). In this chapter, we discuss evidence that in luteinized cultured pig granulosa cells, luteotrophins and cAMP induce an increase in 3β-HSD mRNA levels that can be inhibited by the activation of protein kinase C.

3β-HSD mRNA Response to Gonadotrophins

In our studies, both luteinizing hormone (LH) and hCG induce increases of 3β-HSD mRNA. An increase in 3β-HSD mRNA is observed at 1 h of hCG exposure, and a maximal stimulation of 3-fold relative to controls occurs after 8 h (4). LH at 10 to 1000 ng/mL produces a 3-fold increase in the relative amount of 3β-HSD mRNA (Fig. 1). Actinomycin D, an inhibitor of transcription, blocks the hCG-induced elevation of the message (5), suggesting that hCG effects are primarily due to increased mRNA synthesis as with other hCG-induced genes in luteinized tissue (6). However, the possibility that the hCG effects are mediated in part by altering 3β-HSD mRNA stability cannot be ruled out. The absence of changes in γ-actin mRNA expression indicates that the effects are specific and not a result of a change in overall cellular transcription (5). Cycloheximide, an inhibitor of peptide elongation, has no effect on the 3β-HSD mRNA level in the absence of hCG, but partially blocks induction of 3β-HSD mRNA by hCG (5), suggesting that the hCG effect on 3β-HSD mRNA accumulation depends on the synthesis of protein.

cAMP Pathway Regulation of 3β-HSD mRNA Levels

LH and hCG stimulate formation of the second messenger cyclic adenosine 3',5'-monophosphate (cAMP) (7), which activates cytoplasmic protein kinase A (PKA), whose effects include an increase in steroidogenesis (8). Cholera toxin and forskolin (5), which induce endogenous cAMP, or the cAMP analogs $N^6,2'$-O dibutyryladenosine 3':5'-cyclic monophosphate (Bu$_2$-cAMP) (5) and 8-bromoadenosine 3':5'-cyclic monophosphate (8-br-cAMP) (4) produce an increase in the 3β-HSD mRNA expression. This evidence suggests that gonadotrophins act, at least in part, through cAMP levels to regulate 3β-HSD mRNA levels.

Phosphatidylinositol Pathway Regulation of 3β-HSD mRNA Levels

The phosphatidylinositol pathway also mediates surface ligand signals in luteal tissue. LH (9) and hCG (10) induce an increase in the membrane inositol breakdown and consequent stimulation of the intracellular protein kinase C (PKC) by diacylglycerol (11). We have studied the effect of stimulating PKC with the tumor-promoting phorbol ester phorbol 12-myristate 13-acetate (PMA). From 0.1 to 100 nM, PMA dose-dependently blocks the stimulatory effect of 1-IU/mL hCG on 3β-HSD mRNA expression in granulosa cells in culture (4). PMA alone has no effect on 3β-HSD mRNA levels. The phorbol ester 4α-PDD, which does not activate PKC, elicits no inhibitory effect. PMA also inhibits the stimulatory effect of cholera toxin (4), forskolin (4), 8-br-cAMP (4), LH (Fig. 1), and Bu$_2$-cAMP (Table 1) on 3β-HSD mRNA. Inhibition of 3β-HSD mRNA is observed at concentrations of PMA (1 to 100 nM), which activate PKC-dependent processes in a cell-free system (12) and in ovine luteal cells (13). The diterpene mezerein (100 nM), a non-phorbol ester PKC activator (14), also inhibits hCG stimulation of 3β-HSD mRNA levels (Fig. 2).

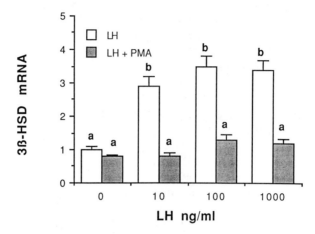

FIGURE 1. Effect of LH and PMA on 3β-HSD mRNA levels in cultured pig granulosa cells. Cells were treated for 6 h. (Values are means relative to the control group, ± SEM of 4 determinations and are representative of 3 experiments; a ≠ b, P < 0.01.)

Conclusion

PKC stimulators block the accumulation of 3β-HSD mRNA that is stimulated by hCG, LH, cAMP analogs, or endogenously elevated cAMP levels, even though PMA itself raises cAMP levels in cultured, luteinized pig granulosa cells (4, 15) and pig corpus luteum (16). The physiological significance is not clear, as LH and hCG each stimulate both PKA and PKC pathways in luteal tissue. PKC might be involved in downregulating the response to chronic luteotrophin exposure.

TABLE 1. Effect of Bu_2-cAMP and PMA on 3β-HSD mRNA expression.

Bu2-cAMP (μM)	No PMA	PMA (100 μM)
0	1.0 ± 0.1	0.9 ± 0.1
10	1.8 ± 0.2 (a)	1.1 ± 0.1 (b)
30	2.3 ± 0.3 (a)	1.2 ± 0.1 (b)
100	2.6 ± 0.3 (a)	1.0 ± 0.1 (b)

Note: Cultured, luteinized pig granulosa cells were treated for 6 h before RNA extraction. Slot-blots (6-μg total RNA) were hybridized to labeled 3β-HSD cDNA and rehybridized to human γ-actin cDNA. Optical densities of the 3β-HSD mRNA autoradiogram were divided by the corresponding values for the γ-actin mRNA. (Values are means relative to the control group, ± SEM of 4 determinations and are representative of 3 experiments; a ≠ b, P < 0.01.)

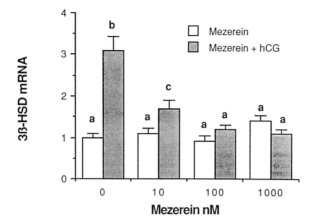

FIGURE 2. Effect of mezerein on hCG stimulated 3β-HSD mRNA levels. Pig granulosa cells were treated for 6 h. (Values are means relative to the control group, ± SEM of 3 determinations and are representative of 3 experiments; a ≠ b and b ≠ c, P < 0.01.)

Acknowledgments. We thank Dr. V. Misra for his help and advice and Drs. F. Labrie and V. Luu-The for providing the 3β-HSD cDNA and aid of many kinds. The research reported in this chapter was supported by a grant from the Medical Research Council of Canada (BDM).

References

1. Samuels LT, Helmreich ML, Lasater MB, Reich H. An enzyme in endocrine tissues which oxidizes Δ⁵-3hydroxy steroids to α,β unsaturated ketones. Science 1951;113:490-1.
2. Jones PBC, Hsueh AJW. Regulation of ovarian 3β-hydroxysteroid dehydrogenase activity by gonadotropin-releasing hormone and follicle-stimulating hormone in cultured rat granulosa cells. Endocrinology 1982;110:1663-71.
3. Jones PBC, Valk CA, Hsueh AJW. Regulation of progestin biosynthetic enzymes in cultured rat granulosa cells: Effects of prolactin, β₂-adrenergic antagonist, human chorionic gonadotropin and gonadotropin releasing hormone. Biol Reprod 1983;29:572-85.
4. Chedrese PJ, Zhang D, The VL, Labrie F, Juorio AV, Murphy BD. Regulation of the mRNA expression of 3β-hydoxy-5-ene steroid dehydrogenase in porcine granulosa cells in culture: A role for the protein kinase C pathway. Mol Endocrinol 1990. Submitted.
5. Chedrese PJ, Luu-The V, Labrie F, Juorio AV, Murphy BD. Evidence for the regulation of 3β-hydroxysteroid dehydrogenase messenger RNA by human chorionic gonadotrophin in luteinized porcine granulosa cells. Endocrinology 1990;126:2228-30.

6. Golos TG, Strauss JF, III. Regulation of low density lipoprotein receptor gene expression in cultured human granulosa cells: Roles of human chorionic gonadotropin, 8-bromo-3'5'cyclic adenosine monophosphate, and protein synthesis. Mol Endocrinol 1987;1:321-6.

7. Marsh JM. The role of cyclic AMP in gonadal steroidogenesis. Biol Reprod 1976;14:30-5.

8. Strauss JF, III, Golos TG, Silavin SL, Soto DA, Takagi K. Involvement of cyclic AMP in the functions of granulosa and luteal regulation of steroidogenesis. In: Haseltine FP, First NL, eds. Meiotic inhibition: Molecular control of meiosis. New York: Alan R. Liss, 1988:201-26.

9. Davis JS, Weakland LL, West LA, Farese RV. Luteinizing hormone stimulates the formation of inositol triphosphate and cAMP in rat granulosa cells: Evidence for phospholipase C generated second messengers in the action of luteinizing hormone. Biochem J 1986;238:597-604.

10. Davis JS, West LA, Weakland LL, Farese RV. Human chorionic gonadotropin activates the inositol 1,4,5-trisphosphate-Ca^{2+} intracellular signalling system in bovine luteal cells. FEBS Lett 1986;208(suppl 2):287-91.

11. Nishizuka Y. The role of protein kinase C in cell surface signal transduction and tumor promotion. Nature 1984;308:693-8.

12. Castagna M, Takai Y, Kaibuchi K, Sano K, Kikkawa U, Nishizuka Y. Direct activation of calcium-activated, phospholipid-dependent protein kinase by tumor promoting phorbol esters. J Biol Chem 1982;257:7847-51.

13. Wiltbank MC, Knickerbocker JJ, Niswender GD. Regulation of the corpus luteum by protein kinase C, I. Phosphorylation activity and steroidogenic action in large and small ovine luteal cells. Biol Reprod 1989;40:1194-200.

14. Miyake R, Tanaka Y, Tsuda T, Kaibuchi K, Kikkawa U, Nishizuka Y. Activation of protein kinase C by non-phorbol tumor promoter, mezerein. Biochem Biophys Res Commun 1984;121:649-56.

15. Murphy BD, Chedrese PJ, Kadaba R. Evidence of cross-talk between protein kinase C and cAMP pathway in porcine granulosa cells [Abstract]. 22nd Annual Meeting of the Society for the Study of Reproduction. Columbia, MO, 1989.

16. Wheeler MB, Veldhuis JD. Facilitative actions of the protein kinase-C effector system on hormonally stimulated adenosine 3',5'monophosphate production by swine luteal cells. Endocrinology 1989;125:2414-20.

30

Control of 3β-HSD mRNA and Activity During the Estrous Cycle in the Bovine Ovary

J. COUËT, C. MARTEL, V. LUU-THE, M.-A. SIRARD, H.F. ZHAO, AND F. LABRIE

Precise programming of the expression of the steroidogenic enzymes in the theca, interstitial, granulosa, and luteal cells of the ovary achieves the physiological pattern of sex steroid secretion observed during the estrous cycle (1, 2). The physiological changes in estrogen and progesterone secretion are accompanied by characteristic morphological modifications reflecting the various stages of the development and growth of ovarian follicles and corpora lutea.

Following cleavage of the side-chain of cholesterol by cytochrome P-450$_{SCC}$, thus leading to the formation of pregnenolone and related Δ^5-3β-hydroxysteroids, a key step in the formation of all classes of steroid hormones is the oxidation and isomerization of the Δ^5-3β-hydroxysteroid precursors into Δ^4-3-ketosteroids. This key step is catalyzed by 3β-hydroxysteroid dehydrogenase/Δ^5-Δ^4 isomerase (3β-HSD) (3, 4), and the 3β-HSD system is present in the gonads (5, 6), adrenal cortex (7), and placenta (4), as well as in several peripheral tissues (8–12). Since 3β-HSD plays a central role in ovarian physiology and reproductive functions, we have taken advantage of the recent cloning and sequencing of human (4) and bovine (5) 3β-HSD cDNA to study the pattern of 3β-HSD mRNA levels and activity in bovine corpora lutea during the estrous cycle.

Results

As illustrated in Figure 1A, bovine luteal 3β-HSD mRNA levels increase progressively from days 1–3 of the luteal phase to reach a maximal value of 65% above control (P < 0.001) on days 10–11 after estrus before decreasing

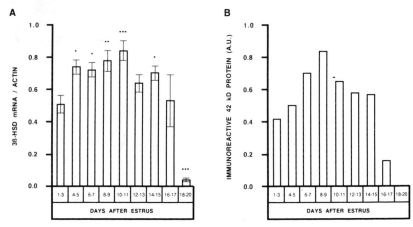

FIGURE 1. *A*: Relative levels of 3β-HSD mRNA in bovine corpora lutea at different stages of the estrous cycle. Total RNA from bovine corpora lutea obtained from the indicated time periods after estrus was extracted by the guanidinium isothiocyanate/ CsCl method. RNA was blotted onto nylon membranes following serial 2-fold dilutions (from 10- to 0.078-μg RNA). Prehybridization and hybridization were performed at 42°C. The ^{32}P-labeled bovine 3β-HSD cDNA or chicken β-actin probes were added at a concentration of 3×10^6 cpm/mL in hybridization buffer. The filters were then washed and exposed to X-ray film for 4 different time intervals. Spot intensities were measured with an image analyzer, and data are expressed as means ± SEM of ratios of 3β-HSD and actin hybridization intensities. (*, P < 0.05; **, P < 0.01; and ***, P < 0.001, experimental versus days 1–3 after estrus.) *B*: Immunoreactive 42-kDa band intensities of bovine corpora lutea crude homogenate at different stages of the estrous cycle. Total protein (150μg) of corpus luteum homogenate of each group was separated by SDS-PAGE. The blot was treated with a rabbit anti-human 3β-HSD serum and labeled with ^{125}I-labeled goat anti-rabbit IgG. The autoradiograph was obtained after exposing the filter to X-ray films for 22 h. The intensities of the 42-kDa immunoreactive protein band were measured with an image analyzer and are shown in arbitrary units.

progressively until days 16–17 before an abrupt fall to 5% of maximal levels measured on days 18–20. Using a polyclonal antiserum raised in rabbits against purified human placental 3β-HSD (4), a predominant 42-kDa immunoreactive band was observed by immunoblot analysis of bovine corpus luteum homogenate (13). In close parallelism with the changes in 3β-HSD mRNA levels described above, the level of immunoreactive 3β-HSD (42-kDa component), as illustrated in Figure 1*B*, increases progressively from days 1–3 to a maximal 100% increase over control on days 8–9 with a progressive decrease thereafter to undetectable levels on days 18–20.

Since there is evidence for multiple 3β-HSDs (14), enzymatic activity was measured in the corpora lutea at the same 9 stages of development using 3 different substrates: pregnenolone, dehydroepiandrosterone (DHEA), and

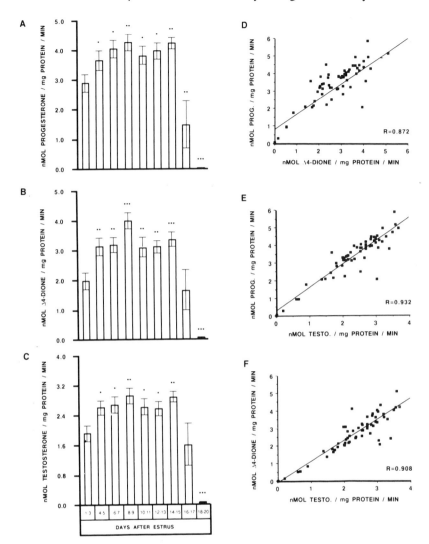

FIGURE 2. *Left panels*: 3β-HSD enzymatic activity in bovine corpora lutea at different stages of the estrous cycle using pregnenolone (*A*), DHEA (*B*), and Δ^5-diol (*C*) as substrates. Bovine corpora lutea homogenate (100 μL) was incubated with 20 μM of the substrate (0.4 μCl), 0.02-mL propylene glycol, 0.88-mL phosphate buffer, and 1-mM NAD⁺ for 15 min at 37°C. Steroids were extracted twice with 2 volumes of CH_2Cl_2 before evaporation and suspension in 0.1-mL $CHCL_3$:methanol (2:1;v/v). Aliquots (20 μL) were chromatographed on TLC plates with $CHCL_3$:acetone (19:1;v/v), and radioactive spots were cut out and counted. (Data are expressed as means ± SEM.) *Right panels*: Correlation of 3β-HSD activity in bovine corpora lutea obtained at various stages of the estrous cycle using pregnenolone (PREG), DHEA, and Δ5-diol as substrates: *D*, PREG vs. DHEA; *E*, PREG vs. Δ^5-DIOL; *F*, DHEA vs. Δ^5-DIOL. (P < 0.0001 for all correlations.)

androst-5-ene-3β,17β-diol (Δ^5-diol). As illustrated in Figure 2A, when pregnenolone was used as substrate, there was a progressive increase in 3β-HSD activity from 2.91 ± 0.29 nM/mg protein/min progesterone formed on days 1–3 to a maximal value of 4.27 ± 0.27 nM/mg protein/min (P < 0.01) on days 8–9 after estrus with levels remaining on a plateau until days 14–15. Thereafter, a dramatic fall was observed up to days 18–20 to values less than 1% of those measured on days 1–3 (P < 0.001). It can also be seen in Figure 2 that almost superimposable results were obtained when DHEA (Fig. 2B) or Δ^5-diol (Fig. 2C) were used as labeled substrates. With DHEA, a maximal value of 103% over control (P < 0.001) was obtained on days 8–9 after estrus, while a value of 51% above control (P < 0.01) was measured on the same days of the luteal phase when Δ^5-diol was the substrate used. As also shown in Figure 2, strong correlations were found when comparing the enzymatic activities obtained with each substrate (P < 0.0001). The correlation between all values of 3β-HSD mRNA levels were also determined relative to corresponding individual enzymatic activities. The calculated correlation coefficients (R) are, respectively, 0.763, 0.731, and 0.785, using pregnenolone, DHEA, and Δ^5-diol as substrates (P < 0.0001). As expected from data on 3β-HSD content and the enzymatic activity described in Figure 2, there is a close correlation between the levels of 3β-HSD immunoreactivity and enzymatic activity measured for each substrate: pregnenolone (R = 0.951), DHEA (R = 0.978), and Δ^5-diol (R = 0.982) (P < 0.0001).

Discussion

Understanding of the pattern of ovarian estrogen and progesterone secretion during the estrous cycle requires precise knowledge of the mechanisms controlling the expression and activity of each steroidogenic enzyme involved. Previous studies have described the enzymatic activity and mRNA levels of two important steroidogenic enzymes, namely, P-450$_{SCC}$ and P-450$_{17\alpha}$ No information, however, was available about 3β-HSD, an essential step in the formation of progesterone as well as all precursors of androgens and estrogens.

In agreement with the marked changes in total steroid biosynthesis measured between the follicular and luteal phases of the cycle, the present data also show that low levels of 3β-HSD activity were measured in bovine ovarian follicles before ovulation (13), these levels being dramatically increased on days 1–3 after estrus. Thereafter, ovarian 3β-HSD mRNA levels increase to maximal values on days 8–11, with an almost complete loss of expression on days 18–20. The present study also shows a close correlation between 3β-HSD mRNA, protein content, and enzymatic activity levels during all stages of the luteal phase.

Such data offer an explanation for the marked changes in progesterone secretion observed during the estrous cycle (1). A large increase in the secretion of progesterone takes place following ovulation and maximal levels are reached 8–10 days after estrus in the bovine species. In parallel, there is a marked increase in P-450$_{SCC}$ activity after ovulation (15) from undetectable levels in bovine ovarian follicles (16). Moreover, the activity of HMG/CoA reductase, a rate-limiting enzyme in cholesterol biosynthesis, is also greatly elevated in corpora lutea (17), thus providing high levels of precursor cholesterol, while the activity of 17α-hydroxylase originally present in theca interna cells decreases to undetectable levels in the corpus luteum (15), thus blocking androgen and estrogen formation and providing all precursors for maximal progesterone secretion.

While some evidence suggests the possible existence of multiple 3β-HSDs (14), the present data show a very high degree of correlation of substrate specificity at all levels of enzymatic activity using the 3 substrates pregnenolone, DHEA, and Δ5-diol. Such data do not exclude the possibility of more than one ovarian 3β-HSD having different substrate specificity, but they offer no evidence for preferential expression of one enzymatic form during the estrous cycle.

Conclusion

The expression of 3β-HSD in the ovary has been suggested as being constitutive (3, 18). The present study clearly indicates that the expression of 3β-HSD is strongly modulated in the ovary during the estrous cycle. The demonstration of a close parallelism between 3β-HSD mRNA levels, protein content, and activity suggests that the formation of progesterone in the corpus luteum is regulated, at least up to a large extent, by changes in 3β-HSD gene expression and/or 3β-HSD mRNA stability.

References

1. Hansel W, Convey EM. Physiology of the estrous cycle. J Anim Sci 1983;57:404-29.
2. Hsueh AJH. Ovarian hormone synthesis, circulation and mechanism of action. In: De Groot LJ, Besser GM, Cahill GF, et al., eds. Endocrinology. 2nd ed; vol 3. 1989.
3. Readhead C, Lobo RA, Kletzky DA. The activity of 3β-hydroxysteroid dehydrogenase and Δ4-5 isomerase in human follicular tissue. Am J Obstet Gynecol 1983;145:491-5.
4. Luu-The V, Lachance Y, Labrie C, et al. Full length cDNA structure and deduced aminoacid sequence of human 3β-hydroxy-5-ene steroid dehydrogenase. Mol Endocrinol 1989;3:1310-2.

5. Zhao HF, Simard J, Labrie C, et al. Molecular cloning, cDNA structure and predicted amino acid sequence of bovine 3β-hydroxy-5-ene-steroid dehydrogenase/Δ4-Δ5-isomerase. FEBS Lett 1989;259:153-7.

6. Ishii-Ohba H, Saiki N, Inano H, Tamaoki BI. Purification and properties of testicular 3β-hydroxy-5-ene-steroid dehydrogenase and 5-ene-4-ene isomerase. J Steroid Biochem 1986;24:753-60.

7. Ishii-Ohba H, Inano H, Tamaoki BI. Testicular and adrenal 3β-hydroxy-5-ene-steroid dehydrogenase and 5-ene-4-ene-isomerase. J Steroid Biochem 1987;27:775-9.

8. Lacoste D, Bélanger A, Labrie F. Biosynthesis and degradation of androgens in human prostatic cancer cell lines. In: Bradlow H, Castagnetta L, d'Aquino S, Labrie F, eds. Steroid formation, degradation and action in peripheral, normal and neoplastic tissues. Ann New York Acad Sci 1990;595:389-91.

9. Abul-Hajj YJ. Metabolism of dehydrogenase administration by hormone-dependant and hormone-independant human breast carcinoma. Steroids 1975;26:488-500.

10. Cameron EM, Baillie AM, Grant JK, Milne JA, Thompson J. Transformation in vitro of [7α-3H] dehydroepiandrosterone to [3H] testosterone by skin from men. J Endocrinol 1966;35:xix-xx.

11. Lax ER, Schriefers H. Δ4-3β-hydroxysteroid dehydrogenase activity in rat liver. Intracellular distribution and sex dependancy. Acta Endocrinol (Copenh) 1981;98:261-6.

12. Jung-Testas I, Hu ZY, Baulieu EE, Robel P. Neurosteroids: Biosynthesis of pregnenolone and progesterone in primary cultures of rat glial cells. Endocrinology 1989;125:2083-91.

13. Couët J, Martel C, Dupont E, et al. Changes in 3β-hydroxysteroid dehydrogenase/Δ5-Δ4 isomerase mRNA, activity and protein levels during the estrous cycle in the bovine ovary. Endocrinology (in press).

14. Hiwatashi A, Hamamoto I, Ichikawa Y. Purification and kinetic properties of 3β-hydroxysteroid dehydrogenase from bovine adrenocortical microsomes. J Biochem 1985;98:1519-26.

15. Rodgers RJ, Waterman MR, Simpson ER. Cytochromes P450scc, P450 17α, adrenoxin and reduced nicotinamide adenine dinucleotide phosphate-cytochrome p450 reductase in bovine follicles and corpora lutea. Changes in specific contents during the ovarian cycle. Endocrinology 1986;118:1366-74.

16. Rodgers RJ, Waterman MR, Simpson ER. Levels of messenger ribonucleic acid encoding cholesterol side-chain cleavage cytochrome P-450, 17α-hydroxylase cytochrome P-450, adrenoxin and low density lipoprotein receptor in bovine follicles and corpora lutea throughout the ovarian cycle. Mol Endocrinol 1987; 1:274-9.

17. Rodgers RJ, Mason JI, Waterman MR, Simpson ER. Regulation of the synthesis of 3-hydroxy-3-methylglutamyl coenzyme A reductase in the bovine ovary in vivo and in vitro. Mol Endocrinol 1987;1:172-80.

18. Gore-Lanston RE, Armstrong DT. Follicular steroidogenesis and its control. In: Knobil E, Neill J, eds. The physiology of reproduction; vol 1. New York: Raven Press, 1988:331.

31

Expression of IGF-I and IGF-I Receptor Gene in the Corpus Luteum

T.G. PARMER, M. ZILBERSTEIN, I. KHAN, C. ALBARRACIN, AND G. GIBORI

Insulin-like growth factors (IGFs) are peptide mitogens that have been implicated in growth and development of the rat ovary. Insulin-like growth factor I (IGF-I) has been shown to affect granulosa cell proliferation and differentiation in vitro (1).Recent investigations indicate that granulosa cells produce IGF-I and IGF-I binding proteins (2) and are a major site of IGF-I mRNA gene expression (1). In addition, binding studies have revealed that granulosa and theca interstitial cells have receptors for IGF-I (3).Thus, IGF-I appears to act not only in an autocrine fashion, but also in a paracrine one as well, by serving as one of several signals through which the granulosa cells may communicate with the nearby theca interstitial cells.

The cells of the corpus luteum are formed by a process involving luteinization and differentiation of the theca and granulosa cells. This process by which cells of the follicle hypertrophy or the mechanisms that cause a luteinized granulosa cell to stop dividing and transform into a highly differentiated steroidogenic cell is not fully understood. Since IGF-I acts primarily on cell growth and differentiation it became of interest to determine whether the corpus luteum is the site of expression and/or action of this growth factor.

Thus, the objectives of this study were to determine *(a)* if the corpus luteum of the pregnant rat expresses the IGF-I and IGF-I receptor genes, *(b)* to examine the tissue specificity of such expression, and *(c)* to determine the developmental expression of IGF-I and IGF-I receptor in the rat corpus luteum during pregnancy.

Materials and Methods

Pregnant Sprague-Dawley rats were purchased from Holtzman Co. (Madison, WI). Liver, uterus, kidney, lung, decidua, and adrenal were removed from day-14 pregnant rats. Whole ovaries were obtained from cycling rats. For developmental studies, corpora lutea were isolated from days 5–21 of pregnancy and 24 h after parturition.

Total cellular RNA was prepared by homogenization in guanidinium thiocyanate (4). Ethidium bromide staining confirmed that the ribosomal RNAs were intact and that equal amounts of RNA were loaded in each lane. For Northern blots 20–40 µg of total RNA per lane were fractionated by electrophoresis on 1.5% agarose/2.2 M formaldehyde gels in 1× 3-morpholinopropanesulfonic acid buffer and blotted to nylon membranes (GeneScreen, DuPont-NEN, Boston, MA) according to manufacturers instructions. For slot-blots, 20 µg of total RNA from each tissue was denatured in 6% formaldehyde and 50% deionized formamide and applied to GeneScreen using a filtration manifold. The rat IGF-I cDNA probe was a 376 base pair (bp) fragment that contained 102 bp of 5'-untranslated region and 224 bp of the coding region (5). The rat IGF-I receptor cDNA probe was a 265-bp fragment containing sequences encoding 15 bases of the 5'-untranslated region and sequences encoding the signal peptide and the first 53 amino acids of the α-subunit (6). Both probes were labeled with [^{32}P]dCTP (3000 Ci/mM; Amersham Co., Arlington Heights, IL) using a random prime labeling kit. Blots were hybridized with cDNA probes in a solution containing 50% formamide, 5× SSPE, 1% sodium dodecyl sulfate, 10× Denhardt's and 100-µg/mL heterologous DNA at 50°C, washed in 2× SSPE and 0.2% SDS, followed by 0.1× SSPE at 50°C and 0.1× SSPE at 60°C. Blots were then exposed to Kodak XAR-2 film (Eastman Kodak, Rochester, NY) for 3–7 days at –7°C with intensifying screens. The same hybridization and washing conditions were used for both probes. Densitometric scanning of autoradiograms of slot blots was conducted using an Ephortec Joyce Loebl Densitometer.

Results

Results of this study show that the corpus luteum of the pregnant rat is a site for IGF-I as well as IGF-I receptor gene expression. Northern blot analysis shows the presence of multiple transcripts for IGF-I in the corpus luteum on day 16 of pregnancy with estimated sizes of 1.0, 1.7, 4.7, and 7.5 kb (Fig. 1). These transcripts are identical to those seen in the liver.

Results shown in Figure 2 indicate that the corpus luteum also expresses mRNA for IGF-I receptor. Northern blot analysis, performed with 40 µg of total RNA, shows the presence of multiple transcripts in the corpus luteum with estimated sizes of 3.1, 5.4, and 11.0 kb.

Developmental studies reveal that luteal IGF-I and IGF-I receptor mRNAs are present in the corpus luteum on all days of pregnancy tested, as well as 24-h postpartum (data not shown).

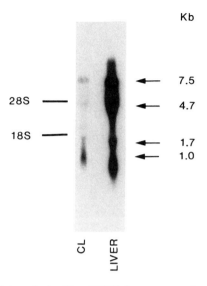

FIGURE 1. Northern blot analysis of total RNA from corpora lutea and liver of day-16 pregnant rat hybridized with rIGF-I cDNA. Each lane contains 20-µg RNA. The numbers to the right of the blot indicate the sizes of specific hybridizing transcripts estimated from sizes of the 28S and 18S ribosomal bands and standards of known size.

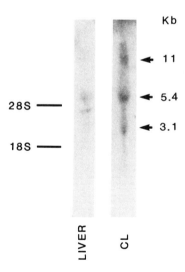

FIGURE 2. IGF-I receptor mRNA in liver and luteal tissue. Total RNA from corpora lutea and liver of day-16 pregnant rats was analyzed by Northern blot using the rIGF-I receptor cDNA. Each lane contained 40-µg total RNA.

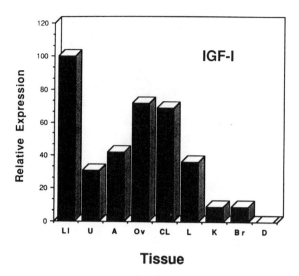

FIGURE 3. Relative expression of IGF-I mRNA from liver (Li), uterus (U), adrenal (A), ovary (Ov), corpus luteum (CL), lung (L), kidney (K), brain (Br), and decidua (D) from day-15 pregnant rats. Autoradiograms of slot-blots were subjected to densitometric analysis.

In comparison to other tissues of the day-15 pregnant rat and to ovaries from cycling rats, the corpus luteum had the third highest amount of message for IGF-I (Fig. 3). IGF-I mRNA was also fairly abundant in the uterus, adrenal, and lung, while low levels were detectable in kidney and brain. No message was seen in the decidua.

Results of the tissue specificity study shown in Figure 4 indicate that the message for IGF-I receptor is abundantly expressed in the corpus luteum as compared to liver, adrenal, ovary, lung, and uterus. No message was detected in decidua and kidney.

Discussion

Results of this investigation have revealed that mRNAs for both IGF-I and IGF-I receptor are abundantly expressed in the corpus luteum of the pregnant rat. The multiple transcripts seen for IGF-I in the corpus luteum were identical to those found in the liver. Hybridization of IGF-I cDNAs to RNA from various rat tissues has demonstrated the presence of these major species (7). The IGF-I gene transcript has been shown to exist in multiple forms due to alternative splicing and promoter sites as well as differences in polyadenylation sites (8). In this study, multiple transcripts were also seen

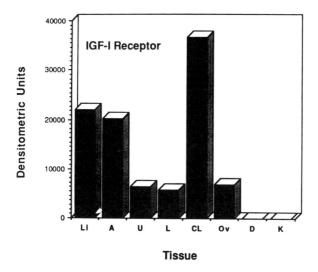

FIGURE 4. Comparison of IGF-I receptor mRNA levels (in densitometric units) from liver (Li), adrenal (A), uterus (U), lung (L), corpus luteum (CL), ovary (Ov), decidua (D), and kidney (K) from day-15 pregnant rats. Autoradiograms of slot-blots were subjected to densitometric analysis.

for IGF-I receptor in the corpus luteum. It has been reported that the human IGF-I receptor gene is transcribed into 7- and 11-kb mRNAs (9). In the rat corpus luteum transcripts at 3.1, 5.4 and 11 kb were detected. The mechanism by which these three size classes of IGF-I receptor mRNA are generated and their significance remains unknown.

In comparison to other tissues of the pregnant rat, the corpus luteum displayed the second highest level of message for IGF-I with the liver being the most abundant. Similar levels of mRNA were seen in ovaries from cycling rats. For IGF-I receptor, the corpus luteum contained the highest level of message, having twice as much mRNA for IGF-I receptor than liver and adrenal and almost five times as much as the ovary. IGF-I mRNA in the ovary has been reported to be granulosa cell-selective (10).

The role of IGF-I in ovarian physiology is still unclear but it may be involved in the regulation of follicular growth and differentiation in vivo. The significance of the abundance of mRNA for both IGF-I and IGF-I receptor in the corpus luteum is of great interest. Luteal cells are highly differentiated cells which undergo hypertrophy with the advance of pregnancy. IGF-I mRNA increases markedly from day 10 of pregnancy. This is a time when the corpus luteum doubles in size. This temporal relationship suggests that the corpus luteum may produce the growth factor responsible for its own growth.

In summary, this study has demonstrated that the corpus luteum of the pregnant rat expresses the genes for both IGF-I and the IGF-I receptor and may, therefore, be a major site of secretion and action of this growth factor in the ovary.

Acknowledgments. We wish to express our sincere appreciation to Dr. D. LeRoith for providing the IGF-I and IGF-I receptor cDNA probes and to Dr. H. Werner for helpful advice and discussions. We also thank Ms. L. Alaniz for photography. The research reported here was supported by NIH grants HD-11119 and HD-12356 (GG) and NIH-NRSA Fellowship HD-7336 (TGP).

References

1. Adashi EY, Resnick C, Hernandez ER, et al. Rodent studies on the potential relevance of insulin-like growth factor (IGF-I) to ovarian physiology. In: Hirshfield AN, ed. Growth factors and the ovary. New York: Serono Symposia, USA/ Plenum Press, 1989:95-105.
2. Hammond JM, Baranao JLS, Skaleris D, et al. Production of insulin-like growth factors by ovarian granulosa cells. Endocrinology 1985;117:2553-5.
3. Adashi EY, Resnick CE, Hernandez ER, et al. Characterization and regulation of specific cell membrane receptors for somatomedin-C/insulin-like growth factor-I in culture and rat granulosa cells. Endocrinology 1988;122:194-201.
4. Chirgwin JM, Przybyla AE, Macdonald RJ, Rutter WJ. Isolation of biologically active ribonucleic acid from sources enriched in ribonuclease. Biochemistry 1979;18:5294-9.
5. Roberts CT, Jr, Lasky SR, Lowe WL, Jr, et al. Molecular cloning of rat insulin-like growth factor I complementary deoxyribonucleic acids: Differential messenger ribonucleic acid processing and regulation by growth hormone in extrahepatic tissues. Mol Endocrinol;1:243-8.
6. Werner H, Woloschak M, Adamo M, et al. Developmental regulation of the rat insulin-like growth factor I receptor gene. Proc Natl Acad Sci USA 1989; 86:7451-5.
7. Shimatsu A, Rotwein D. Mosaic evolution of insulin-like growth factors: Organization, sequence and expression of the rat insulin-like growth factor I gene. J Biol Chem 1987;262:7894-900.
8. Daughaday WH, Rotwein P. Insulin-like growth factors I and II. Peptide, messenger ribonucleic acid and gene structures, serum and tissue concentrations. Endocr Rev 1989;10:68-91.
9. Roberts CT, LeRoith D. Molecular aspects of insulin-like growth factors, their binding proteins and receptors. Bailliere's Clin Endocrinol Metab 1988;2: 1069-85.
10. Hernandez ER, Hurwitz A, Adashi EY. Rat ovarian IGF-II gene expression is theca-interstitial cell exclusive: Hormonal regulation of IGF-II and type II IGF receptors gene expression [Abstract]. Endocrinology 1990;127:1067A.

32

Expression of IGF-I and IGF-I Receptor Gene in Transformed Luteal Cells

M. ZILBERSTEIN, T.G. PARMER, S. NELSON, M.P. MCLEAN,
L. HARLOW, N. GLEICHER, J.Y. CHOU, AND G. GIBORI

We have recently demonstrated that the rat corpus luteum synthesizes both insulin-like growth factor I (IGF-I) and IGF-I receptor mRNAs (1). IGF-I is a mitogenic factor known for its stimulatory effect on cell proliferation (2). In certain cells and specifically rat granulosa cells, IGF-I also causes cellular differentiation and maturation. Therefore, in the granulosa cells, IGF-I may have a dual function as modulator of growth and differentiation (3). The primary culture of rat luteal cells and their long-term maintenance have been difficult. Low cellular yields have limited the possibilities for the study of gene regulation in luteal cells. In order to circumvent the shortcomings of primary cultures, various attempts have been made to immortalize epithelial cells from normal tissues and cell cultures that will retain a spectrum of tissue-specific traits and function. Recently, we have been able to characterize a temperature-sensitive rat granulosa cell line (4) that subsequently allowed the cloning of the rat IGF-I receptor cDNA (5). The goal of this investigation was to immortalize luteal cells and establish a cell line that expresses IGF-I and IGF-I receptors in order to study their respective gene regulation.

Materials and Methods

Luteal cells were isolated from corpus luteum of day-14 pregnant rats according to the method described by Nelson et al. (6) and purified to homogeneity by flow cytometry. Cells were cultured in mixed media (1:1 McCoy 5A and Ham F-12, Cellgro Mediatech, Washington, DC), supplemented with 5%

fetal calf serum. After plating of 24 h, the cells were washed twice and infected with the SV40 tsA 255 mutant virus. The cultures were then maintained at 33°C. The first colonies appeared after 3 months of culture and were harvested by trypsin/EDTA treatment as described before (4, 8).

Detection of 3β-HSD was done by hystochemical staining of cells fixed in 1% paraformaldehyde in PBS. After one h, fixation cells were incubated at 37°C overnight in the presence of etiocholanone, NADH, and nitro blue tetrazolium. They were then fixed again in 1% glutaraldehyde in Brenner Broth and counterstained with eosin.

Total cellular RNA was prepared by homogenization in guanidinium thiocyanate and by centrifugation through a CsCl gradient. For slot-blots analysis 20 μg of total ACLA1 cells, RNA denatured in 6% formaldehyde and 50% deionized formamide, were applied to Genescreen using a filtration manifold. The rat IGF-I cDNA probe was a 376-bp HindIII/EcoRI fragment (9). The rat IGF-I receptor cDNA probe was 265-bp fragment containing sequences encoding 15 bases of the 5'-untranslated region and sequences encoding the signal peptide as well as the first 53 amino acids of the α-subunit (5). Both probes were labeled with [^{32}P]dCTP (3000 Ci/mM, Amersham Co., Arlington Heights, IL), using a random prime labeling kit. Blots were hybridized with cDNA probes in solution containing 50% formamide, 5× SSPE, 1% sodium dodecyl sulfate, 10× Denhardt's solution, and 100 μg/mL heterogenous DNA at 50°C, washed in 2× SSPE and 0.2% SDS, followed by 0.1× SSPE at 50°C and 0.1× SSPE at 60°C. Blots were then exposed to Kodak XAR-2 film for 3–7 days at –70°C with intensifying screens. Densitometric scanning of autoradiograms of slot-blots was conducted using an Ephortec Joyce Loebl Densitometer.

Results

Three months after infection of rat luteal cells with tsA 255 virus the ACLA1 colony was harvested. The cells were passed when they reached confluence, and after 41 passages, they still kept their morphology and heat sensitivity. To demonstrate that the cloned ACLA1 cells are indeed temperature sensitive for maintenance of cell proliferation, their growth was recorded at both temperatures after two-week incubation (Fig. 1). While primary luteal cells do not divide in culture, ACLA1 cells rapidly multiplied at the permissive temperature (33°C) to form multilayers. When shifted to the nonpermissive temperature (40°C), cell division ceased, and cells grew as monolayer. The morphology of ACLA1 also changed as they assumed a nontransformed phenotype of wide cytoplasmatic cells (Fig. 2). ACLA1 cells retained their epithelial nature at both temperatures. Almost every cell at both temperatures exhibited the expression of cytokeratin in the cytoplasm (Fig. 3). ACLA1

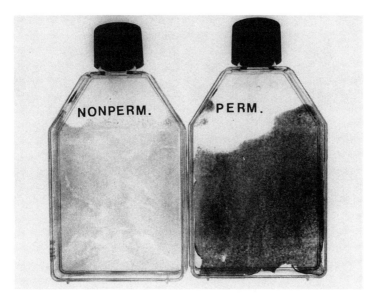

FIGURE 1. Growth characteristics of ACLA1 cells. ACLA1 cells at concentration of 1 million cells per flask were plated in 75-cm^2 tissue culture flasks. After 2 days at 33°C, one of the flasks was shifted to 40°C, and one flask stayed at 33°C. Incubation continued for 12 more days, and the medium was changed every day. At the end of the experiment, the cells were washed 3 times, fixed, and stained. Increased ability to grow on plastic and increased saturation density at the permissive temperature is shown by darker staining. (Nonperm = nonpermissive 40°C; perm = permissive 33°C.)

cells produced small amounts of progesterone and demonstrated aromatase activity (data not shown). They also expressed 3β-HSD activity, as shown in Figure 4. These findings attest to the luteal origin of ACLA1 cells.

ACLA1 cells expressed IGF-I mRNA at both temperatures. Northern blot analysis of IGF-I mRNA in transfected luteal cells revealed two major hybridization bands with estimated size of 7.5 kb and 11 kb and two additional minor bands (data not shown). Slot-blot analysis of IGF-I mRNA obtained from these ACLA1 cells, grown at 33°C and 40°C, is shown in Figure 5.

Recently we have demonstrated the existence of specific IGF-I binding sites on luteal cells (I. Khan, S. Nelson, E.Y. Adashi, and G. Gibori, unpublished data). It became, therefore, of interest to examine the expression of IGF-I receptor in these luteal-derived cells. Total RNA, prepared from ACLA1 cells at both temperatures, hybridized with ^{32}P-labeled rat IGF-I receptor cDNA, revealed a major band of 11 kb. As shown in Figure 6, IGF-I receptor mRNA is also expressed in ACLA1 cell at both temperatures.

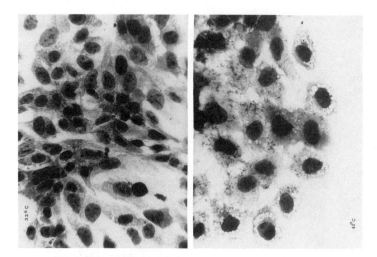

FIGURE 2. Morphological characteristic of ACLA1 cells. ACLA1 cells were plated on coverslips at concentration of 10^5 cells. The cells were incubated for a week at either 33°C *(left panel)* or 40°C *(right panel)*. At the end of the incubation period, the cells were fixed and stained with hematoxylin and eosin. Photomicrographs of ACLA1 cell (35×) are shown.

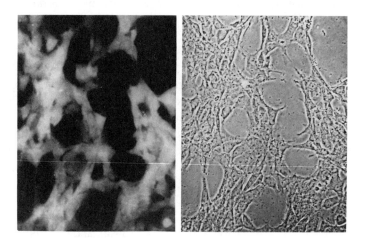

FIGURE 3. Immunofluorescence for cytokeratin in ACLA1 cells. Cells were grown at 33°C for 7 days on coverslips at the initial concentration of 10^5 cells before staining. The microphotographs (35×) taken in dark field *(left panel)* and light field *(right panel)*.

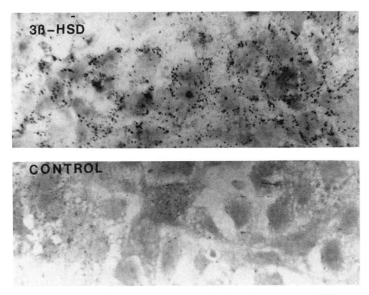

FIGURE 4. 3β-HSD activity in ACLA1 cells grown at 40°C.

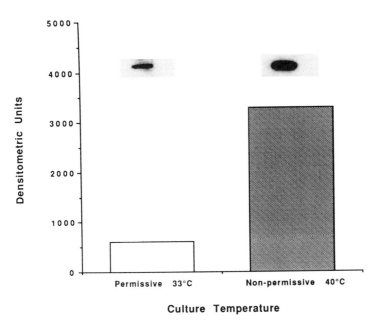

FIGURE 5. Slot-blot analysis of IGF-I mRNA in ACLA1 cells. Autoradiograms were subjected to densitometric analysis.

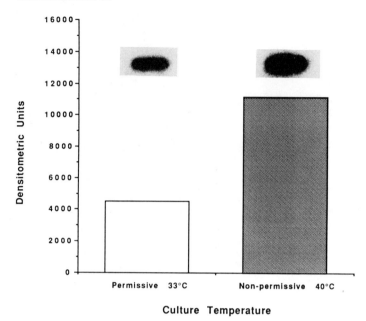

FIGURE 6. Slot-blot analysis of IGF-I receptor mRNA in ACLA1 cells as in Figure 5.

Discussion

It has been recently suggested that IGF-I might have a role in luteal cells (9), similar to that in granulosa cells (3). The primary culture of rat luteal cells is difficult and does not allow the study of gene expression due to low yield. The cloned ACLA1 cells are conditionally transformed; they extensively divide and express the transformed phenotype at the permissive temperature (33°C). At the nonpermissive temperature (40°C), the cells cease to divide, lose their ability to form multilayers, and form a monolayer of large cells. ACLA1 cells retain their epithelial nature, express limited steroidogenic capabilities under the conditions tested so far, and also retain the ability to express both IGF-I and IGF-I receptor genes. ACLA1 cells feature the advantages of a temperature-sensitive cell line that has a built-in internal control for the study of cell proliferation and differentiation processes (7). We therefore suggest ACLA1 cells for further studies of such mechanisms, relevant to epithelial cells and specifically to corpus luteum cells. The establishment of ACLA1 cells will enable us to study IGF-I and IGF-I receptor gene expression and regulation in an epithelial cell model that retains some of the original luteal cell traits; ACLA1 cells produce small amounts of progesterone and demonstrate both aromatase and 3β-HSD activity. The temperature-sensitive nature of ACLA1 cells secures unlimited number of cells of luteal origin and confers adequate internal controls.

Acknowledgments. We express sincere appreciation to Dr. D. LeRoith for the IGF-I and IGF-I receptor cDNA probes and thank Ms. Linda Alaniz for photography and Janice Gentry for typing the manuscript. Supported by NIH grant HD-11119 (GG) and Foundation for Reproductive Medicine, Inc., Chicago (MZ).

References

1. Parmer TG, Khan I, Albarracin C, Zilberstein M, LeRoith D, Gibori G. Expression of IGF-I and IGF-I receptor gene in the corpus luteum [Abstract]. VIII Ovarian Workshop. Serono Symposia, USA, Maryville, TN, 1990. (*See* Chapter 31, this volume.)
2. Clemmons DR, Van Wyk JJ. Somatomedins: Physiological control and effects on cell proliferation. In: Baserga R, ed. Handbook of experimental pharmacology. New York: Springer-Verlag, 1981;57:161-208.
3. Adashi EY, Resnick CE, D'Ercole AJ, Svoboda ME, Van Wyk JJ. Insulin like growth factors as intraovarian regulators of granulosa cell growth and function. Endocr Rev 1985;6:400-20.
4. Zilberstein M, Chou JY, Lowe WL, Jr, et al. Expression of insulin-like growth factor I and its receptor by SV40-transformed rat granulosa cells. Mol Endocrinol 1989;3:1467-88.
5. Werner H, Woloschak M, Adamo M, Shen-Orr Z, Roberts CT, Jr, LeRoith D. Developmental regulation of the rat insulin-like growth factor I receptor gene. Proc Natl Acad Sci USA 1989;86:7451-5.
6. Nelson S, Jaytalak PG, Hunzicker-Dunn M, Gibori G. Characterization of two luteal cell types from the pregnant rat corpus luteum. Biol Reprod 1987;36:135A.
7. Chou JY. Differentiated mammalian cell lines immortalized by temperature-sensitive tumor viruses. Mol Endocrinol 1989;3:1511-4.
8. Chou JY. Establishment of rat liver lines and characterization of their metabolic and hormonal properties: Use of temperature-sensitive SV40 virus. Methods Enzymol 1985;109:385-96.
9. Roberts CT, Jr, Lasky SR, Lowe WL, Jr, Seamon WT, LeRoith D. Molecular cloning of rat insulin-like growth factor I complementary deoxyribonucleic acids: Differential messenger ribonucleic acid processing and regulation by growth hormone in extrahepatic tissues. Mol Endocrinol 1987;1:243-8.
10. McArdle CA, Holtorf AP. Oxytocin and progesterone release from bovine corpus luteal cells in culture: Effect of insulin-like growth factor I, insulin and prostaglandins. Endocrinology 1989;124:1278-86.

33

Relationships of Oocyte Quality and IGF-I in Follicular Fluid During the Estrual Period in Cattle and Effects of Pre-Estrual Progestins

T. WISE, J.M. GRIZZLE, AND R.R. MAURER

Two techniques are predominantly utilized to synchronize beef animals to estrus for artificial insemination or in vitro fertilization of oocytes: *(a)* prostaglandin-induced corpus luteum regression, which results in estrus and ovulation in 48–60 h, and *(b)* implanting/injecting progestins for 5–20 days, which upon removal of silastic implants and clearance of progestin, results in estrus and ovulation. Both techniques produce comparable results in reference to estrus and ovulation, but conception and fertility are generally reduced with progestins (1, 2, 3). Follicular progesterone concentrations and the time when progesterone concentrations increase and fall are important in the maturation and quality of oocytes (4, 5). Insulin-like growth factor I (IGF-I) may have a role in regulating follicular progesterone concentrations (6, 7, 8, 9) and subsequent oocyte quality. The objectives of this study were to *(a)* elucidate possible differences in oocyte quality between prostaglandin- and progestin-synchronized estrus in heifers and *(b)* establish relationship of follicular IGF-1 to oocyte quality, follicular development, and progestin effects as influenced by treatments.

Materials and Methods

Cyclic crossbred heifers were randomly assigned to 3 treatments consisting of *(a)* prostaglandin-induced corpora lutea regression (n = 30) to synchronize to estrus, *(b)* silastic progestin (Norgestomet) implants for 8 days, which, upon removal, results in estrus (n = 30), or *(c)* prostaglandin-synchronized animals, which were administered a silastic progestin implant 12 h prior to prostaglandin injection (n = 25). All animals were superovulated with follicle stimulating hormone (FSH) by the method of Wise et al. (10). Subsequently, animals were ovariectomized at 12, 36, 48, 60, or 72 h after prostaglandin injection or progestin implant removal. After ovariectomy, follicular diameter was measured, follicular fluid aspirated, and follicles flushed with heparinized phosphate buffered saline. Oocytes were located in the follicular fluid or saline flush and evaluated for quality (viable or degenerate). In follicles ≤4-mm diameter, follicular fluid was pooled within ovary and syringe-rinsed to collect oocytes. Oocytes were evaluated under a dissecting microscope and stained for later examination. Follicular fluid was centrifuged to remove debris and frozen for later analysis for IGF-I by radioimmunoassay (11, 12), as validated for cattle. The within- and between-assay coefficient of variation was 8.5% and 14%, respectively. Data were analyzed by analysis of variance in which treatment, time, follicle size, and interactions were tested for differences. Oocyte viability was evaluated with Chi-square analysis.

Results

Concentrations of IGF-I significantly decreased in follicular fluid with time after prostaglandin injection or progestin implant removal (Fig. 1) and as follicle size increased in all treatments (Fig. 2). The interaction of treatment × time revealed that IGF-I concentrations were high 12-h after prostaglandin injection, but had declined 60% by 36 h and remained low throughout the rest of the sampling period in the prostaglandin-synchronized animals. Oocyte quality in prostaglandin-synchronized animals followed the trends of IGF-I, and by 36 h, 70–80% of oocytes evaluated were viable, and numbers of degenerative oocytes remained low throughout the estrual period (Table 1). In the progestin synchronized (Fig. 1, *top*) and prostaglandin synchronized with progestin implant treatments (Fig. 1, *bottom*), IGF-I concentrations were still high at 36 h and gradually decreased to 60 h. In progestin-synchronized animals, oocyte quality was 60% degenerate at 12 h, then increased to 80–90% good at 36–60 h; but by 72 h, oocyte quality had fallen (30% degenerate). Results from oocyte evaluation in prostaglandin-synchronized animals receiving progestin implants was intermediate to the other two treatments. Changes in IGF-I and oocyte quality in progestin-treated animals seem to indicate an asynchrony of endocrine and maturational events that might produce lower fertility/conception rates.

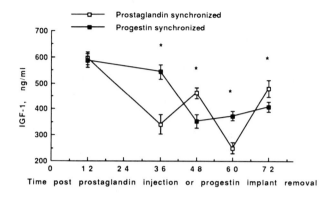

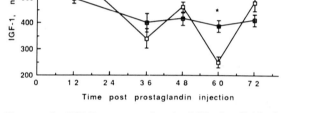

FIGURE 1. Changes in IGF-I concentration in follicular fluid after prostaglandin injection and progestin implant removal *(top)* and prostaglandin injection in conjunction with progestin implant *(bottom)*. (* = IGF-I concentrations decreased with time [P < 0.01] in conjunction with significant time × treatment interaction.)

Discussion

The ability of IGF-I to stimulate synthesis of side-chain cleavage enzyme and mRNA synthesis (9, 13) supports a role for IGF-I being a local regulator in progesterone synthesis. Follicular changes in progesterone content and oocyte development are related (5, 14), and increased progestins during the preovulatory period may result in high percentage of degenerate oocytes due to some aspect of asynchrony of endocrine and paracrine events (Table 1; Figs. 1, 2). Overall increased IGF-1 concentrations in follicular fluid of progestin synchronized animals in comparison to prostaglandin-synchronized animals (442 ± 1.0 vs. 407 ± 1.0, P < 0.05, respectively) in conjunction with increased numbers of degenerate oocytes during the estrual period in

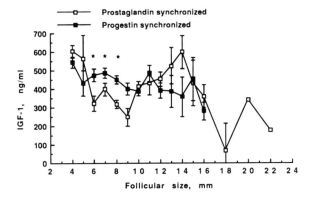

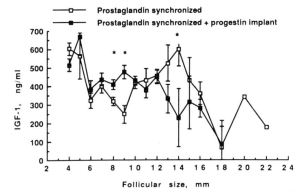

FIGURE 2. Changes in IGF-I concentration from various sizes of follicles in animals synchronized to estrus by prostaglandin (PG) and progestin *(top)* or prostaglandin and prostaglandin plus a progestin implant *(bottom)*. (* = IGF-I concentrations decreased with increases in follicular size (P < 0.01) in conjunction with a significant size × treatment interaction.)

TABLE 1. Percent degenerate oocytes during estrual period.

| Treatment | Time (post prostaglandin injection or post progestin implant removal) | | | | |
	12 h	36 h	48 h	60 h	72 h
Prostaglandin synchronization[a]					
	29.9 ± 3.9 (87)	23.7 ± 7.5 (59)	11.3 ± 5.1 (106)	24.1 ± 3.3 (112)	22.6 ± 4.1 (102)
Progestin synchronization					
	61.6 ± 4.7[b] (73)	12.6 ± 3.7[b] (87)	16.7 ± 4.0 (84)	24.4 ± 3.0 (164)	28.0 ± 2.3[b] (229)
Prostaglandin synchronization plus progestin implant					
	34.1 ± 3.0 (129)	15.3 ± 3.9 (85)	20.0 ± 4.0 (85)	26.6 ± 3.8 (109)	36.6 ± 4.2[b] (93)

[a]Mean ± SEM (number of observations).

[b]Treatment comparisons within time (P < 0.05); prostaglandin vs. progestin or prostaglandin plus progestin methods of estrous synchronization.

progestin synchronized animals may explain why fertility is reduced when synthetic progestins are utilized to synchronize farm animals to estrus.

Acknowledgments. The authors acknowledge D. J. Taubenheim and J. Boyum for their technical support and L. Parnell for stenographic assistance.

References

1. Chenault JR, McAllister JF, Kasson CW. Synchronization of estrus with melengestrol acetate and prostaglandin $F_{2\alpha}$ in beef and dairy heifers. J Anim Sci 1990;68:296-303.
2. Hansel W, Donaldson LE, Wagner WC, Brunner MA. A comparison of estrous synchronization methods in beef cattle under feedlot conditions. J Anim Sci 1966;25:497-503.
3. Zimbelman RG, Smith LW. Control of ovulation in cattle with melengestrol acetate, II. Effects on follicular size and activity. J Reprod Fertil 1966;11: 193-202.
4. Callesen H, Greve T, Hyttel P. Preovulatory endocrinology and oocyte maturation in superovulated cattle. Theriogenology 1986;25:71-86.
5. Wise T, Süss U, Maurer RR. The relationships of oocyte quality and follicular fluid prolactin and progesterone in superovulated beef heifers with and without Norgestomet implants. In: Mahesh VB, Dhindsa DS, Anderson E, Kalra SP, eds. Regulation of ovarian and testicular function. New York: Plenum Press, 1987: 697-701.
6. Spicer LJ, Echternkamp SE, Canning SF, Hammond JM. Relationship between concentrations of immunoreactive insulin-like growth factor-I in follicular fluid and various biochemical markers of differentiation of bovine antral follicles. Biol Reprod 1988;39:573-80.
7. Adashi EY, Resnick CE, D'Ercole J, Svoboda ME, Van Wyk JJ. Insulin-like growth factors as intraovarian regulators of granulosa cell growth and function. Endocr Rev 1985;6:400-20.
8. Hammond JM, Hsu CJ, Klindt J, Tsang BK, Downey BR. Gonadotropins increase concentrations of immunoreactive insulin-like growth factor-1 in porcine follicular fluid in vivo. Biol Reprod 1988;38:304-8.
9. Magoffin DA, Kurtz KM, Erickson GF. Insulin-like growth factor-I selectively stimulates cholesterol side-chain cleavage expression in ovarian theca-interstitial cells. Mol Endocrinol 1990;4:489-96.
10. Wise T, Vernon MW, Maurer RR. Oxytocin, prostaglandin E and F, estradiol, progesterone, sodium and potassium in preovulatory follicles either developed normally or stimulated by follicle stimulating hormone. Theriogenology 1986; 26:757-78.
11. Copeland KC, Underwood LE, Van Wyk JJ. Induction of immunoreactive somatomedia-C in human serum by growth hormone: Dose response relationships and effect on chromatographic profiles. J Clin Endocrinol Metab 1980;50:690-7.

12. Chatelain PG, Van Wyk JJ, Copeland KC, Blethen SL, Underwood LE. Effect of in vitro action of serum porteases on exposure to acid on measurable immunoreactive somatomedin-C in serum. J Clin Endocrinol Metab 1982;56:376-83.

13. Veldhuis JD, Rodgers RJ, Dee A, Simpson ER. The insulin-like growth factor, somatomedin C, induces the synthesis of cholesterol side-chain cleavage cytochrome P-450 and adrenodoxin in ovarian cells. J Biol Chem 1986;261: 2499-2502.

14. Xie S, Broermann DM, Nephew KP, Ottobre JS, Day ML, Pope WF. Changes in follicular endocrinology during final maturation of porcine oocytes. Dom Endocrinol 1990;7:75-82.

34

Thecal Cell Luteinization In Vitro: Role of Insulin and IGF-I

H. Engelhardt, R.E. Gore-Langton,
and D.T. Armstrong

The cells of the theca interna contribute to the corpus luteum in most mammalian species, but little is known about the regulation of the luteinization process in these cells. We have developed a culture system for porcine thecal cells in which androstenedione is the major steroid product in the first 24 h of culture, after which androgen production declines and progesterone production increases, such that total steroidogenesis actually increases with time in culture (1). Because LH is required for this process, we refer to it as "in vitro luteinization." Insulin markedly enhances the effect of LH on progesterone production in luteinized cells, but required concentrations of insulin (maximally effective at 1 µg/mL) suggest that this effect is likely mediated through insulin-like growth factor I (IGF-I) receptors. In porcine thecal from large follicles, progesterone production is stimulated by IGF-I in 72-h cultures (2), and IGF-I binding sites are present on freshly isolated cells (3). To date, changes in IGF-I responsiveness with time in culture have not been studied in thecal cells.

It is now generally accepted that the somatomedins act as paracrine or autocrine messengers, rather than by endocrine mechanisms. Most tissues have been shown to contain mRNA for IGF-I (4) and to be capable of IGF-I synthesis (5). In prepubertal pigs, follicular fluid concentrations of IGF-I increase 2-fold 72–96 h after injection of PMSG, while serum concentrations remain constant (6). This suggests that IGF-I may act as a paracrine/autocrine mediator of early luteinization. The purposes of this study were to (a) compare the effects of insulin and IGF-I on progesterone production in luteinized porcine thecal cells and (b) determine whether thecal cells secrete factors that could mimic the effect of exogenous IGF-I.

Materials and Methods

Thecal cells were prepared from abattoir material using a modification of the technique described by Hunter and Armstrong (7). Briefly, theca interna from medium-sized (3–6 mm) follicles of prepubertal gilts were scraped free of granulosa cells and enzymatically dissociated. Aliquots of 150,000 cells were incubated in 1 mL of DMEM:F12 (1:1) containing antibiotics in 24-well plates at 37°C in 5% CO_2 in air. Unless otherwise noted, medium was harvested and replaced daily; therefore, day-1 steroid production refers to accumulation over the first 24 h of culture. Samples of medium were assayed without extraction for progesterone (8). DNA was assayed by the fluorometric technique of Karsten and Wollenberger (9), with the modifications of Louis and Fritz (10). LH (USDA-bLH-B5) was used at a maximally stimulatory dose of 250 ng/mL. Porcine insulin was obtained from Gibco (Burlington, Ont.); fetal bovine serum (Cellect Silver) from Flow Laboratories (Mississauga, Ont.); and human recombinant IGF-I from Boehringer-Mannheim (Montreal). Results are presented as means ± SEM of triplicate or quadruplicate cultures.

Results

Insulin (1.0 μg/mL), in combination with LH (250 ng/mL) and 1% heat-inactivated fetal bovine serum, caused a dramatic stimulation of progesterone production, which was not associated with an increase in cellular DNA (Fig. 1). Previous studies have shown that 1% serum is optimal for this synergism (1). Thus this concentration of serum has been used in all of the following experiments. The effects of insulin and IGF-I were assessed in luteinized cells (LH at 250 ng/mL, day 3 of culture). A comparison of dose-response curves (Fig. 2, *top*) showed that although these peptides had similar effects, the dose of IGF-I required for maximal stimulation of progesterone production was ~25-fold lower than that for insulin. Responsiveness to insulin/IGF-I increased with time in culture, such that there was either no effect or moderate stimulation in day-1 cultures, but by day 3, insulin or IGF-I caused up to 10-fold increases in progesterone production over controls (cultured with LH and 1% serum; Fig. 2, *bottom*).

To investigate the possibility that theca-derived autocrine factors could mimic the IGF-I effect, total 3-day accumulation of progesterone was compared in cultures subjected to daily changes of medium, versus those allowed to "condition" their own medium (left undisturbed for 3 days). In cultures subjected to daily medium changes, 3-day progesterone production was the sum of progesterone concentrations in medium harvested on days 1, 2, and 3.

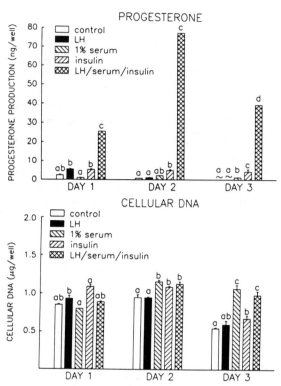

FIGURE 1. Effect of insulin (1.0 μg/mL), LH (250 ng/mL), and 1% serum on progesterone production *(top)* and cellular DNA *(bottom)* in porcine thecal cells. Cells were cultured at 150,000 cells/well as described in text. (Bars with different letters within a day are significantly different; P < 0.01.)

Due to variability of results, this experiment has been repeated 5 times, and the two patterns of responses that have emerged are shown in Figure 3. In experiment 1 *(left)*, in the absence of IGF-I, allowing cells to condition their own medium increased 3-day progesterone accumulation 15-fold over cultures subjected to daily medium changes; whereas in the presence of IGF-I (50 ng/mL), conditioning resulted in only a 30% increase in progesterone accumulation. In experiment 2 *(right)*, in the absence of IGF-I, conditioning again increased progesterone production relative to medium-changed controls (9-fold), but even with maximal IGF-I, conditioning increased progesterone production 3.8-fold relative to medium-changed controls. In addition, progesterone accumulation was nearly 3-fold higher in conditioned cultures without exogenous IGF-I than in medium-changed cultures with maximal IGF-I (second bar vs. third bar).

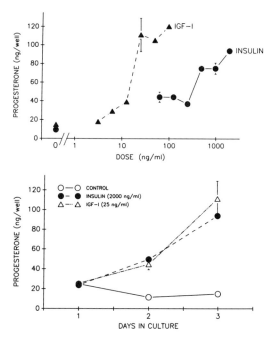

FIGURE 2. Relative potencies of insulin and IGF-I in stimulation of progesterone production in day-3 cultures of luteinized thecal cells *(top)*, and changes in responsiveness to insulin and IGF-I with time in culture *(bottom)*. All cells received LH (250 ng/mL) and 1% serum.

Discussion

Insulin and IGF-I, in the presence of LH, were highly potent stimulators of progesterone production in luteinized thecal cells. These peptides have been reported to augment gonadotropin-stimulated steroidogenesis in other porcine thecal cell systems (2, 11, 12), as well as in a number of other gonadal cell types, including porcine Leydig cells (13, 14), and rat theca interstitial cells (15, 16). Insulin and IGF-I have been shown to have effects at multiple subcellular sites, both proximal and distal to cAMP generation. In rat granulosa cells, IGF-I was found to increase both adenylate cyclase activity and cAMP-supported steroidogenesis, without increasing FSH binding (17). In porcine Leydig and granulosa cells, IGF-I was reported to increase [^{125}I]hCG binding (13, 14, 18). In porcine granulosa cells, Veldhuis and Rodgers (19) have shown that IGF-I can augment progestin biosynthesis by increasing both cholesterol side-chain activity and uptake of low-density lipoprotein.

In the present study, the maximal responses to insulin and IGF-I were similar, but IGF-I was effective at much lower concentrations, suggesting that insulin was acting through IGF-I receptors. Although specific receptors for both insulin and IGF-I have been demonstrated on steroidogenic cells (20, 21), those studies did not determine whether insulin exerted its effects through its own receptors or IGF-I receptors. In studies using porcine Leydig cells, Bernier and coworkers (13) found that the steroidogenic response to insulin was biphasic: The first plateau was reached with 10–25 ng/mL insulin, at which point steroid production was lower than that obtained with the same concentration of IGF-I; a second plateau was reached with 5–10 µg/ mL insulin, with steroidogenesis being substantially higher than the maximal response with IGF-I. These results were interpreted as evidence that insulin acted through its own receptors at nanomolar concentrations and through IGF-I receptors at higher concentrations.

Follicular fluid concentrations of IGF-I change in response to gonado- tropin treatment in vivo, while serum IGF-I levels are constant (6). These results suggest, but do not prove, that the IGF-I was produced within the ovary. Porcine granulosa cells, under the control of gonadotropins and growth factors, have been reported to produce IGF-I (22), but the possibility of thecal cells as the source of ovarian IGF-I has not been addressed. Under the culture conditions used in the present study (150,000 cells/mL), any autocrine factors would be highly diluted, and beneficial effects of condition- ing the medium would have to outweigh any negative effects of either depletion of nutrients or product inhibition due to accumulation of progester- one (23). Even so, in some experiments (Fig. 3, *left*) conditioning of cultures

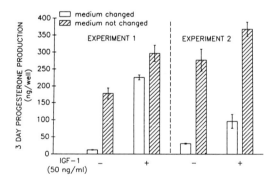

FIGURE 3. Effect of "conditioning" on progesterone production in the absence and presence of IGF-I. In each experiment, medium was either harvested and replaced daily *(open bars)*, or not changed, allowing cells to condition their own medium over 3 days *(striped bars)*. In medium-changed cultures, the response was the sum of progesterone produced on days 1–3, whereas in conditioned cultures, the response was the total accumulation of progesterone over the 3-day period.

without IGF-I increased progesterone production to 79% of that observed in medium-changed cultures given IGF-I daily (second bar vs. third bar). These results would be consistent with the hypothesis that thecal cells produced IGF-I or a factor that mimicked its effects. However, even in the presence of IGF-I, conditioning greatly enhanced progesterone production in other experiments (Fig. 3, *right*), suggesting that thecal cells produced factors other than IGF-I, which enhanced progesterone production. The variation between batches of cells in the conditioning effect probably reflects differential ability of the cells to produce these autocrine factors, which may help to explain the varying steroidogenic performance encountered by researchers using abattoir tissue.

These studies have shown that IGF-I is a potent stimulator of LH-induced progesterone production in luteinized thecal cells and that these cells appear to produce autocrine factors, which, in concert with LH and 1% serum, not only mimic the stimulatory effect of IGF-I, but also enhance progesterone production in the presence of maximal IGF-I concentrations.

References

1. Engelhardt H, Gore-Langton RE, Armstrong DT. Luteinization of porcine thecal cells in vitro [Abstract]. Biol Reprod 1989;40:38.
2. Caubo B, DeVinna RS, Tonetta, SA. Regulation of steroidogenesis in cultured porcine theca cells by growth factors. Endocrinology 1989;125:321-6.
3. Caubo B, Tonetta SA. Binding sites for IGF-I identified on theca cells from large porcine follicles. In: Hirshfield AN, ed. Growth factors and the ovary. New York: Plenum Press, 1989:169-74.
4. Mathews LS, Norstedt G, Palmiter RD. Regulation of insulin-like growth factor I gene expression by growth hormone. Proc Natl Acad Sci USA 1986;83:9343-7.
5. D'Ercole AJ, Stiles AD, Underwood LE. Tissue concentrations of somatomedin C: Further evidence for multiple sites of synthesis and paracrine or autocrine mechanisms of action. Proc Natl Acad Sci USA 1984;81:935-9.
6. Hammond JM, Hsu C-J, Klindt J, Tsang BK, Downey BR. Gonadotropins increase concentrations of immunoreactive insulin-like growth factor-1 in porcine follicular fluid in vivo. Biol Reprod 1988;38:304-8.
7. Hunter MG, Armstrong DT. Oestrogens inhibit steroid production by dispersed porcine thecal cells. Mol Cell Endocrinol 1987;50:165-70.
8. Leung PCK, Armstrong DT. A mechanism for the intraovarian action of estrogen on androgen production. Biol Reprod 1979;21:1035-42.
9. Karsten U, Wollenberger A. Improvements in the ethidium bromide method for direct fluorometric estimation of DNA and RNA in cell and tissue homogenates. Anal Biochem 1977;77:464-77.
10. Louis BG, Fritz IB. Follicle-stimulating hormone and testosterone independently increase the production of androgen-binding protein by Sertoli cells in culture. Endocrinology 1979;104:454-61.

11. Barbieri RL, Makris A, Ryan KJ. Effects of insulin on steroidogenesis in cultured porcine ovarian theca. Fertil Steril 1983;40:237-41.

12. Morley P, Calaresu FR, Barbe GJ, Armstrong DT. Insulin enhances luteinizing hormone-stimulated steroidogenesis by porcine theca cells. Biol Reprod 1989;40:735-43.

13. Bernier M, Chatelain P, Mather JP, Saez JM. Regulation of gonadotropin receptors, gonadotropin responsiveness, and cell multiplication by somatomedin-C and insulin in cultured pig Leydig cells. J Cell Physiol 1986;129:257-63.

14. Perrard-Sapori M-H, Chatelain PG, Jaillard C, Saez JM. Characterization and regulation of somatomedin-C/insulin-like growth factor 1 (Sm-C/IGF-I) receptors on cultured pig Leydig cells. Eur J Biochem 1987;165:209-14.

15. Cara JF, Rosenfeld RL. Insulin-like growth factor I and insulin potentiate luteinizing hormone-induced androgen synthesis by rat ovarian thecal-interstitial cells. Endocrinology 1988;123:733-9.

16. Magoffin DA, Erickson GF. An improved method for primary culture of ovarian androgen-producing cells in serum-free medium: Effect of lipoproteins, insulin, and insulin like growth factor-I, IV. Cell Dev Biol 1988;24:862-70.

17. Adashi EY, Resnick CE, Hernandez ER, et al. Insulin-like growth factor-I as an amplifier of follicle-stimulating hormone action: Studies on mechanism(s) and site(s) of action in cultured rat granulosa cells. Endocrinology 1988;122:1583-91.

18. Amsterdam A, May JV, Schomberg DW. Synergistic effect of insulin and follicle-stimulating hormone on biochemical and morphological differentiation of porcine granulosa cells in vitro. Biol Reprod 1988;39:379-90.

19. Veldhuis JD, Rodgers RJ. Mechanisms subserving the steroidogenic synergism between follicle-stimulating hormone and insulin-like growth factor I (Somatomedin C). J Biol Chem 1987;262:7658-64.

20. Lin T, Haskell J, Vinson N, Terracio L. Characterization of insulin and insulin-like growth factor I receptors of purified Leydig cells and their role in steroidogenesis in primary culture: A comparative study. Endocrinology 1986;119:1641-7.

21. Penhoat A, Chatelain PG, Jaillard C, Saez JM. Characterization of insulin-like growth factor I and insulin receptors on cultured bovine adrenal fasciculata cells. Role of these peptides on adrenal cell function. Endocrinology 1988;122:2518-26.

22. Mondschein JS, Hammond JM. Growth factors regulate immunoreactive insulin-like growth factor-I production by cultured porcine granulosa cells. Endocrinology 1988;123:463-8.

23. Caffrey JF, Nett TM, Abel JH, Jr, Niswender GD. Activity of 3β-hydroxy-Δ⁵-steroid dehydrogenase/Δ⁵-Δ⁴-isomerase in the ovine corpus luteum. Biol Reprod 1979;20:279-87.

35

Decreased Ovulation Rate Associated with Increased mRNA for Inhibin α-Subunit in the Domestic Hen

SHU-YIN WANG AND PATRICIA A. JOHNSON

There are several major changes in ovarian function associated with aging in the domestic hen that possibly contribute to the decline in egg production (1). Among these changes, a decrease in ovulation rate is one of the most significant factors. We hypothesized that the gonadal hormone inhibin may regulate the rate of follicular recruitment and, hence, ovulation in the hen. The domestic hen possesses a unique hierarchy of follicles, with the largest destined to ovulate on the next day, the second largest on the following day, and so on. Williams and Sharp (2) observed that the average weight of the largest preovulatory follicle in old hens was approximately 50% greater than that in young hens. In addition, old hens possess fewer follicles in the hierarchy, with a greater distinction in size among the preovulatory follicles compared to young hens.

Inhibin has been shown to be involved in the regulation of the rate of follicular development in mammals by exerting a negative feedback effect on follicle stimulating hormone (FSH) at the pituitary gland (3, 4). Inhibin has been found to be produced in the greatest quantity by the largest follicles in the rat (5) and ovine (6) ovary. There are few reports characterizing inhibin in birds. In a heterologous system using rat pituitaries, preparations of chicken testes (7) and hen ovarian follicle cell-conditioned media (8) selectively suppressed FSH secretion. If the situation in avians is similar to that in mammals, one would predict that inhibin production by ovarian follicles is related to the size of the follicle. As mentioned previously, the most mature follicles of older hens are larger than those of young hens of comparable maturity. Perhaps increased inhibin production by the largest follicles of older hens is responsible for the decrease in rate of ovulation with aging. We pursued this question by examining expression of the mRNA for the α-subunit of inhibin in the granulosa layer of young and old hens.

Materials and Methods

Young and old hens (white leghorns; Babcock B300) were maintained on a light:dark (12:12) schedule in a temperature-controlled facility. Young hens (laying 2–4 week) were killed at the age of 5 months. The average laying sequence for young hens was 21 days. Old hens (laying 4–5 months) were killed at the age of 8 months and had an average laying sequence of 5–7 days. The 5 largest preovulatory follicles were removed immediately and placed in ice-cold Krebs-Ringer bicarbonate buffer (pH 7.4). The granulosa cell layer from each follicle was isolated and stored at $-70°C$ until use (n = 4 pools of 4–5 follicles).

Total RNA was prepared according to the method described by Chomczynski and Sacchi (9). For validation of the size of the hybridized hen mRNA, polyadenylated RNA (mRNA), isolated by subjecting the total RNA to oligo-dT cellulose columns (Collaborative Research Inc, MA) from hen granulosa layers and from pig ovaries was compared by Northern analysis. For Northern blots, mRNA (5 µg) or total RNA (20 µg) was subjected to electrophoresis in 1.5% agarose gel containing formaldehyde and transferred to a nylon membrane (Genescreen Plus). After baking for 2 h, the blots were prehybridized overnight at 42°C and then hybridized with the ^{32}P-labeled α-inhibin probe for 16 h. The probe for the inhibin α-subunit was a full-length porcine cDNA (1350 bp) provided by Dr. K. Mayo (Northwestern University). Blots were washed twice in 2× SSC (pH 7.4) at room temperature for 5 min, then twice in 2× SSC/1% SDS at 60°C for 30 min, and finally twice in 0.1× SSC at room temperature for 30 min. The blots were exposed to Kodak XAR films with an intensifying screen at $-70°C$ for 24 h. RNA standards (16S and 23S; Pharmacia) were used as size markers. Equality of RNA loading among wells was verified by methylene blue staining. For slot-blots, total RNA (2, 4, 6, and 8 µg) was loaded onto Genescreen Plus using a slot-blot apparatus (Minifold II, Schleicher and Schuell). The slot-blot was baked and hybridized as described for Northern blots, and subsequently the autoradiogram was quantitated by densitometry. Data were analyzed by the general linear models procedure of SAS, and the differences between groups were tested by Fisher's protected LSD.

Results

Northern blot analysis of the pig ovary and hen granulosa layer mRNA is shown in Figure 1. A single band of α-inhibin mRNA could be seen in both pig ovary and hen granulosa mRNA preparations. The size of the mRNA was 1.7 kb for the hen and 1.5 kb for the pig. Total RNA from follicles of young and old hens was also assessed by Northern analysis (Fig. 2). When total RNA was

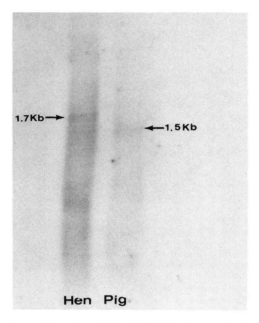

FIGURE 1. Comparison of the size of the mRNA for the α-subunit of inhibin in hen granulosa tissue and pig ovary. Northern blot was prepared using 5 μg mRNA/gel lane and was hybridized with ^{32}P-labeled porcine cDNA α-inhibin.

used, an additional band was detected at 3.9 kb, even with stringent washing conditions. Densitometric analysis of slot-blots from the same group of RNA samples is illustrated in Figure 3. A dose-related increase in signal intensity with increasing doses of RNA was found in both young and old hens. However, the overall specific activity of mRNA for the α-subunit of inhibin for old hens was significantly greater than that of young hens (P < 0.05).

Discussion

There are few reports characterizing inhibin in the hen. The studies that have been reported used heterologous assay systems to assess in vivo (7) and in vitro (8, 10) production of inhibin. The inhibin α-subunit cDNA (1350 bp) from porcine ovary has been shown to detect a mRNA (1.5 kb) encoding the α-subunit of inhibin in both porcine ovary and human placenta (11). We have used this cDNA to probe preparations of hen granulosa layer mRNA and have found a single band of hybridization (12). A recent report (13) indicated that human α-inhibin cDNA detects a message for rooster inhibin at approximately 1.3 kb. In the present study, we used the porcine probe and

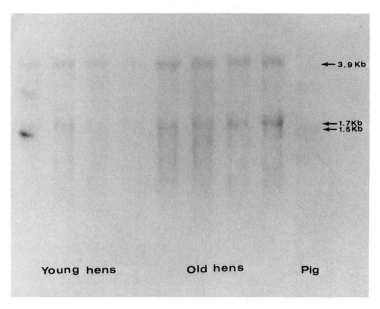

FIGURE 2. Northern blot analysis of the α-inhibin mRNA in young and old hens. The blot was prepared using 20 μg total RNA/gel lane and was hybridized with ^{32}P-labeled porcine cDNA for α-inhibin.

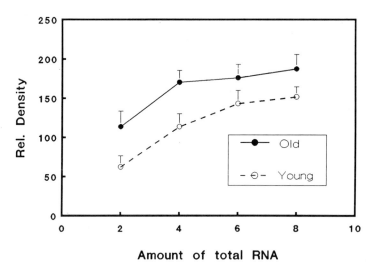

FIGURE 3. Results of densitometric analysis of slot-blot of total RNA in young and old hens. Each point represents the mean of results from 4 animals. mRNA for α-inhibin in the granulosa tissue of old hens is significantly greater than that in young hens at all doses ($P < 0.05$).

detected a major species of mRNA in hen granulosa mRNA preparations, which is slightly larger (1.7 kb) than that in the pig. However, when we probed total RNA preparations from follicles of young and old hens with the cDNA for the porcine α-subunit of inhibin, we observed 2 major bands. Without excluding the possibility of the existence of other size-species of inhibin mRNA, it seems likely that the additional band found in the total RNA preparation may be cross-hybridization of the probe with noninhibin mRNA or ribosomal RNA. The Northern blot shown in Figure 2 indicates that the amount of α-subunit inhibin message was greater in old hens than in young hens. This finding is confirmed by densitometric analysis of the slot-blot, which indicates that the average amount of α-inhibin message in the granulosa layer of the preovulatory follicles of old hens was greater than that in young hens (P < 0.05). This relationship is dose-related up to 8 μg of RNA per slot. Due to the fact that the size of the largest ovarian follicle of old hens is approximately 50% greater than that of young hens, one can predict that the total amount of RNA extracted from the granulosa layer would be greater in old hens as well. Therefore, the increase in specific activity (amount/μg RNA) of expressed inhibin α-subunit gene that we found in old hens would be magnified in terms of the total amount of mRNA for the α-subunit of inhibin being expressed. Results in this study suggest that the larger follicles of old hens may produce more inhibin that is ultimately responsible for the decreased rate of follicle recruitment and ovulation. Since the degree of similarity of the cDNA for the α-subunit of inhibin between the pig and hen is not currently known, a goal of our future research is to obtain a clone for the cDNA of the α-subunit of inhibin in the hen.

Acknowledgments. This work was supported (in part) by a grant from the Cornell Biotechnology Program, which is sponsored by the New York State Science and Technology Foundation, a consortium of industries, the U.S. Army Research Office, and the NSF.

References

1. Bahr JM, Palmer SS. The influence of aging on ovarian function. Crit Rev Poult Biol 1989;2:103-10.
2. Williams JB, Sharp PJ. Ovarian morphology and rates of ovarian follicular development in laying broiler breeders and commercial egg producing hens. Br Poult Sci 1978;19:387-95.
3. Steinberger A, Steinberger E. Secretion of an FSH-inhibiting factor by cultured Sertoli cells. Endocrinology 1976;99:918-21.
4. Schwartz NB, Channing CP. Evidence for ovarian "inhibin": Suppression of the secondary rise in serum follicle stimulating hormone levels in oestrous rats by injection of porcine follicular fluid. Proc Natl Acad Sci USA 1977;74:5721-4.

5. Woodruff TK, D'Agostino J, Schwartz NB, Mayo KE. Dynamic changes in inhibin messenger RNAs in rat ovarian follicles during the reproductive cycle. Science 1988;239:1296-9.

6. Tsonis CG, Quigg H, Lee VWK, Leversha L, Trounson AO, Findlay JK. Inhibin in individual ovine follicles in relation to diameter and atresia. J Reprod Fertil 1983;67:83-90.

7. Bandivdekar AH, Moodbidri SB, Sheth AR. FSH receptor binding activity associated with low molecular weight inhibin from sheep, human, rat and chicken. Experientia 1984;40:994-5.

8. Akashiba H, Taya K, Sasamoto S. Secretion of inhibin by chicken granulosa cells in vitro. Poult Sci 1988;67:1625-31.

9. Chomczynski P, Sacchi N. Single-step method of RNA isolation by acid guanidinium thiocyanate-phenol-chloroform extraction. Anal Biochem 1987; 162:156-9.

10. Tsonis CG, Sharp PJ, McNeilly AS. Inhibin bioactivity and pituitary cell mitogenic activity from cultured chicken ovarian granulosa and thecal/stromal cells. J Endocrinol 1988;116:293-9.

11. Mayo KE, Cerelli GM, Spiess J, et al. Inhibin α-subunit cDNAs from porcine ovary and human placenta. Proc Natl Acad Sci USA 1986;83:5849-53.

12. Johnson PA. Presence and regulation of messenger RNA for the α-subunit of inhibin in the granulosa layer of preovulatory follicles of the domestic hen. Biol Reprod 1989;40(suppl 1):119.

13. Lewis WM, Muster KM, Martin TL, et al. Evidence for inhibin in roosters. Biol Reprod 1989;40(suppl 1):109.

36

Changes in Concentrations of Inhibin α- and β$_A$-Subunit mRNAs During Maturation of Ovulatory Follicles in the Pig

H.D. GUTHRIE, R.M. ROHAN, C.E. REXROAD, JR., AND B.S. COOPER

In the pig, preovulatory follicle maturation is accompanied by increased immunoreactive plasma inhibin (1), decreased plasma FSH (1, 2), and increased atresia of nonovulatory follicles (2). Preovulatory follicles may be the major source of inhibin because granulosa cells cultured from large follicles, >5 mm in diameter, produced more inhibin than those from small follicles, <5 mm (3, 4). Inhibin production is putatively regulated by gonadotropins, androgens, and growth factors. This study was conducted to investigate changes in inhibin subunit mRNA concentration during preovulatory follicle maturation.

Materials and Methods

Spontaneous preovulatory follicle maturation was blocked after luteolysis in cyclic female pigs by top dressing a progesterone agonist, altrenogest, on their morning feed. Preovulatory follicle maturation was initiated by terminating administration of altrenogest. Ovaries were collected at slaughter from 5 pigs each on days 1, 3, 5, and 7 after the last feeding of altrenogest. A total of 133 individual follicles were dissected, classified as small (3–5 mm in diameter) or large (>5 mm), aspirated for fluid, homogenized in guanidinium thiocyanate, and stored at –70°C until the RNA was isolated by CsCl gradient ultracentrifugation (5). RNA was also extracted from the granulosa cells and the remaining theca shell of 11 additional large follicles and from 12 ovulated follicles. After CsCl isolation, RNA was phenol-chloroform extracted, ethanol precipitated, redissolved in water, quantified by optical density at 260 nM, and stored at −70°C. The integrity of mRNA isolated from some follicle samples was determined by Northern blot analysis. The mean A_{260}/A_{280} absorbance ratio for follicle RNA was 1.8, the mean concentration of RNA was 1250 μg/g of follicle wet weight, and the amount of RNA/follicle ranged from 11 to 190 μg.

The α-subunit mRNA probe was a 1.3 kb insert of a porcine inhibin α-subunit cDNA (6). The $β_A$-subunit probe was cloned directly from ovine genomic DNA by the polymerase chain reaction and corresponded to nucleotides 952–1295 of the cDNA described previously (7). Probes were labeled with [^{32}P]dCTP by random priming (Pharmacia). Standard mRNA for porcine α- and $β_A$- ovine subunits were prepared separately by in vitro transcription of cDNA probes recloned into Bluescribe vector (Stratagene). The α mRNA standard was 1.5 kb in length and $β_A$ mRNA was .52 kb in length.

RNA was bound to nylon membranes (Zeta-Probe, Bio-Rad) in a solution of 10-mM NaOH and 1-mM EDTA using a 96-well dot-blot microfiltration apparatus. Aliquots of each follicle sample (containing 1 μg of total RNA) were assigned at random to well locations on one of three membranes and replicated twice. Subunit mRNA standard curves (containing 6.9 to 221 pg for α and 2.7 to 21.6 pg for $β_A$, each brought up to 1 μg in liver RNA) were blotted in duplicate on each membrane. Membranes were prehybridized in 1.5× SSPE, 50% formamide, 0.1% SDS, 10× Denhardt's solution, and 300 μg/mL salmon sperm DNA at 45°C. Hybridization was in the same solution with the addition of 10% dextran sulphate. Hybridized membranes were washed in a solution of 0.1× SSC and 1.0% SDS at 60°C for α-subunit and 65°C for $β_A$-subunit mRNA. Membranes were stripped by boiling in a solution of 0.1× SSC and 1.0% SDS and rehybridized with a different probe.

Hybridized membranes were exposed to Kodak XAR film with Kodak X-Omatic screens at −70°C. Autoradiographic images were scanned on a Bio-Rad Model 620 video optical densitometer and quantified using Bio-Rad 2D-Analyst II computer software. Equations for regression of optical density on mRNA content of the diluted mRNA standards were used to calculate the mRNA concentrations for individual samples on each membrane and were expressed as pg of mRNA/μg of total RNA. The α- and $β_A$-subunit mRNA concentrations for each sample was the mean of the values from two different membranes.

Follicular fluid estradiol-17β was determined by radioimmunoassay (2). Concentrations of inhibin subunit mRNA and estradiol-17β were statistically analyzed by least squares analysis of variance. Linear relationships of inhibin subunit mRNAs, estradiol-17β, and follicle diameter were determined by correlation analysis.

Results

α mRNA and estradiol-17β concentrations (Table 1) were greater ($P < 0.05$) in large follicles recovered on days 3 and 5 than in small follicles recovered on day 1. α mRNA and estradiol-17β concentrations were less ($P < 0.05$) in large follicles recovered on day 7 than in large follicles recovered on days 3 and 5. Mean β_A mRNA concentration was approximately 2 pg/µg on days 1, 3, and 5 and decreased ($P < 0.05$) to nondetectable levels on day 7. α mRNA concentration was positively correlated (Table 2) with follicle diameter and β_A mRNA

TABLE 1. Concentrations of inhibin subunit mRNAs in follicle tissue and estradiol-17β in follicular fluid.

Day Sampled	Follicle Size[a]	No.	α (pg of mRNA/µg total RNA)[b]	β_A (pg of mRNA/µg total RNA)[b]	Estradiol-17β (ng of steroid/ml)[b]
1	Small	34	56.5 (16.1)	1.98 (.69)	29.0 (9.2)
	Large	0			
3	Small	16	74.4 (41.4)	1.77 (.90)	160.9 (92.9)
	Large	17	139.0 (47.1)	2.23 (.96)	243.9 (90.5)
5	Small	4	4.8 (4.8)	.03 (.03)	15.6 (14.7)
	Large	29	143.7 (4.9)	2.41 (.90)	512.0 (88.7)
7	Small	1	5.9	0	1.0
	Large	32	40.4 (11.1)	0	48.6 (31.8)

[a]Small size is 3–5 mm and large is >5 mm in diameter.
[b]Mean, with SEM in parentheses.

TABLE 2. Linear correlation coefficients for associations among concentrations of inhibin subunit mRNA, estradiol-17β and follicle diameter.

Item	Day Sampled/Number of Follicles 1/34	3/33	5/33	7/33
α				
Diameter	.532**	.689***	.473**	.125
β_A	.777***	.754***	.486**	
Estradiol-17β	.346	.814***	.728***	.059
β_A				
Diameter	.397*	.398*	−.054	
Estradiol-17β	.131	.617***	.503**	
Estradiol-17β				
Diameter	.591***	.514**	.443*	−.215

Note: Statistical levels of significance: * = $P < 0.05$; ** = $P < 0.01$; *** = $P < 0.001$.

concentration on days 1, 3, and 5, but not on day 7. β_A mRNA was positively correlated with follicle diameter on days 1 and 3, but not on day 5. Estradiol-17β concentration was positively correlated with α and β_A mRNA on days 3 and 5 and positively correlated with follicle diameter on days 1, 3, and 5.

Granulosa cells and theca shells from 5 large follicles recovered on days 3 and 5 had mean α mRNA concentrations of 203 and 64 and β_A mRNA concentrations 3.8 and 0.18 pg/μg of total RNA, respectively. Granulosa cells and theca shells from 6 large follicles recovered on day 7 had mean α mRNA concentrations of 175 and 13 pg/μg, respectively, and β_A was not detectable in either cell type. Twelve ovulated follicles from one gilt on day 7 had an α mRNA mean of 63 pg/μg, and β_A mRNA was not detectable.

Discussion

This study demonstrates that α mRNA increased in porcine preovulatory follicles before the preovulatory LH surge. Preovulatory follicle maturation was demonstrated by increased estradiol-17β production and follicle size between days 1 and 5 after the last feeding of altrenogest. The concentration of the α mRNA appeared to follow a pattern similar to that of estradiol-17β. The increase in α mRNA in preovulatory follicles reflects the increase in inhibin secretion during luteolysis in the pig (1). Others have shown that production of inhibin by porcine granulosa cells was greater by cells from large than from small follicles (3, 4).

The regulation of β_A-subunit gene expression differed from that of the α-gene. The concentration of α mRNA increased almost 3-fold before the LH surge, while the concentration of β_A mRNA did not increase during preovulatory maturation. In follicles collected from pigs, the concentration of α mRNA was higher than the concentration of β_A mRNA. Correcting for the different sizes of the standard mRNAs for the two subunits, the molar ratio of the concentration ratio of α:β_A mRNA in large follicles recovered on days 3 and 5 was approximately 20:1. In agreement with our results, the intensity of α mRNA bands on Northern blots of total porcine ovarian RNA (7) and bovine (8) follicle RNA was greater than the intensity of β_A mRNA bands. This is in contrast to ewe follicles, which contain nearly equivalent amounts of mRNA for the two subunits (9).

In transfected cells, a high ratio of α-to-β mRNA was necessary to produce inhibin as opposed to the β/β-homodimer, activin (10). A similar excess of α mRNA may be necessary for inhibin production in pig follicles. The excess of α mRNA during preovulatory follicle maturation indicates that the pig, like the cow (11), may contain monomeric α-subunit in follicular fluid and ovarian venous plasma. The function of excess α mRNA or peptide requires investigation.

Estrus and the preovulatory surge begin late on day 5 or on the morning of day 6 after the last feeding of altrenogest. Therefore, follicles on day 7 were recovered 24–40 h after the onset of the preovulatory LH surge. Decreased follicle fluid estradiol-17β and increased progesterone concentrations on day 7 indicated that follicles had luteinized; one pig had ovulated. Decreased α and β$_A$ mRNA suggests that the preovulatory LH surge decreased expression of inhibin subunit genes. The preovulatory LH surge in the rat induces a similar dramatic decline of ovarian α and β$_A$ mRNA (12).

The physiological mechanisms that initiate increased secretion of inhibin during luteolysis in the pig are unknown. Roles for FSH and LH are indicated by their ability to stimulate inhibin production by cultured granulosa cells (4, 13). The structure of the promotor of the rat α-subunit gene suggests regulation by gonadotropins through a cAMP- and phorbol ester-response element (14). The promotor for β$_B$-subunit gene in the rat was similar to promoters in growth-related genes containing potential binding sites for transcription factor Spl (14). Transcription of the β$_B$-subunit gene was not markedly increased by gonadotropins (14). However, during preovulatory follicle maturation, FSH secretion decreased and remained low until the preovulatory LH surge (1, 2). A transient increase in LH secretion during luteolysis in pigs was found in some experiments (1) but not in others (2). Exposure to gonadotropins before the decline in progestins, either natural or induced, may be sufficient to initiate preovulatory follicle maturation and permit increased inhibin production in response to low levels of plasma gonadotropins. In summary, the results of this study suggest that physiological regulation of inhibin production is imposed at the level of transcription in porcine follicles.

References

1. Hasegawa Y, Miyamoto K, Iwamura S, Igarashi M. Changes in serum concentrations of inhibin in cyclic pigs. J Endocrinol 1988;118:211-9.
2. Guthrie HD, Bolt DJ. Changes in plasma follicle-stimulating hormone, luteinizing hormone, estrogen and progesterone during growth of ovulatory follicles in the pig. Dom Anim Endocrinol 1990;7:83-91.
3. Anderson LD, Hoover DJ. Hormonal control of inhibin secretion. In: Channing CP, Segal SJ, eds. Advances in experimental medicine and biology; vol 47. New York: Plenum Press, 1982:53-78.
4. Michel U, Jarry H, Metten M, Wuttle W. Inhibin production by porcine granulosa and luteal cells: Development and biological validation of a RIA. Acta Endocrinol (Copenh) 1989;120:511-8.
5. Davis LG, Dibner MD, Battey JF. Basic methods in molecular biology. New York: Elsevier, 1986.
6. Mayo KE, Cerelli GM, Spiess J, et al. Inhibin alpha-subunit cDNAs from porcine ovary and human placenta. Proc Natl Acad Sci USA 1986;83:5849-53.

7. Mason AJ, Hayflick JS, Ling N, et al. Complementary DNA sequences of ovarian follicular fluid inhibin show precursor structure and homology with transforming growth factor Beta. Nature 1985;318:659-63.

8. Rodgers RJ, Stuchbery SJ, Findlay JK. Inhibin mRNAs in ovine and bovine follicles and corpora lutea throughout the estrous cycle and gestation. Mol Cell Endocrinol 1989;62:95-101.

9. Rohan RM, Guthrie HD, Rexroad CE, Jr. Measurement of inhibin RNA in ovarian follicles of the ewe following treatment with gonadotropins [Abstract]. 71st Annual Meeting of the Endocrine Society. Seattle, WA, 1989.

10. Mason A. Structure and recombinant expression of human inhibin and activin. In: Hodgen GD, Rosenwax Z, Spieler J. Proceedings of CONRAD International Workshop on Nonsteroidal Gonadal Factors: Physiological roles and possibilities in contraceptive development. Norfolk, VA: The Jones Institute Press, 1989: 19-29.

11. Knight PG, Beard AJ, Wrathall JHM, Castillo. Evidence that the bovine ovary secretes large amounts of monomeric inhibin α subunit and its isolation from bovine follicular fluid. J Mol Endocrinol 1989;2:189-200.

12. Woodruff TK, D'Agostino J, Schartz NB. Decreased inhibin gene expression in preovulatory follicles requires primary gonadotropin surges. Endocrinology 1989;124:2192-9.

13. Bicsak TA, Tucker EM, Cappel S, et al. Hormonal regulation of granulosa cell inhibin biosynthesis. Endocrinology 1986;119:2711-9.

14. Feng Z-M, Li Y-P, Chen C-LC. Analysis of the 5'-flanking regions of rat inhibin α- and β-B-subunit genes suggests two different regulatory mechanisms. Mol Endocrinol 1989;3:1914-25.

37

Expression of *Jun*/AP-1 Superfamily Genes and Cell Cycle-Related Genes in Mitotically Active Rat Granulosa Cells

BEVERLY C. DELIDOW, JOHN LYNCH, BRUCE A. WHITE, AND JOHN J. PELUSO

The growth and differentiation of ovarian granulosa cells (GCs) are regulated both directly and indirectly by the pituitary gonadotropins, follicle stimulating hormone (FSH), and luteinizing hormone (LH) (1). However, the effects of gonadotropins on GC proliferation are not as well-characterized as those on differentiation, because while GCs differentiate readily in culture (2), they rarely exhibit the rapid and extensive growth response seen in vivo (3). In a wide variety of other cell types, cell-cycle traverse is associated with the expression of a defined set of genes. Among the earliest genes expressed in response to a proliferative signal are proto-oncogenes of the *fos/jun* superfamily, known as AP-1 (4). The products of these genes are transcription factors that act together to regulate the expression of other genes. Expression of the c-*myc* proto-oncogene is also rapidly induced in mitogen-stimulated cells (5). The exact function of c-*myc* is not known, but it is necessary for proliferation of several cell lines (6, 7), and it has been suggested that *myc* may be directly involved in DNA synthesis (8). We have shown that GnTH administration leads to the rapid induction of c-*myc* and c-*fos* in granulosa cells (GCs) of immature rats at the RNA and protein levels and that this response precedes an increase in DNA synthesis (9). This suggests that gonadotropins regulate GC proliferation at the level of gene expression.

While c-*myc* and AP-1 family genes are expressed early in the cell cycle (G_0/G_1); the products of other genes are active later. Proliferating cell nuclear antigen (PCNA, formerly called "cyclin"), an auxilliary protein of DNA polymerase Δ (10), functions during the S-phase (11). During mitosis itself, the recently described cdc2/histone H1 kinase becomes active. Cdc2 is a protein serine-specific kinase required for completion of mitosis (12, 13) and is present in the cells of all eukaryotes studied to date. The expression of both these genes has been shown to be regulated during the mammalian cell cycle (10, 14). There is no information on their expression in GCs.

We have expanded our investigation of the molecular response of GCs to gonadotropins challenge to include a number of cell cycle-related genes: c-*myc*, c-*fos*, c-*jun*, *jun* B, PCNA, and cdc2.

Materials and Methods

Ovary Perifusion. Immature female Wistar rats (24–26 days of age) were killed by cervical dislocation, and the ovaries were removed, trimmed, and placed into culture chambers. Chambers containing 4 ovaries were perifused with medium 199 in the presence or absence of FSH (NIADDK, 200 RP-1 U/mL) and insulin (Iletin, 0.2 U/mL). For measurement of DNA synthesis, 10 µCi/mL [^{3}H]thymidine (Research Products International, 45 Ci/mM) was included in the medium of some experiments. Each treated group was pair matched with its control. Perifusion was carried out in a 37°C water bath, at a flow rate of 6 mL/h, using an Ismatec peristaltic pump (Cole-Parmer). One control and one treated group was removed from perifusion after 15, 30, and 60 min, and the ovaries were placed into 1 mL of cold sterile saline. Granulosa cells were expressed by puncturing the ovaries repeatedly with a 25-g needle and then pelleted by microcentrifugation. For measurement of DNA synthesis, the GCs of each ovary were expressed in to 1 mL of saline and treated as individual samples.

[^{3}H]Thymidine Incorporation. Cell pellets were resuspended in 300-µL saline and 150-µL aliquots were harvested onto Filtermat filters. Incorporated radioactivity was measured by liquid scintillation counting of the dried filters. Data were normalized to cell number, measured using a hemocytometer.

RNA Isolation and Measurement by Quantitative PCR. Cell pellets were resuspended in 1 mL of 4.2-M guanidine isothiocyanate, 0.025-M Na citrate (pH 7.0), 0.5% Sarkosyl, and 0.1-M β-mercaptoethanol. They then sonicated for 10 sec (VirSonic 50, Virtis Co., Gardiner, NY, setting "10"). Carrier *E. coli* tRNA (10 µg) was added to the samples, and each was layered over 875 µL of 1 gm/mL CsCl in 100-mM EDTA. RNA was pelleted by centrifugation (40,000 rpm, for 3 h, 16°C, Beckman TLS-55 rotor). The RNA pellets were drained dry, then resuspended in 400-µL TES (10-mM Tris, pH 7.4, 1-mM EDTA, 0.2% SDS), and phenol-CHCl$_3$ extracted before ethanol precipitation (15).

RNA samples were centrifuged (15,000 rpm for 30 min, 4°C, Beckman TLA-45 rotor), and the pellets resuspended in 10 µL of TE plus 1µL (40 U)

RNasin (Promega). Each sample was reverse transcribed for 1 h, 37°, in 50 μL containing 125 μM each dATP, dGTP and dTTP; 62.5-μM dCTP + 0.25-μCi [^{32}P]dCTP (3000 Ci/mM, Amersham), 4-μg oligo-dT 18-20 (Pharmacia), 500-U MMLV reverse transcriptase (BRL), 50-mM Tris (pH 8.3), 75-mM KCl, 3-mM MgCl$_2$, and 10-mM DTT. PCR was performed using Amplitaq Taq DNA polymerase (Perkin-Elmer Cetus) according to manufacturer's instructions. Equal amounts of sample cDNAs were PCR amplified 25–30 cycles in reactions containing 2.5-U Amplitaq, 200-μM of each dNTP, except dCTP (100 μM + 0.4 – 0.8-μCi [^{32}P]dCTP), and 100 pM each of 5' and 3' primers. The reaction products were visualized by acrylamide gel electrophoresis, followed by ethidium bromide staining. For quantification of bands, the gels were dried onto filter paper and autoradiographed on Kodak X-Omat film. Band densities were measured by scanning densitometry using a Gilford Response spectrophotometer. Under these conditions, band intensity is directly proportional to the amount of cDNA amplified and the amount of specific mRNA in the original sample (15).

The following oligonucleotide primers were used. Each primer pair was chosen based on sequences published in GenBank, and spans an intron where possible, in order to distinguish genomic DNA amplification from that of cDNA. Cdc2 primers were chosen to be complementary to a region completely conserved between the human and yeast sequences. c-*jun* and *jun* B primers were chosen by comparison of the human and murine sequences, choosing regions of minimal homology between the *jun*'s themselves; nucleotide positions refer to the murine sequences. All other sequences are from rat genes.

rat c-*myc* (16): 5', 2717-2736; 3', 4286-4310; 545 bp fragment
rat c-*fos* (17): 5', 613-633; 3', 1305-1329; 717 bp fragment
c-*jun* (18, 19): 5', 767-786; 3', 1092-1111, 355 bp fragment
jun B (19, 20): 5', 374-393; 3', 915-934, 561 bp fragment
rat PCNA (11): 5', 574-593; 3', 770-789; 216 bp fragment
cdc2 (12): 5', 530-549; 3', 654-673; 144 bp fragment

Results and Discussion

In the GCs of ovaries perifused with control media, all 6 mRNAs underwent gradual changes (Figs. 1 and 2), in keeping with the modest rate of DNA synthesis. In GCs of ovaries perifused with FSH/insulin, the levels of all 6 mRNAs changed rapidly. The levels of c-*myc* and c-*fos* mRNAs began to rise at 15 min and were induced 4- to 5-fold by 30 min in perifusion (Fig. 1; c-*myc*, 5.12-fold; c-*fos*, 4.46-fold). The most striking increase occurred in c-*jun* mRNA, which was induced 9-fold by 15 min and rose to nearly 20-fold the control level by 30 min (Fig. 1). Levels of the related *jun* B mRNA were only

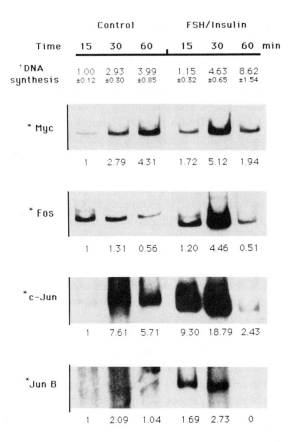

FIGURE 1. Relative levels of c-*myc*, c-*fos*, c-*jun* and *jun* B mRNAs in control and FSH/insulin-treated granulosa cells in vitro. mRNA levels were measured by quantitative PCR at 15, 30, and 60 min of perifusion and are expressed as the fold-increase over the 15-min control value. Data from one experiment are shown; a second experiment gave comparable results. GC DNA synthesis was measured by incorporation of [^{3}H]thymidine into precipitable counts in separate experiments and is also expressed as the fold-increase over 15-min controls (n = 6-8).

moderately elevated (2.73-fold). By 60 min, all had dropped back towards control levels. The levels of PCNA and cdc2 mRNAs were also rapidly induced by FSH/insulin treatment, but to a lesser degree (Fig. 2, 1.5- to 2-fold), and they returned quickly to control levels. As occurs in vivo (9), GC DNA synthesis was highly stimulated (over 8-fold) by FSH/insulin at 60 min.

It is noteworthy that c-*jun* expression is highly stimulated by FSH/insulin, while *jun* B is induced only moderately. It has been suggested that these two transcription factors may differ in their regulation of gene expression, either

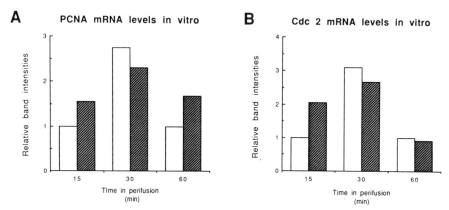

FIGURE 2. Relative mRNA levels of PCNA and cdc2/histone H1 kinase in granulosa cells of perifused ovaries. *A:* Effect of FSH/insulin on PCNA mRNA levels in granulosa cells of perifused ovaries. *B:* Effect of FSH/insulin on cdc2 mRNA levels in granulosa cells of perifused ovaries. Granulosa cell mRNA levels were measured by quantitative PCR at 15, 30, and 60 min of perifusion culture. Results of 2 experiments are shown. (Open bars = controls; shaded bars = FSH/insulin.)

as *jun/jun*, or as *jun/fos*, dimers (20, 21). Our data demonstrate an association between c-*fos* and c-*jun* mRNA expression and GC DNA synthesis. In primary cultures of Sertoli cells, which cannot be stimulated to proliferate, FSH treatment leads to an increase in c-*fos* expression associated with differentiation (22). If subsets of AP-1-responsive genes are differentially regulated, depending on which members of the *jun*/AP-1 family are co-expressed, this offers a mechanism whereby the gonadotropin signal may be able to stimulate either proliferation or differentiation of GCs, depending upon the complement of AP-1 factors available.

Granulosa cells of immature rats proceed through the cell cycle at a modest pace in vivo (9) and in perifusion culture (Figs. 1, 2). This progression is accompanied by moderate levels of cell cycle-related gene expression. When GCs are stimulated by PMSG in vivo, or by FSH/insulin in vitro, there is a rapid (within 15 min) induction of both early response genes (c-*jun*, c-*fos* and c-*myc*) and of genes whose products are active during the S and M-phases of the cell cycle (PCNA and cdc2). These changes in mRNA levels are followed by a substantial increase in DNA synthesis at 60 min. These data suggest that gonadotropin control of GC proliferation is exerted at the molecular level by induction of genes active at several points in the cell cycle. Given that untreated GCs progress slowly through the cell cycle, it is likely that gonadotropins act to both speed the response of cycling GCs and to recruit even more cells into proliferation, thus producing a large increase in DNA synthesis. By stimulating expression of genes active at various points in the cycle, it is also possible for gonadotropins to elicit a uniform proliferative response from a population of unsynchronized cells. This may allow gonadotropins to stimulate many more GCs than simply that subpopulation in G_0/G_1 and may be important in generating the rapid burst of growth that occurs in growing small antral follicles (3).

References

1. Hirschfield AN, ed. Growth factors and the ovary. New York: Plenum Press, 1989.
2. Richards JS, Jahnsen T, Hedin L, et al. Ovarian follicular development: From physiology to molecular biology. Recent Prog Horm Res 1987;43:231-76.
3. Peluso JJ. Role of the peripubertal pattern of FSH, LH and prolactin in regulating in vitro steroidogenesis and follicular growth. J Reprod Fertil 1989;86: 705-11.
4. Rauscher FJ III, Voulalas PJ, Franza BR Jr, Curran T. *Fos* and *jun* bind cooperatively to the AP-1 site: Recognition in vitro. Genes Dev. 1989;2:1687-99.
5. Armelin HA, Armelin MCS. The interactions of peptide growth factors and oncogenes. In: Guroff G, ed. Oncogenes, genes and growth factors. New York: John Wiley and Sons, 1987:331-73.
6. Heikkila R, Schwab G, Wickstrom E, et al. A c-*myc* antisense oligodeoxynucleotide inhibits entry into S-phase but not progress from G_0 to G_1. Nature 1987; 328:445-9.
7. Holt JT, Redner RL, Nienhius AW. An oligomer complementary to c-*myc* mRNA inhibits proliferation of HL-60 promyelocytic cells and induces differentiation. Mol Cell Biol 1988;8:963-73.
8. Studzinski GP, Brelvi ZS, Feldman SC, Watt RA. Participation of c-*myc* protein in DNA synthesis of human cells. Science 1986;234:467-70.
9. Delidow BC, White BA, Peluso JJ. Gonadotropin induction of c-*fos* and c-*myc* expression and deoxyribonucleic acid synthesis in rat granulosa cells. Endocrinology 1990;126:2302-6.
10. Morris GF, Mathews MB. Regulation of proliferating cell nuclear antigen during the cell cycle. J Biol Chem 1989;264:13856-64.
11. Matsumoto K, Moriuchi T, Koji T, Nakane PK. Molecular cloning of cDNA coding for rat proliferating cell nuclear antigen (cyclin). EMBO J 1987;6:637-42.
12. Lee MG, Nurse P. Complementation used to clone a human homologue of the fission yeast cell cycle control gene cdc2⁺. Nature 1987;327:31-5.
13. Riabolwol K, Draetta G, Brizuela L, Vandre D, Beach D. The cdc2 kinase is a nuclear protein that is essential for mitosis in mammalian cells. Cell 1989;57:393-401.
14. Lee MG, Norbury CJ, Spurr NK, Nurse P. Regulated expression and phosphorylation of a possible mammalian cell-cycle control protein. Nature 1988;333: 676-9.
15. Delidow BC, Peluso JJ, White BA. Quantitative measurement of mRNAs by polymerase chain reaction. Gene Anal Techn 1989;6:120-4.

16. Hayashi K, Makino R, Kawamura H, Arisawa A, Yoneda K. Characterization of rat c-*myc* and adjacent regions. Nucleic Acids Res 1987;15:6419-36.
17. Curran T, Gordon MB, Rubino KL, Sambucetti LC. Isolation and characterization of the c-*fos* (rat) cDNA and analysis of post-translational modification in vitro. Oncogene 1987;2:79-84.
18. Ryder K, Lau LF, Nathans D. A gene activated by growth factors is related to the oncogene v-*jun*. Proc Natl Acad Sci USA 1988;85:1487-91.
19. Shutte J, Viallet J, Nau M, et al. *Jun* B inhibits and c-*fos* stimulates the transforming and trans-activating activities of c-*jun*. Cell 1989;59:987-97.
20. Lamph WP, Wamsley P, Sassone-Corsi P, Verma IM. Induction of proto-oncogene *jun*/AP-1 by serum and TPA. Nature 1988;334:629-31.
21. Chiu R, Angel P, Karin M. *Jun* B differs in its biological properties from, and is a negative regulator of, c-*jun*. Cell 1989;59:979-86.
22. Hall SH, Joseph DR, French FS, Conti M. Follicle-stimulating hormone induces transient expression of the protooncogene c-*fos* in primary Sertoli cell cultures. Mol Endocrinol 1988;2:55-61.

38

Prolactin Regulation and Developmental Expression of a 37,000 M$_r$ Protein in the Corpus Luteum

CONSTANCE T. ALBARRACIN AND GEULA GIBORI

Prolactin (PRL), a polypeptide hormone secreted by the anterior pituitary, has a diverse array of actions. In mammals, it acts on both the mammary gland and corpus luteum. In the mammary gland, PRL stimulates the expression of milk proteins, increasing both casein gene transcription and mRNA half life (1, 2). In the corpus luteum, PRL is essential for optimal growth and steroidogenesis resulting in the maintenance of high progesterone levels required for the normal progression of pregnancy (3). The corpus luteum thus provides a model that is highly and specifically responsive to PRL, allowing the systematic study of PRL action. In addition, progesterone levels provide a measurable focal endpoint of PRL action in the corpus luteum.

Although the physiological roles of PRL have been well established, our knowledge of the cellular and molecular action of PRL in general and of the corpus luteum in particular is very limited. The precise nature of the post-receptor events leading to the biological effects of PRL remains highly speculative. In this study, we have examined the changes in protein synthesis that accompany PRL stimulation of luteal steroidogenesis and growth, using both an in vivo approach and luteal cell culture.

Materials and Methods

For the in vivo experiments, pregnant Sprague-Dawley rats (Holtzman Co., Madison, WI) were hypophysectomized on day 3 of pregnancy and injected subcutaneously with either vehicle or ovine PRL (NIADDK oPRL-18; 30 IU/mg) in 50% polyvinylpyrrolidone (PVP), pH 9.0, twice daily (125 µg in 0.25 mL/injection) for 3–4 days. For the ontogeny experiments, corpora lutea were obtained from days 5–21 of pregnancy. Luteal tissue was homogenized in buffer containing 50-mM Tris-HCl (pH 7.4), 1-mM EDTA, 1-mM phenyl-methylsulfonyl fluoride, 1-mM dithiothreitol, and 250-mM sucrose. Subcellular fractions were obtained by differential centrifugation (4). Proteins were separated on either 7.5–15% gradient or 10% SDS polyacrylamide gels (5). Isoelectric focusing of cytosolic proteins was performed with a pH range of 4.5 to 8, using the system of O'Farrell (6). Blood samples were obtained by cardiac puncture under light ether anesthesia. Serum progesterone was assayed by RIA as previously described (7).

To examine the luteal content of a 37-kDa protein (37K), separated proteins were transferred to nitrocellulose. The blots were blocked with 1–3% gelatin in TBS for 1 h and then incubated for 2–5 h with a 1:2000 dilution of antibody to the 37K (8). Immunoreactive proteins were detected using either ^{125}I-labeled protein A (2×10^5 cpm/mL) (ICN, Irvine, CA) or alkaline phosphatase-labeled secondary antibody (Stratagene, CA).

For the in vitro experiments, luteal cells obtained from day-3 pregnant rats were cultured in Ham's F12:McCoy's 5A (Sigma Chemical Co., St. Louis, MO) with 10% fetal calf serum for the first 24 h and with 1% Nutridoma (Boehringer Mannheim, IN) thereafter.

Results

PRL treatment of hypophysectomized rats caused a substantial decrease in the luteal content of a 37-kDa protein and a concomitant increase in progesterone levels (Fig. 1). These results indicate that the luteal content of this 37-kDa protein is markedly regulated by PRL and appears to be inversely related to progesterone production by the corpus luteum.

Two-dimensional analysis of luteal proteins obtained from hypophysectomized rats not treated with PRL (Fig. 2) indicates that the 37-kDa band resolves into 5 different isoelectric species with one major variant (pI 6.15). To establish whether these different species were isoforms of the same protein, we developed a polyclonal antibody highly specific to the major isoelectric variant (8). On Western blot, this antibody recognized only the #3 protein (37 kDa) and none of the other species indicating that the minor proteins are not variants of the 37K.

To examine the intracellular localization of this protein, nuclear, mitochondrial, microsomal, and cytosolic fractions were obtained by differential centrifugation. Western blot analysis of these luteal fractions using the 37K antisera indicate that although the 37K is found predominantly in the cytosol, it is also relatively abundant in both mitochondrial and microsomal fractions (Fig. 3). PRL treatment reduced the 37K content to undetectable levels in each subcellular fraction in which it was detected.

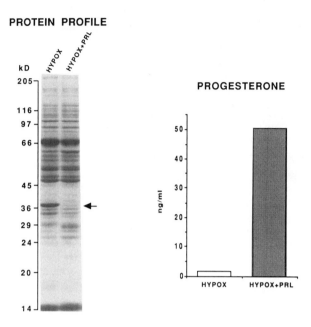

FIGURE 1. Effect of prolactin on luteal proteins. Rats were hypophysectomized and treated with PRL (Hypox + PRL) or vehicle (Hypox) as described. Luteal proteins were centrifuged at 100,000 × g centrifugation to obtain the cytosolic fraction. Protein samples were separated by SDS-PAGE on 7.5–18% gradient gels *(left panel)*. Each treatment group has at least 4 rats. Arrow represents the 37-kDa protein whose content is decreased by PRL treatment. The right panel represents serum progesterone levels.

Luteal cell cultures indicated that the cellular content of the 37K is decreased by a high dose of PRL (1000 ng/mL) (Fig. 4) within 6 h and that this inhibitory effect is sustained throughout 5 days of culture. This inhibition appears to be an all or none effect and is not observed at lower concentrations of PRL.

To examine the developmental expression of the PRL-regulated 37K, luteal proteins were obtained from rats between days 5 to 21 of pregnancy. Equal amounts of cytosolic proteins were loaded on SDS polyacrylamide gels and immunoblottted using the 37K antisera. The results shown in Figure 5 indicate that the 37K is abundantly expressed at the end of pregnancy, when progesterone secretion by the corpus luteum is markedly decreased.

Discussion

In summary, we have shown, by both in vivo and in vitro methods, that PRL causes a rapid and remarkable downregulation of the expression of a 37,000

PROTEIN PROFILE

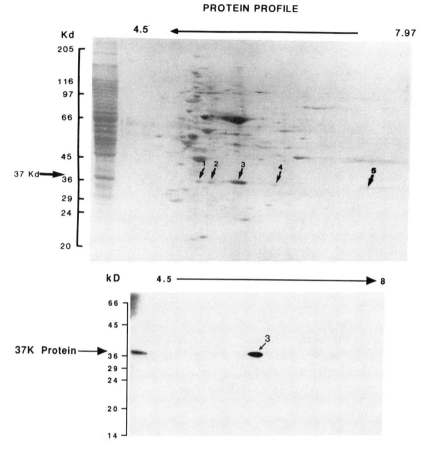

FIGURE 2. Two-dimensional analysis of the 37-kDa protein and immunoblotting using the 37-kDa antisera. Cytosolic luteal proteins taken from non-PRL treated rats were resolved by isoelectric focusing followed by SDS-PAGE in the second dimension. Proteins were transferred onto nitrocellulose and stained with fast green *(top)*. Arrows represent isoelectric species of the 37-kDa band. Immunoblotting *(bottom)* was done using the 37-kDa antisera. Immunoreactive proteins were detected using [^{125}I]protein A and subsequent autoradiography.

M_r protein (37 kDa) in the rat corpus luteum. We have developed a specific antibody to this PRL-regulated protein (pI 6.15) and demonstrated that the 37-kDa protein is abundantly expressed in corpora lutea undergoing luteolysis. The inhibitory effect of PRL on this protein is temporally related to PRL stimulation of progesterone synthesis. Whether the downregulation of this protein is necessary for the normal process of steroidogenesis and

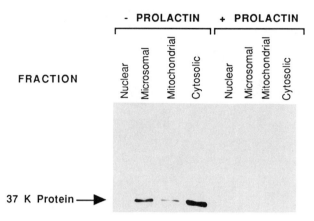

FIGURE 3. Subcellular localization of the 37-kDa protein. Nuclear, mitochondrial, microsomal, and cytosolic fractions were obtained from corpora lutea of hypophysectomized rats, nontreated and treated with PRL, and Western blot analysis was performed using an alkaline phosphatase-labeled secondary antibody.

whether PRL stimulation of progesterone biosynthesis occurs as a result of a decrease in the luteal content of this protein remain to be investigated. However, it is clearly evident from the results of this investigation that the 37K is an excellent marker for PRL action in the corpus luteum.

Although the identity of the 37K has not been determined, possible candi-

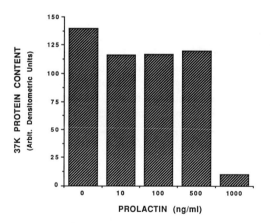

FIGURE 4. Time-course and dose-response of the 37-kDa protein to PRL treatment. Luteal cells were cultured with PRL (0-1000 ng/mL) for 6 h. Western blot analysis of cellular proteins was performed as described in Figure 3, and immunoreactive proteins were quantitated by densitometry.

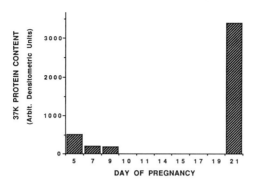

FIGURE 5. Ontogeny of the 37-kDa protein during pregnancy. Luteal cytosolic proteins were obtained from pregnant rats on days 5–21 of pregnancy. Western blotting analysis was done as described in Figure 3.

dates for this protein include 20α-hydroxysteroid dehydrogenase (20α-HSD). This enzyme is a 36,000 M$_r$ cytosolic protein (9) whose activity is known to be be inhibited by PRL (10). Although we have failed to detect 20α-HSD activity in the 37K, its expression throughout pregnancy closely parallels the ontogeny of 20α-HSD activity in the rat ovary, being highly expressed at the end of pregnancy when the ability of the corpus luteum to produce progesterone is markedly reduced (11). The cloning of this protein, presently in progress in our laboratory, should provide more definitive answers regarding its identity and function in the corpus luteum.

Acknowledgments. We wish to acknowledge the technical assistance of Linda Alaniz. This research was supported by NIH grant HD-11119 (GG).

References

1. Guyette WA, Matusik RJ, Rosen JM. Prolactin-mediated transcriptional and post-transcriptional control of casein gene expression. Cell 1979;17:1013-23.
2. Matusik RJ, Rosen JM. Prolactin regulation of casein gene expression: Possible mediators. Endocrinology 1980;106:252-9.
3. Rothchild, I. The regulation of the mammalian corpus luteum. Recent Prog Horm Res 1980;37:183-298.
4. Fleischner S, Kervina M. Subcellular fractionation of rat liver. Methods Enzymol 1974;3:6-41.
5. Laemmli UK. Cleavage of structural proteins during the assembly of the head of bacteriophage T4. Nature 1970;227:680-5.

6. O'Farrell PH. High resolution two-dimensional electrophoresis of proteins. J Biol Chem 1975;250:4007-21.

7. Gibori G, Antczak E, Rothchild I. The role of estrogen in the regulation of luteal progesterone secretion in the rat after day 12 of pregnancy. Endocrinology 1977; 100:1483-95.

8. Albarracin CT, Gibori G. Inhibitory action of prolactin on a protein specific to the corpus luteum [Abstract]. Biol Reprod 1990;A292:138.

9. Pongsawasdi P, Anderson B. Kinetic studies of rat ovarian 20α-hydroxysteroid dehydrogenase. Biochem Biophys Acta 1984;799:51.

10. Lamprecht SA, Lindner HR, Strauss, JF III. Induction of 20α-hydroxysteroid dehydrogenase in rat corpora lutea by pharmacological blockade of pituitary prolactin secretion. Biochem Biophys Acta 1959;187:133-43.

11. Wiest WG, Kidwell WR, Balogh K, Jr. Progesterone catabolism in the rat ovary: A regulatory mechanism for progestational potency during pregnancy. Endocrinology 1968;82:844-59.

39

Baboon Corpus Luteum Relaxin: Absence of Effect on Luteal Cell Progesterone Production

FIRYAL S. KHAN-DAWOOD

Relaxin is a polypeptide hormone with structural similarities, both in amino acid sequence and at the DNA level, to insulin and insulin-like growth factors (1). Until recently it has been recognized to be a hormone of pregnancy; its main function is considered to relate to the preparation of the birth canal prior to parturition. However, Dallenbach and Dallenbach-Hellweg (2) demonstrated its presence using immunofluorescence methods in not only human placenta and decidua but also in the nonpregnant endometrium. Immunohistochemical studies also suggest that the ovary of the cycle as well as of pregnancy may also be a source of relaxin (3, 4, 5). Thus, in the nonpregnant woman, relaxin was identified in the corpus luteum and endometrium in the secretory phase, but not in the proliferative phase. Our data indicates that there is a net production of the hormone into the ovarian vein from an ovary containing the corpus luteum (6). The mean relaxin concentration was 0.41 U ± 0.09 (U ± SE) µg/L (n = 8). In contrast, relaxin was not detectable in the corresponding peripheral plasma or the contralateral venous drainage from an ovary without a corpus luteum. More recently, we have shown that the mid- to late-luteal phase human corpus luteum has a substantial capacity for hormone biosynthesis using DNA/RNA hybridization methodology to assess the presence of relaxin gene transcripts (7). Thus, the objective of the present study was to examine the effect of relaxin on luteal cell progesterone production using baboon *(Papio anubis)* ovarian tissue.

Materials and Methods

Corpora lutea were obtained from 6 adult female baboons with well-defined menstrual cycles and weighing between 14 and 17 kg. Blood samples were drawn for plasma progesterone in parallel with observations of the sex skin turgescence; the day of ovulation was taken as the last day of maximal turgescence. Thus, luteectomy or ovariectomy was performed 9 days after ovulation was detected to obtain the mid-luteal phase corpora lutea. The study was approved by the Institutional Review Board for Animal Experimentation and was carried out in accordance with the principles and procedures described in "Guidelines for the Care and Use of Experimental Animals" as approved by the National Institutes of Health.

The preparation of dispersed cells has been extensively described elsewhere (8). Each corpus luteum was finely minced and cells were dissociated in Ham's F-10 medium containing 10% bovine serum albumin, 20-nM HEPES, 0.02% calcium lactate, 100-μ/mL penicillin, 100 μg/mL streptomycin, 0.25-μg of fungizone, 100-μg DNase, 150 μg trypsin inhibitor, and 800-U collagenase/gram of tissue. After several treatments at 37°C, the cells were suspended in media without the dissociating enzymes, and aliquots were counted in a hemocytometer. Viability of each cell preparation was determined (9). The final volume of the suspension was adjusted with medium to obtain 50,000 cells per 100 μL. The cells (50 k) were incubated in quadruplicate for each experimental point, and incubations were carried out in air at 37°C for 3 h with 0.1–500-ng relaxin or with 10-IU of hCG and relaxin (0.1–500 ng). At the end of the incubation period, media and cells were frozen at –70°C until assayed for progesterone and 17α-hydroxyprogesterone. Total progesterone (media and cells) was assayed by a specific radioimmunoassay as previously described (10), using antisera raised against progesterone-11-oxime bovine serum albumin conjugate. Total 17α-hydroxyprogesterone was also determined using commercially available reagents (Radioassay Systems Laboratories, Inc., Carson, CA). The antiserum was raised in rabbits immunized against 17α-hydroxyprogesterone, 7α-carboxymethyl thioether bovine serum albumin conjugate. The antiserum shows less than 2% cross-reaction with 17α-hydroxypregnenolone, 1.2% with 11-deoxycortisol, and 0.1% with progesterone. The radioactive ligand was tritiated 17α-hydroxyprogesterone. The intra- and interassay coefficents of variation were 6.8% and 14%, respectively.

Statistical Analysis. All comparisons for the effect of relaxin and relaxin with hCG were made against the respective controls when no hCG or relaxin was added. Comparisons were also made between any two different experimental points when evaluating the optimum conditions for the in vitro luteal cell progesterone production. Difference between these comparisons was tested for statistical significance using both the paired Student's *t*-test and the analysis of variance. P-values were derived from a 2-value table, and a P-value of more than 0.05 was considered not significant. All values were normalized to 100-K cells.

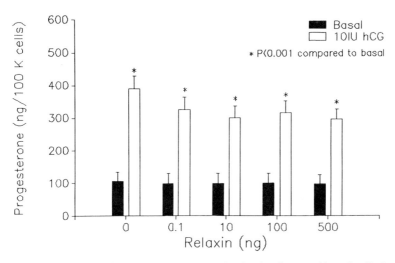

FIGURE 1. Effect of relaxin on progesterone production by dispersed luteal cells from mid-luteal phase corpora lutea (mean ± SEM; n = 5).

Results

An incubation time of 3 h was chosen from preliminary studies in which 50,000 cells/well were incubated at 37°C for 1, 2, 3, and 4 hours. Total basal progesterone concentration in the cells was 9.1 ± 0.22 ng per 50,000 cells, and a 5-fold increase was obtained at 3 h with no further increase at 4 h. With the addition of 10 IU of hCG, the cells responded by increasing the progesterone production 3-fold at 1 h when compared to basal progesterone. With hCG stimulation, progesterone output continued to increase further and significantly for up to 3 h of incubation. Although progesterone production did not increase any further at 4 h, the number of cells that were viable at 4 h was similar (75–80%) to those at 3 h. Thus a 3-h incubation was used in further experiments.

When the effect of hCG was examined, maximum progesterone production was seen with 1-IU hCG/mL. No further increase was seen if the concentration was increased to 10- or 100-IU hCG. Thus, 10-IU hCG was employed in all experiments.

In the mid-luteal phase corpora lutea in this study (Fig. 1), in the absence of relaxin, hCG-stimulated progesterone production was 3-fold higher (397.5 ± 100 ng/100-K cells) than basal progesterone production of 113.7 ± 25 ng/100-K cells. There was no significant change in either basal progesterone production with 0.1 ng (98.78 ± 12 ng/100-K cells) and 500 ng (87.71 ± 20 ng/100-K cells) relaxin or hCG-stimulated progesterone production,

324.2 ± 20 ng/100-K cells and 290.4 ± 14 ng/100-K cells, respectively. A similar effect was seen in 17α-hydroxyprogesterone production.

Discussion

In our previous studies, we have shown that relaxin-mRNA is not expressed equally throughout the human menstrual cycle ovarian tissue. In early luteal tissue, no relaxin transcript was detectable using DNA/RNA hybridization methodology. However, there was a progressive increase in levels from days 21–30, such that the late luteal phase of the menstrual cycle demonstrated quantitatively as much relaxin-mRNA as in the pool of samples from pregnancy. Hence the reason for examining the effect of relaxin in mid-luteal phase corpus luteum progesterone production. However, as postulated, this peptide does not appear to have any effect on the major activity of the corpus luteum; that is, in the synthesis and production of progesterone. However, it may modulate the activities of other peptides in the corpus luteum. Relaxin increases endometrial aromatase activity (11), while oxytocin inhibits primate luteal cell progesterone production (8). The human luteal tissue oxytocin content correlates positively with secretion of progesterone and 17α-hydroxyprogesterone into the ovarian vein (12). Relaxin itself inhibits oxytocin release from the neurohypophysis (13). Thus, these two peptides appear to act opposite to each other and may therefore be paracrine or autocrine modulators of primate luteal cell steroidogenesis. This suggestion is consistent with increased secretion of relaxin and progesterone, but decreased secretion of oxytocin by the corpus luteum of early pregnancy (6). Relaxin produced by the corpus luteum may downregulate the production of luteal oxytocin and thereby turn off the intraluteal luteolytic action of oxytocin and progesterone production. The exact role of relaxin in the nonpregnant primate corpus luteum remains to be elucidated.

Acknowledgments. The author is grateful to Dr. D.O. Sherwood who generously provided the porcine relaxin for these studies, and thanks Lisa Holmquist for her excellent technical assistance, and is indebted to the staff of the Biological Resources Laboratories for indispensable assistance with the baboons.

References

1. Sherwood OD. In: Knobil E, Neill J, eds. The physiology of reproduction. New York: Raven Press, 1988:585-673.

2. Dallenbach FD, Dallenbach-Hellweg G. Immunohistologische untersuchungen zur lokalization des relaxins in menschlicher placenta und decidua. Virchows Arch [A] 1964;337:301-7.
3. Balboni GC, Denkova R, Vannelli GB, Zecchi S. In: Bigazzi M, Greenwood FC, Gaspari F, eds. Biology of relaxin and its role in the humans. Amsterdam: Excerpta Medica:216-8.
4. Yki-Jarvinen H, Wahlstrom T, Seppala M. Immunohistochemical demonstration of relaxin in the genital tract of pregnant and non-pregnant women. J Clin Endocrinol Metab 1983;57:451-4.
5. Yki-Jarvinen H, Wahlstrom T, Teuhunen A, Koskimies AI, Seppala M. In Vitro Fertil Embryo Transfer 1984;1:180-2.
6. Khan-Dawood FS, Goldsmith LT, Weiss JG, Dawood MY. Human corpus luteum secretion of relaxin, oxytocin and progesterone. J Clin Endocrinol Metab 1989;68:627-31.
7. Ivell R, Hunt N. Khan-Dawood FS, Dawood MY. Expression of the human relaxin gene in the corpus luteum of the menstrual cycle and in the prostate. Mol Cell Endocrinol 1989;66:251-5.
8. Khan-Dawood FS, Huang J-C, Dawood MY. Baboon corpus luteum oxytocin: An intragonadal peptide modulator of luteal function. Am J Obstet Gynecol 1988;158:882-91.
9. Tennant JR. Evaluation of the trypan blue technique for the determination of cell viability. Transplantation 1964;2:685-94.
10. Dawood MY, Fuchs F. Estradiol and progesterone in the maternal and fetal circulation in the baboon. 1980;22:179-84.
11. Tseng L, Mazella J, Chen G. Effect of relaxin on aromatase activity in human endometrial cells. Endocrinology 1987;120:2220-6.
12. Dawood MY, Khan-Dawood FS. Human ovarian oxytocin. Its source and relationship to steroid hormones. Am J Obstet Gynecol 1986;154:756-63.
13. O'Byrne KT, Eltringham L, Clarke G, Summerlee AJS. Effects of porcine relaxin on oxytocin release from the neurohypophysis in the anaesthetized lactating rat. J Endocrinol 1986;109:393-7.

40

Relaxin Secretion by the Primate Corpus Luteum During Simulated Early Pregnancy in Hyperstimulated Menstrual Cycles

J.S. OTTOBRE, R.L. STOUFFER, C.A. VANDEVOORT, AND A.C. OTTOBRE

Peripheral concentrations of immunoreactive relaxin are generally undetectable during the nonfertile menstrual cycle in humans (1, 2) and rhesus monkeys (3, 4), but become measurable during pregnancy (2, 3, 5–7). The major source of relaxin in primates is the corpus luteum (CL)(5, 8–10). Chorionic gonadotropin (CG) induces relaxin secretion in nonpregnant primates (4, 11, 12) and thus appears to be a primary stimulus for such induction during early pregnancy. Relaxin is thought to play a role in uterine quiescence during pregnancy (13) and may be an important component for successful pregnancy maintenance.

Ovarian hyperstimulation, often part of in vitro fertilization protocols, frequently results in deficient luteal function (14, 15). It is not known if such deficiencies impair timely relaxin secretion during early pregnancy. Furthermore, increasing relaxin secretion in primates is associated with declining progesterone production during simulated early pregnancy (SEP) induced with human CG (4, 11). This relationship has not been examined in hyperstimulated cycles. The objectives of this study were to characterize the pattern of serum relaxin during SEP in hyperstimulated cycles and to relate relaxin patterns to those of serum estradiol and progesterone. Comparison of the timing and sequelae of relaxin release during SEP in hyperstimulated and natural menstrual cycles would permit detection of an impairment associated with deficiencies in luteal function.

Materials and Methods

Aspects of the following animal protocol have been described previously (14). Adult, female rhesus monkeys, housed at the Oregon Regional Primate Research Center, were checked daily for menses, and menstrual records were maintained (onset of menses = day 1 of the menstrual cycle). Animals exhibiting regular cycles of approximately 28 days were used in the current study. Blood samples were collected daily by saphenous venipuncture at 8:00 A.M. (before any scheduled hormone injection) from day 1 of the cycle until the next onset of menses. The serum was stored at $-20\,^{\circ}$C until assayed for hormone levels. Concentrations of progesterone, estradiol-17β, and relaxin in serum samples were determined via radioimmunoassay (4, 16, 17). Beginning at menses, monkeys (n = 6) received intramuscular (im) injections of follicle stimulating hormone (hFSH, Metrodin, Serono, Randolph, MA, 30 IU twice daily, days 1 to 6) followed by human menopausal gonadotropin (hMG, Pergonal, Serono, 30-IU hFSH/30-IU hLH twice daily, days 7 to 9). This treatment regimen elicits the growth and maturation of multiple follicles that are capable of ovulating (18). On day 10, hCG (1000 IU, APL, Ayerst Laboratories, Rouses Point, NY) was given to mimic the LH surge (luteal phase day 0). Follicle aspiration was performed 27 h later by the Department of Surgery to collect oocytes that were fertilized in vitro (18). Beginning on day 9 of the luteal phase (i.e., near the typical time of implantation) hCG was injected im twice daily (8:00 A.M. and 5:00 P.M.) in doses increasing daily throughout a 6-day treatment interval (15, 30, 45, 90, 180, and 360 IU/dose twice daily). The protocol was similar to that used previously by this laboratory to invoke patterns of circulating CG and progesterone that mimic those during early pregnancy in rhesus monkeys. However, the treatment interval was shortened from 10 to 6 days to minimize the production of antibodies to hCG. Some of the progesterone data have been reported previously (14), but are included here for the purposes of comparison and completeness.

Results

Serum concentrations of relaxin, progesterone, and estradiol in 4 monkeys that received the hCG regimen during the luteal phase of hyperstimulated cycles are depicted in Figure 1. Based on serum progesterone and estradiol, the CL of hyperstimulated cycles were functionally short-lived. Whereas a natural menstrual cycle has a luteal phase that is 14–16 days (19), serum progesterone and estradiol were near baseline by day 9 of the luteal phase in hyperstimulated cycles. Despite this deficiency, CL were very responsive, in terms of steroid and relaxin production, to CG treatment of SEP. Serum progesterone and estradiol were substantially elevated throughout SEP and

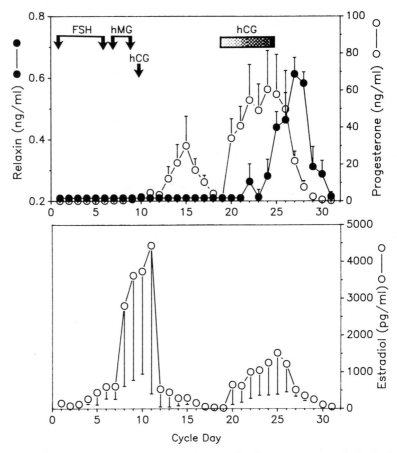

FIGURE 1. Peripheral concentrations ($\bar{x} \pm$ SE; n = 4) of progesterone and relaxin *(top panel)* and estradiol-17β *(bottom panel)* during hyperstimulation of follicular development followed by simulated early pregnancy (day 1 = onset of menses). Notations above the graph indicate treatments and intervals of hyperstimulation and simulation of early pregnancy. For superovulation, monkeys were given hFSH beginning at menses (30 IU twice daily, days 1 to 6), human menopausal gonadotropin (hMG, 30-IU hFSH/30-IU hLH twice daily, days 7 to 9), and hCG (1000 IU, day 10). For simulation of early pregnancy, hCG was injected twice daily beginning near the typical time of implantation (day 9 of the luteal phase) in doses increasing daily (as depicted by the increase in shading in the bar above the treatment interval; 15, 30, 45, 90, 180, and 360 IU/dose).

did not decrease until after cessation of CG treatment. Serum relaxin was detectable 4.25 ± 0.75 days after the initiation of CG treatment and rose continuously to peak levels 3–4 days after cessation of CG treatment.

Contrary to what was observed during SEP in the natural cycle (4), the initial detection and early rise in serum relaxin was not accompanied by a decline in serum progesterone during SEP in the hyperstimulated cycle. There were positive and significant (P < 0.05) correlations between serum relaxin and either serum progesterone or estradiol during CG treatment of SEP and during the period from cessation of CG treatment to menses. Correlation coefficients ranged from 0.42 to 0.73. Therefore, serum progesterone and estradiol sometimes varied with serum relaxin, and there was no evidence for negative relationships. Relaxin was only detectable during the luteal phase after CG treatment and was not detectable during the follicular phase (i.e., <0.2-ng/mL serum), despite hyperstimulation of follicular development.

The remaining 2 monkeys in this experiment failed to respond to the hCG treatment simulating early pregnancy. One of these monkeys had a spontaneous LH surge 2 days before the ovulatory dose of hCG. As a result, the ovulatory dose of hCG was administered during luteal development and may have rendered the CL somewhat refractory to rescue by CG later. The other monkey had very low serum levels of progesterone (<1 ng/mL by days 8–9 of the luteal phase) at the time of initiation of SEP. Menses began 1 day after initiating SEP in this monkey. Serum progesterone, estradiol, and relaxin did not increase in these 2 monkeys during SEP.

Discussion

During the hyperstimulated follicular phase in the current study, serum relaxin was undetectable (<0.2-ng/mL serum). These data are similar to those of Nixon et al. (12), who failed to detect relaxin even in the ovarian vein of rhesus monkeys after 12 days of follicular stimulation. In a woman superovulated for two consecutive cycles, levels of relaxin were detectable in the late follicular phase just prior to and during ovulation induction (20). Relaxin concentrations detected in that study were near the limit of detectability in the current study. It is possible that subtle rises in serum relaxin during the follicular phase of hyperstimulated monkeys may occur, but are of low magnitude.

When CG treatments were administered to nonpregnant rhesus monkeys during the natural cycle, in doses and times that simulated early pregnancy, immunoreactive relaxin was detected in the serum beginning 6.6 ± 1.4 days after the initiation of CG treatment (4). In the current study, during SEP in hyperstimulated cycles, serum relaxin was detected 4.25 ± 0.75 days after the initiation of CG treatment. The apparent earlier detection of serum relaxin in the current study may be due to the presence of multiple CL in hyperstimulated monkeys versus a single CL during natural cycles. Multiple CL would be expected to secrete more relaxin collectively than a single CL and would likely achieve a level of detectability sooner. These data clearly indicate that CL of hyperstimulated cycles are capable of timely relaxin release during early pregnancy, despite functional deficiencies prior to initiation of rescue by CG. Thomas et al. (20) initiated repeated hCG treatments following superovulation of a woman in 3 consecutive cycles. This regimen, which appeared to begin early in the luteal phase prior to reduced steroid secretion, also resulted in prolonged luteal function and elevations in serum relaxin and progesterone.

We observed previously, as has been noted in other species, that increased relaxin secretion seemed to be associated with functional luteolysis during SEP in natural cycles of rhesus monkeys (4). In the current study, the rise in serum relaxin was not accompanied by a decline in serum progesterone during SEP in hyperstimulated cycles. In addition, serum progesterone and relaxin were not negatively correlated. From these observations, it can be inferred that a decline in luteal progesterone production is not required for augmentation of relaxin release in the primate.

Acknowledgments. We are grateful to Dr. O.D. Sherwood and Dr. B.G. Steinetz for their assistance in development of the relaxin radioimmunoassay and their donations of assay reagents. The generous donations of second antibody from Dr. D.R. Deaver, hCG (APL) from Wyeth-Ayerst Laboratories, and Pergonal and Metrodin from Serono Laboratories are gratefully acknowledged. We also thank Brenda Houmard for her scientific contributions. This work was supported by grants from the National Institutes of Health (HD-21319, HD-18185/IVF-EE Core, RR-00163). Certain salaries and additional research support were provided by state and federal funds appropriated to the Ohio Agricultural Research and Development Center, The Ohio State University. This is ORPRC Publication No. 1727.

References

1. O'Byrne EM, Carriere BT, Sorensen L, Segaloff A, Schwabe C, Steinetz BG. Plasma immunoreactive relaxin levels in pregnant and nonpregnant women. J Clin Endocrinol Metab 1978;47:1106-10.
2. Quagliarello J, Szlachter N, Steinetz BG, Goldsmith LT, Weiss G. Serial relaxin concentrations in human pregnancy. Am J Obstet Gynecol 1979;135:43-4.
3. Weiss G, Steinetz BG, Dierschke DJ, Fritz G. Relaxin secretion in the rhesus monkey. Biol Reprod 1981;24:565-7.
4. Ottobre JS, Nixon WE, Stouffer RL. Induction of relaxin secretion in rhesus monkeys by human chorionic gonadotropin: Dependence on the age of the corpus luteum of the menstrual cycle. Biol Reprod 1984;31:1000-6.
5. Weiss G, O'Byrne EM, Steinetz BG. Relaxin: A product of the human corpus luteum of pregnancy. Science 1976;194:948-9.
6. O'Byrne EM, Steinetz BG. Radioimmunoassay (RIA) of relaxin in sera of various species using an antiserum to porcine relaxin (39377). Proc Soc Exp Biol Med 1976;152:272-6.

7. Quagliarello J, Steinetz BG, Weiss G. Relaxin secretion in early pregnancy. Obstet Gynecol 1979;53:62-3.
8. Mathieu P, Rahier J, Thomas K. Localization of relaxin in human gestational corpus luteum. Cell Tissue Res 1981;219:213-6.
9. Nixon WE, Reid R, Abou-Hozaifa BM, Williams RF, Steinetz BG, Hodgen GD. Origin and regulation of relaxin secretion in monkeys: Effects of chorionic gonadotropin, luteectomy, fetectomy, and placentectomy. In: Greenwald GS, Terranova PF, eds. Factors regulating ovarian function. New York: Raven Press, 1983:427-31.
10. Castracane VD, D'Eletto R, Weiss G. Relaxin secretion in the baboon *(Papio cynecephalus)*. In: Greenwald GS, Terranova PF, eds. Factors regulating ovarian function. New York: Raven Press, 1983:415-9.
11. Quagliarello J, Goldsmith L, Steinetz B, Lustig DS, Weiss G. Induction of relaxin secretion in nonpregnant women by human chorionic gonadotropin. J Clin Endocrinol Metab 1980;51:74-7.
12. Nixon WE, Schenken RS, Reid R. Relaxin response to ovarian hyperstimulation during the menstrual cycle in monkeys [Abstract]. 65th Annual Meeting. Endocrine Society, 1983.
13. Sherwood OD. Relaxin. In: Knobil E, Neill JD, eds. The physiology of reproduction. New York: Raven Press, 1988:585-673.
14. VandeVoort CA, Hess DL, Stouffer, RL. Luteal function following ovarian stimulation in rhesus monkeys for in vitro fertilization: Atypical response to human chorionic gonadotropin treatment simulating early pregnancy. Fertil Steril 1988;49:1071-5.
15. Olson JL, Rebar RW, Schreiber JR, Vaitukaitus JL. Shortened luteal phase after ovulation induction with human menopausal gonadotropin and human chorionic gonadotropin. Fertil Steril 1983;39:284-91.
16. Resko JA, Norman RL, Niswender GD, Spies HG. The relationship between progestins and gonadotropins during the late luteal phase of the menstrual cycle in rhesus monkeys. Endocrinology 1974;94:128-35.
17. Resko JA, Ploem JG, Stadelman HL. Estrogens in fetal and maternal plasma of the rhesus monkey. Endocrinology 1975;97:425-30.
18. Wolf DP, VandeVoort CA, Meyer-Haas GR, et al. In vitro fertilization and embryo transfer in the rhesus monkey. Biol Reprod 1989;41:335-46.
19. Zeleznik AJ, Hutchison J. Luteotropic actions of LH on the macaque corpus luteum. In: Stouffer RL, ed. The primate ovary. New York: Plenum Press, 1987;163-74.
20. Thomas K, Loumaye E, Ferin J. Relaxin in non-pregnant women during ovarian stimulation. Gynecol Obstet Invest 1980;11:75-80.

41

Physiological Role of Endogenously Derived PGF$_{2\alpha}$ in Regulation of Corpus Luteum Function in the Rat

JAN OLOFSSON, LARS HEDIN, LASSE LARSON,
ENSIO NORJAVAARA, AND GUNNAR SELSTAM

Prostaglandins are considered to be local hormones with rapid metabolism acting near their site of synthesis (1). There are two processes in ovarian function where prostaglandins are implicated to have an important regulatory role, namely, ovulation and luteolysis. All the active endocrine cells of the different compartments in the ovary (e.g., granulosa cells, theca cells, interstitial cells, and luteal cells) are capable of prostaglandin production (2). In most mammalian species, prostaglandin F$_{2\alpha}$ (PGF$_{2\alpha}$) is recognized to have a decisive role in the functional regression of the corpus luteum. This minireview will concentrate on the physiological importance of endogenously derived PGF$_{2\alpha}$ in regulation of luteal function in the rat.

The rat is extremely well adapted for a dynamic reproduction. The adult female rat exhibits estrous cycles with ovulations every fourth to fifth day with subsequent formation of corpora lutea with very short luteal life-span (2–3 days). However, these corpora lutea, which are considered to be nonfunctional since they cannot support a decidual reaction, will be rescued to a prolonged life-span if mating occurs on the estrus day of the cycle. The functional duration of these corpora lutea is prolonged almost to that of the length of gestation (22–23 days) if conception is achieved and to 12–14 days if the mating is nonfertile (3). The luteal phase of the sterile-mated adult pseudopregnant rat can be further extended by manipulation of the uterus. Thus, both uterine decidualization or extirpation of the uterine horns, if performed on day 5 of pseudopregnancy, prolongs the functional duration of the corpora lutea to approximately 18–20 days (4).

Luteolytic Role of PHF$_{2\alpha}$

Administration of PGF$_{2\alpha}$ or PGF$_{2\alpha}$-analogues induces functional luteolysis in most species, including the rat. The cellular mechanism behind this is not completely understood. One important step in the mechanism of PGF$_{2\alpha}$-induced luteolysis is the antigonadotropic effect of PGF$_{2\alpha}$ on the cyclic adenosine 3', 5'-monophosphate (cAMP) system and steroidogenesis (5, 6). The action on the cAMP system is due to an inhibition of the adenylate cyclase activity, whether stimulated by luteinizing hormone (LH) or β-adrenergic agonists (7, 8), and this inhibition increases with luteal age (7). For the rat, we have also shown that the inhibitory effect is mediated by an impairment of the stimulatory regulatory guanine nucleotide binding component (N$_s$-protein) of the adenylate cyclase system (9). This impairment has a rapid onset, lasts for hours, and is responsible for the antigonadotropic effect. Furthermore, the LH-receptor seems to be sensitive to impaired N$_s$-protein function and decreases later in amount, thereby making functional luteolysis irreversible (10). Since PGF$_{2\alpha}$ can induce an increased formation of inositol 1,4,5-triphosphate and diacylglycerol (11), the changes seen in the phosphatidyl inositol system, or possibly other activators of protein kinase C, may be involved in the PGF$_{2\alpha}$-induced luteolysis (12). Also other biochemical events take place during both spontaneous and PGF$_{2\alpha}$-induced luteolysis, such as an alteration in progesterone metabolism by an induction of 20α-hydroxysteroid dehydrogenase (13, 14), resulting in a decreased progesterone:20α-dihydroprogesterone ratio (15). Later structural changes such as rigidification of the luteal cellular membrane (16) and possibly the decreased blood flow (17) may also be ascribed to PGF$_{2\alpha}$-mediated luteolysis.

Origin of Endogenous PGF$_{2\alpha}$

At present, there are two hypotheses as to where the luteolytic PGF$_{2\alpha}$ is originated and how it reaches the corpus luteum. One suggests that PGF$_{2\alpha}$ is released from the uterus and is transferred by the blood in an endocrine mode (18) and the other proposes that PGF$_{2\alpha}$ is locally produced by the luteal cells in a paracrine/autocrine mode (19). The regulatory role of the uterus in the cessation of luteal function has mainly been focused on uterine production of PGF$_{2\alpha}$ since in most nonprimate species hysterectomy prolongs the luteal life-span. In the rat, as for other species, it has been demonstrated that the concentrations of PGF$_{2\alpha}$ in the uterus and uterine vein increases towards the end of the luteal period (13, 20). However, the anatomical basis for a countercurrent mechanism of transfer of PGF$_{2\alpha}$ is not as elaborate in the rat as in domestic ruminants (21). Since the different compartments of the ovary have the capacity to synthesize prostaglandins, we considered it of importance to investigate the possibility of an ovarian source of luteolytic $PGF_{2\alpha}$ in the rat. The main objectives were to relate the endogenous content and synthetic capacity of prostaglandins in the corpus luteum during different functional states as well as to investigate a possible role of the uterus in regulating levels of luteal prostaglandins.

Biosynthesis of Prostaglandins in the Corpus Luteum

During early and mid-pseudopregnancy, the content of the key enzyme in the cyclo-oxygenase pathway, prostaglandin endoperoxide synthase (PGS) is 3- to 6-fold higher in the uterus than in the ovarian compartment (Fig. 1), but on day 13, this ratio of PGS content is reversed (i.e., the content of PGS is 2-fold higher in the corpus luteum than in the uterus). Furthermore, the levels of PGS in the corpus luteum on this day are approximately doubled when compared to other days of the luteal phase. In the remainder of the ovary, which mainly contains corpora lutea of earlier estrous cycles and follicles at

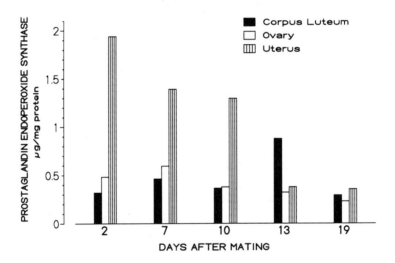

FIGURE 1. Solubilized tissue protein extracts were assayed for content of prostaglandin endoperoxide synthase (PGS) by Western and spot-immunoblotting techniques (22), using a previously characterized antibody (23). Corpora lutea, remainder of ovaries, and uteri obtained from sterile-mated adult pseudopregnant rats on different days of the pseudopregnant cycle and post-luteolytic period, indicated as days after mating, were pooled, homogenized, and solubilized protein fractions were assayed for PGS with dot-blotting technique. Dots were visualized by autoradiography and scanned for densitometric values. Amount of PGS was quantitated by calculation from standard curves of pure ovine PGS run in parallel.

TABLE 1. Effects of luteinizing hormone (LH, 10 µg/mL) on secretion of progesterone, PGF$_{2\alpha}$, and PGE$_2$ in individual corpora lutea on different days of luteal life-span.

Hormone	Days after Mating				
	2	7	10	13	19
Progesterone					
Control	102 ± 14	356 ± 52[a]	182 ± 26[a]	60 ± 16[a]	17 ± 4[a]
LH	157 ± 33[b]	626 ± 110[a, b]	400 ± 75[a, b]	211 ± 71[a, b]	20 ± 3[a]
PGF$_{2\alpha}$					
Control	1.13 ± 0.10	1.10 ± 0.11	1.38 ± 0.07[a]	0.93 ± 0.15[a]	0.57 ± 0.31
LH	1.27 ± 0.21	1.23 ± 0.19	1.18 ± 0.12	1.64 ± 0.33[b]	0.46 ± 0.11[a]
PGE$_2$					
Control	2.21 ± 0.36	2.22 ± 0.39	2.83 ± 0.20[a]	1.49 ± 0.24[a]	0.57 ± 0.15[a]
LH	2.24 ± 0.46	1.91 ± 0.20	2.72 ± 0.56	2.85 ± 0.64[b]	0.39 ± 0.07[a]

Note: Individual corpora lutea were incubated in 1.5-mL HEPES-MEM buffer at 37 °C under 100% oxygen for 120 min whereafter aliquots of media were assayed by radioimmunoassay. Values are presented as pM/mg tissue wet weight, mean ± SEM for 5–10 rats.
[a]Within each parameter, significantly different (P < 0.05) vs. previous day of pseudopregnancy.
[b]For LH-stimulated groups, significantly different (P < 0.05) vs. controls of the same day.

different stages of development, the levels of PGS remains fairly unchanged throughout pseudopregnancy. The synthetic capacity of PGF$_{2\alpha}$ and progesterone and the response to stimulation by LH in isolated corpora lutea incubated in vitro are shown in Table 1. The highest basal synthetic capacity of PGF$_{2\alpha}$ was found, concomitantly with a decline in synthesis of progesterone on day 10 of pseudopregnancy.

Although LH is capable of stimulating luteal progesterone synthesis on all days during the luteal phase, except for the post-luteolytic day 19, increments in synthesis of PGF$_{2\alpha}$ were only detected on day 13 of pseudopregnancy. Interestingly, on this day, when circulating levels of LH are elevated (24), synthesis of both PGF$_{2\alpha}$ and PGE$_2$ reached the same levels as on day 10 in response to LH. Taken together, these findings show that the corpus luteum of pseudopregnancy is capable of de novo biosynthesis of PGF$_{2\alpha}$ and that this synthesis is increasing towards the end of the luteal phase.

In Vivo Luteal Tissue Levels of PGF$_{2\alpha}$

The principal pattern in luteal synthetic capacity of PGF$_{2\alpha}$ is reflected in elevated in vivo tissue content of PGF$_{2\alpha}$ during the late luteal phase and luteolytic period, while levels of prostaglandins in the remainder of the ovary

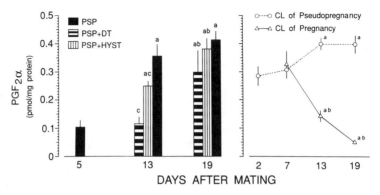

FIGURE 2. Tissue levels of PGF$_{2\alpha}$ in corpora lutea of intact adult pseudopregnant rats (PSP), decidual-tissue bearing pseudopregnant rats (PSP + DT) and hysterectomized pseudopregnant rats (PSP + HYST) on different days after mating with vasectomized (pseudopregnancy) or fertile (pregnancy) male rats. Animals were killed by decapitation, ovaries were quickly excised, and submerged in ice-chilled 14-µM indomethacin. Corpora lutea were identified under a stereomicroscope, dissected away from the ovaries, and snap-frozen in liquid nitrogen. PGF$_{2\alpha}$ was determined by radioimmunoassay after homogenization and extraction procedures. Values are presented as mean ± SEM for 5–9 rats. *Left panel*: a = significantly different (P < 0.05) vs. day 5 of control PSP rats; b = significantly different (P < 0.05) vs. day 13 within the same treatment group; and c = significantly different (P < 0.05) vs. control PSP rats of same luteal age. *Right panel*: a = significantly different (P < 0.05) vs. day 7 of pseudopregnancy or pregnancy; and b = significantly different (P < 0.05) vs. all other groups. (From Olofsson J, Norjavaara E, Selstam G, In vivo levels of prostaglandin F2α, E2 and prosacyclin in the corpus luteum of pregnant and pseudopregnant rats, Biol Reprod 1990, and Olofsson J, Norjavaara E, Effects of hysterectomy and uterine decidualization on in vivo levels of prostaglandins in the corpus luteum of adult pseudopregnant rats, Biol Reprod 1990, with permission.)

remain unchanged throughout pseudopregnancy (25, 26). Thus, a 3.5-fold increase from day 5 to day 13 of pseudopregnancy is registered (Fig. 2). Interestingly, the elevated content of PGF$_{2\alpha}$ (approximately 40 nM) during the luteolytic period is within range of the in vitro concentrations previously reported to inhibit the stimulatory effect of LH and catecholamines (6–8). Furthermore, it is apparent that both the decidual tissue of the nonpregnant uterus and pregnant uterus can exert a suppressive influence on luteal PGF$_{2\alpha}$ (Fig. 2). Noteworthy in this context, on day 19, while pregnancy continues but the influence of the non-pregnant decidual tissue is diminished, the luteal PGF$_{2\alpha}$ levels in pregnant animals are continuously declining. In contrast, in decidual-tissue pseudopregnant rats, the content of PGF$_{2\alpha}$ increases to a similar level as in intact pseudopregnant rats during the luteolytic period.

Moreover, it is evident that hysterectomy does not inhibit the increase of PGF$_{2\alpha}$ associated with luteal curtailment (Fig. 2), since the levels of PGF$_{2\alpha}$ are

2.5-fold increased on day 13 compared to day 5 of pseudopregnancy and further increased on day 19. During both in vitro (Table 1) and in vivo (25–27) conditions, levels of luteal PGE$_2$ are higher than PGF$_{2\alpha}$ and there is a high correlation between these two prostaglandins. The elevated synthesis of PGE$_2$ is most likely to ensure further PGF$_{2\alpha}$ formation by PGE$_2$-9-keto-reductase, an enzyme present in the rat ovary (28), which converts PGE$_2$ to PGF$_{2\alpha}$.

Summary and Conclusions

We have demonstrated that spontaneous luteolysis in the rat is accompanied by an increased luteal content of PGS and an increased capacity of prostaglandin synthesis. The elevated synthesis, possibly augmented by LH, will result in increased luteal tissue concentrations of PGF$_{2\alpha}$, capable of inducing luteolysis. Furthermore, it appears that a signal secreted from the decidual tissue and/or the feto-placental unit, directly or indirectly, will regulate synthesis of PGF$_{2\alpha}$ and thereby ensure an extended period of progesterone production. An intriguing possibility is that luteolysis remains an intrinsic property of the corpus luteum and that the influence of the uterus is to mediate the signal that brings about maternal recognition of pregnancy and an ensuing luteal function.

References

1. Smith WL. Prostaglandin biosynthesis and its compartmentation in vascular smooth muscle and endothelial cells. Annu Rev Physiol 1986;48:251-62.
2. Curry TE, Bryant C, Haddix AC, Clark MR. Ovarian prostaglandin endoperoxide synthase: Cellular localization during the rat estrous cycle. Biol Reprod 1990; 42:307-16.
3. Hilliard J. Corpus luteum function in guinea pigs, hamsters, rats, mice and rabbits. Biol Reprod 1973;203-21.
4. Andersson LL, Bland KP, Melampey RM. Comparative aspects of uterine-luteal relationships. Recent Prog Horm Res 1969;25:57-104.
5. Lahav M, Freud A, Lindner HR. Abrogation by prostaglandin F2α of LH-stimulated cyclic AMP accumulation in isolated rat corpora lutea of pregnancy. Biochem Biophys Res Commun 1976;68:1294-1300.
6. Thomas JP, Dorflinger LJ, Behrman HR. Mechanism of the rapid anti-gonadotropic action of prostaglandins in cultured luteal cells. Proc Natl Acad Sci USA 1978;75:1334-8.
7. Khan MI, Rosberg S, Lahav M, et al. Studies on the mechanism of action of the inhibitory effect of prostaglandin F2α on cyclic AMP accumulation in rat corpora lutea of various ages. Biol Reprod 1979;21:1175-83.
8. Ahrén K, Norjavaara E, Rosberg S, Selstam G. Prostaglandin F2α inhibition of epinephrine stimulated cyclic AMP and progesterone production by rat corpora lutea of various ages. Prostaglandins 1983;25:839-51.

9. Norjavaara E, Rosberg S. Mechanism of action of prostaglandin F2α-induced luteolysis: Evidence for a rapid effect on the guanine nucleotide binding regulatory component of adenylate cyclase in rat luteal tissue. Mol Cell Endocrinol 1986;48:97-104.

10. Behrman HR, Luborsky-Moore JL, Pang CY, Wright K, Dorflinger LJ. Mechanisms of PGF2α action in functional luteolysis. Adv Exp Med Biol 1979; 112:557-75.

11. Raymond V, Leung PC, Labrie F. Stimulation by prostaglandin F2α of phosphatidic acid-phosphatidylinositol turnover in rat luteal cells. Biochem Biophys Res Commun 1983;116:39-46.

12. Sender Baum MS, Rosberg S. A phorbol ester, phorbol 12-myristate 13-acetate, and a calcium ionophore, A23187, can mimic the luteolytic effect of prostaglandin F2α in isolated rat luteal cells. Endocrinology 1987;120:1019-26.

13. Doebler JA, Wickersham EW, Anthony A. Uterine prostaglandin F2α content and 20α-hydroxysteroid dehydrogenase activity of individual ovarian compartments during pseudopregnancy in the rat. Biol Reprod 1981;24:871-8.

14. Lamprecht SA, Herlitz HV, Ahrén KEB. Induction by PGF2α of 20α-hydroxysteroid dehydrogenase in first generation corpora lutea of the rat. Mol Cell Endocrinol 1975;3:273-82.

15. Lau IF, Saksena SK, Chang MC. Serum concentration of progestins, estrogens, testosterone and gonadotropins in pseudopregnant rats with special reference to the effect of prostaglandin F2α. Biol Reprod 1979;20:575-80.

16. Carlson JC, Buhr MM, Riley JC. Alterations in the cellular membranes of regressing rat corpora lutea. Endocrinology 1984;114:521-6.

17. Norjavaara E, Olofsson J, Gåfvels M, Selstam G. Redistribution of ovarian blood flow after injection of human chorionic gonadotropin and luteinizing hormone in the adult pseudopregnant rat. Endocrinology 1987;107-14.

18. Horton EW, Poyser NL. Uterine luteolytic hormone: A physiological role for prostaglandin F2α. Physiol Rev 1976;56:595-651.

19. Rothchild I. The regulation of the mammalian corpus luteum. Recent Prog Horm Res 1981;37:183-298.

20. Weems CW. Prostaglandins F in uterine and ovarian compartments and in plasma from the uterine vein, ovarian artery and vein, and abdominal aorta of pseudopregnant rats with and without deciduomata. Prostaglandins 1979;17: 873-90.

21. Ginther OJ. Internal regulation of physiological processes through local venoarterial pathways: A review. J Anim Sci 1974;39:550-64.

22. Huet J, Sentenac A, Fromageot P. Spot-immunodetection of conserved determinants in eukaryotic RNA polymerases. Study with antibodies to RNA polymerases subunits. J Biol Chem 1982;257:2613-8.

23. Hedin L, Gaddy-Kurten D, Kurten R, DeWitt DL, Smith WL, Richards JS. Prostaglandin endoperoxide synthase in rat ovarian follicles: Content, cellular distribution, and evidence for hormonal induction preceding ovulation. Endocrinology 1987;121:722-31.

24. Welschen R, Osman J, Dullaart J, De Greef WJ, Uilenbroek JTJ, DeJong FH. Levels of follicle-stimulating hormone, luteinizing hormone, oestradiol-17β and

progesterone, and follicular growth in pseudopregnant rat. J Endocrinol 1974;64:37-47.

25. Olofsson J, Selstam G. Changes in corpus luteum content of prostaglandin F2α and E in the adult pseudopregnant rat. Prostaglandins 1988;35:31-40.

26. Olofsson J, Norjavaara E, Selstam G. In vivo levels of prostaglandin F2α, E2 and prosacyclin in the corpus luteum of pregnant and pseudopregnant rats. Biol Reprod 1990.

27. Olofsson J, Norjavaara E. Effects of hysterectomy and uterine decidualization on in vivo levels of prostaglandins in the corpus luteum of adult pseudopregnant rats. Biol Reprod 1990.

28. Watson J, Shepherd TS, Dodson KS. Prostaglandin E-2-9-ketoreductase in ovarian tissues. J Reprod Fertil 1979;57:489-96.

42

Expression and Tissue Specificity of an Abundant 32-kDa Protein Found in the Large Luteal Cell of the Pregnant Rat

T.G. PARMER, M.P. MCLEAN, S. NELSON, AND G. GIBORI

The large luteal cell of the pregnant rat has recently been shown to contain an abundant phosphoprotein with a molecular weight of 32 kDa (32K) (1). Protein analysis by SDS-PAGE showed this protein to be absent from the small luteal cell population as well as other endocrine tissues, such as the liver and placenta. Further study indicated that the 32K is localized to the microsomal fraction, is absent from the cytosol, and is not a secreted protein. Two-dimensional SDS-PAGE revealed that the 32K band resolves into 3 protein species, with the major protein having an isoelectric point (pI) ≥ 8.5. In addition, the content of this protein is enhanced by estradiol treatment. In the pregnant rat, the cells of the corpus luteum undergo specific stages of differentiation characterized by a dramatic hypertrophy beginning at midpregnancy. This increase in size is due to estradiol, the bulk of which is synthesized and secreted by the large luteal cell (2, 3). Whether estrogen regulation of cell hypertrophy is mediated by a specific protein(s) is not known. In addition, the origin of the large and small luteal cell types remains uncertain. The possibility that the small luteal cells originate from the theca interna, while the large cells arise from the granulosa cells has often been proposed (5–7). Since the 32K is present only in the large luteal cell, it may be used to determine the origin of this cell type.

The aim of this investigation, therefore, was to develop a more powerful probe for the 32K and examine the tissue specificity and developmental expression of this unique large luteal cell-specific protein.

Materials and Methods

For antibody production, corpora lutea from day-14 to -15 pregnant Sprague-Dawley rats (Holtzman Co., Madison, WI) were used as the source of the 32-kDa protein. Briefly, microsomal fractions were prepared as described below, separated on SDS-PAGE (7.5–18% gradient gels) and transferred to nitrocellulose. The nitrocellulose blot was stained with Ponceau S, and a single band, at 32,000 M_r was cut from the blot and destained in sterile water. The band was then dissolved in 0.5-mL DMSO, then an equal amount of Freund's adjuvant (complete adjuvant for the first injection and incomplete for subsequent injections) was added, and the mixture was emulsified. New Zealand white male rabbits (Hazelton Labs., Philadelphia, PA) were sedated and injected at multiple sites on the back intradermally. Booster injections were given every 3–4 weeks, blood was obtained and screened for the presence of antibody by Western blot.

All tissues examined were removed from day-14 to -15 pregnant rats. For the ontogeny study, corpora lutea were obtained from day-3 to -21 pregnant rats. Microsomal fractions were prepared by differential centrifugation (4). Equal amounts of protein (100 μg) were separated by SDS-PAGE (7.5–18% gradient gels) and transferred to nitrocellulose. Antral and preovulatory follicles were isolated as previously described (1). Briefly, pregnant intact rats were treated with either 1.5-IU hCG (iv) or vehicle (saline) twice a day on days 12 and 13 of pregnancy. Follicles and corpora lutea were isolated on day 14. Subcellular tissue fractions were obtained by differential centrifugation. 50 μg of protein were separated by SDS-PAGE and transferred to nitrocellulose.

For Western blot analysis, 3% BSA was used to block nonspecific binding. The 32K was identified using a 1:1000–2000 dilution of the 32K antisera. Immunoreactive proteins were detected using a secondary antibody conjugated with either horseradish peroxidase or alkaline phosphatase.

For immunocytochemistry small and large luteal cells were separated by elutriation (3), cultured on glass coverslips, fixed with 3% formaldehyde, and permeabilized with 1% Triton X-100. Nonspecific antigenic sites were blocked with 1% BSA for 1 h. Each coverslip was then incubated with either 32K antisera or with preimmune serum (1:20 dilution) for 12 h. Cells were washed and then incubated for 1 h with fluorescein-conjugated goat anti-rabbit IgG (1:20 dilution). The stained cells were washed, mounted on microscope slides, and observed with a Nikon Microphot FXA microscope.

Results

The polyclonal antisera generated to the 32-kDa protein was highly specific and recognized only this protein by Western blot analysis (Fig. 1). Immunocy-

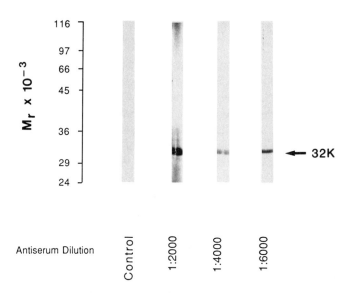

FIGURE 1. Specificity of the 32K antisera. Microsomal proteins were isolated from corpora lutea of day-14 pregnant rats as described in text. 100 μg of protein were separated by SDS-PAGE (7.5–18% gradient gels) and transferred to nitrocellulose. Western blot analysis was performed using 3 dilutions of the 32K antibody.

tochemical observations on small and large cells with the 32K antibody confirm the finding that the 32K is specific to the large cell of the corpus luteum (data not shown). Essentially no reactivity was observed in small cells.

To examine the developmental expression of this large luteal cell-specific protein, Western blot analysis was performed on microsomal fractions obtained from rats between days 3 and 21 of pregnancy. The results (Fig. 2) indicate that this protein is barely detectable until day 11, reaches a peak on days 14–15, and remains elevated through day 21.

To further investigate the tissue specificity of the 32K, microsomal proteins were isolated from liver, heart, skeletal muscle, brain, adrenal, and corpora lutea from day-14 pregnant rats, separated by SDS-PAGE, and immunoblotted with the 32K antibody. The results (Fig. 3) indicate that the 32K is an ovarian-specific protein since it is not present in liver, heart, muscle, or brain nor is it present in other steroidogenic tissues, such as the adrenal or placenta (not shown). However, immunoblotting techniques clearly indicate that the 32K is expressed in the follicle (Fig. 4), although the level of expression is not as abundant as in the corpus luteum. Interestingly, the content of the 32K decreases in the preovulatory follicle (hCG treated) as compared to the antral follicle (vehicle) in the day-14 pregnant rat (Fig. 4).

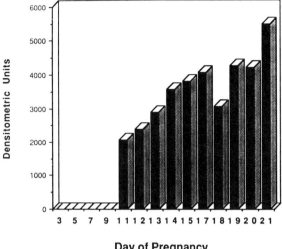

Day of Pregnancy

FIGURE 2. Ontogeny of the 32-kDa protein during pregnancy. Equal amounts of microsomal proteins (100 μg) were separated on SDS-PAGE. Western blot analysis was performed using antisera to the 32K. Content of the 32K from days 3 to 21 of pregnancy is presented in densitometric units.

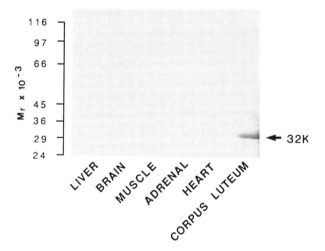

FIGURE 3. Western blot analysis of liver, brain, skeletal muscle, adrenal, heart, and corpus luteum from day-14 pregnant rats. Equal amounts of microsomal protein (100 μg) were separated by SDS-PAGE (7.5–18% gradient gels) and transferred to nitrocellulose. Western blot analysis was performed using antisera to the 32K.

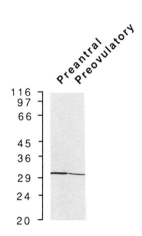

FIGURE 4. Effect of hCG on the content of the 32-kDa protein in the follicle of day-14 pregnant rats. Rats were treated with hCG as described in text. Equal amounts of protein (50 μg) were separated by SDS-PAGE (7.5–18% gradient gels) and transferred to nitrocellulose. Western blot analysis was performed using 32K antisera.

Discussion

A highly specific polyclonal antibody has been generated to the 32K luteal protein. Immunoblotting as well as immunocytochemical techniques have shown that the 32K protein is present only in the follicle and large luteal cells of the corpus luteum of the pregnant rat and not in other steroidogenic tissues. The findings of this investigation are important for several reasons. Use of an antibody to the 32K has allowed for the detection of this protein in the preantral follicle. Since the level of expression of the 32K decreases as the follicle matures and decreases further to undetectable levels in the early corpus luteum, the 32K will be an important marker for studying the process by which the theca and granulosa cells luteinize and differentiate into luteal cells.

In the corpus luteum the 32K protein reaches a peak on days 14–15 and remains elevated through day 21. During midpregnancy, the cells of the corpus luteum undergo hypertrophy and this increase in size is due to estradiol formed locally by the corpus luteum. Since the expression of the 32K has been shown to be up-regulated by estradiol (1) results of this study further support the idea that the 32K may be involved in estradiol's stimulation of large luteal cell growth and differentiation.

Acknowledgments. The authors express their appreciation to Dr. M.L. Boice and Ms. P. Mavrogianis for their helpful discussions on antibody production.

They also thank Ms. L. Alaniz for photography. Supported by NIH grants HD-11119 (GG) and NIH-NRSA Fellowship HD-7336 (TGP).

References

1. McLean MP, Nelson S, Parmer T, et al. Identification and characterization of an abundant phosphoprotein specific to the large luteal cell. Endocrinology 1990; 126:1796-1805.
2. Gibori G, Khan I, Warshaw ML, et al. Placental derived regulators and the complex control of luteal cell function. Recent Prog Horm Res 1988;44:377-429.
3. Nelson S, Jayatilak PG, Hunzicker-Dunn M, Gibori G. Characterization of two luteal cell types from the pregnant rat corpus luteum [Abstract]. Biol Reprod 1987;36:135.
4. Fleischner S, Kervina M. Subcellular fractionation of rat liver. Methods Enzymol 1974;31:6-41.
5. Donaldson L, Hansel W. Histological study of bovine corpora lutea. J Dairy Sci 1965;48:905-9.
6. O'Shea JD, Cran DG, Hay MF. Fate of the theca interna following ovulation in the ewe. Cell Tissue Res 1980;210:305-19.
7. Alila HW, Hansel W. Origin of different cell types in the bovine corpus luteum as characterized by specific monoclonal antibodies. Biol Reprod 1984;31:1015-25.

43

Endometrial Secretory Products: Regulation of Hormonal Responsiveness of Rabbit Luteal Cells In Vitro

JOSEPHINE B. MILLER

In the rabbit, hysterectomy prolongs progesterone secretion from about 18 days to about 22 days (1, 2), which suggests that both uterine and nonuterine (probably ovarian) mechanisms lead to luteal regression. If hysterectomized rabbits are treated with exogenous estradiol, the luteotropic hormone in this species (2), corpora lutea do not regress by day 22, and progesterone secretion remains elevated for greater than 33 days (1). More recent work (3) suggests that there are at least 3 uterine modulators of the corpus luteum: factor 1, secreted between days 10 and 11 of pseudopregnancy is associated with a reduction in progesterone secretion; factor 2, produced between days 11 and 13, prevents the "luteolytic effect" of factor 1; and factor 3 secreted after day 13, is associated with the final phase of luteal regression and correlates temporally with uterine PGF_2 secretion (4). Since inhibition of prostaglandin synthesis with indomethacin does not mimic the effect of hysterectomy in this animal model (3), we have proposed that factors 1 and 2, which are released at mid-pseudopregnancy, are crucial in signaling the initiation of luteal regression. In addition, 2D SDS polyacrylamide gel electrophoresis of proteins secreted by the endometrium during days 10–13 of pseudopregnancy revealed that the uterus undergoes dramatic changes in protein synthetic characteristics during this critical time of pseudopregnancy. Between days 10 and 11, at the time when uterine luteolytic activity was observed, there was a prominent loss of a group of acidic proteins of about 45,000 Da, pI 5.5–6.0, and a more variable reduction in another group of proteins of approximately 30,000 Da, pI of 4.0–4.5. Between days 11–13, there was the appearance of, or the intensification of, two groups of proteins:

one of approximately 40,000 Da, pI 6.5, and the other of approximately 30,000 Da with a neutral pI. Thus, the 45,000-Da proteins correlate with the time frame of uterine luteolytic activity indicated from in vivo studies and suggests that luteolysis may result from the loss of a substance that conveys estrogen responsiveness. In addition, the appearance or intensification of several groups of proteins after day 10 correlates with the luteotropic substance postulated from in vivo studies. The purpose of this research was, therefore, to identify and characterize these proteins, which are potential regulators of estradiol's action on the rabbit corpus luteum. To this end, a luteal cell culture system has been developed to monitor the activity of uterine regulatory substances.

Materials and Methods

New Zealand white rabbits were injected with 50-IU hCG to initiate pseudopregnancy (day 0). A 1-cm estradiol capsule was implanted sc at the base of the neck (1, 2) in rabbits used for the preparation of endometrial-conditioned media. On the designated day of pseudopregnancy, animals were killed with a saturated barbiturate solution, and the tissue was removed and transported to the laboratory in sterile media.

Preparation of Endometrial-Conditioned Media. Uteri, removed on days 8–13 of pseudopregnancy, were trimmed of adhering fat and cut open longitudinally. Endometrium was stripped from the uterus using forceps, placed in sterile media, and cut into 1- to 2-mm pieces. Tissue was incubated (25-mg tissue/mL media) in MEM containing glucose (4 mg/mL), insulin (0.8 U/mL), and nonessential amino acids as described by Fazleabas and Verhage (5). After a 24-h incubation, the media was harvested, centrifuged (100 × g for 15 min) to remove cellular debris, extensively dialyzed (12–14,000 M_r cutoff) against 10-mM Tris (pH 8.2), and filter sterilized.

Preparation and Incubation of Luteal Cell Slices. Corpora lutea were removed on days 8 and 11 of pseudopregnancy, minced and incubated for 4, 24, or 48 h in MEM alone or MEM containing *(a)* 5, 10, or 25% endometrial-conditioned media, *(b)* estradiol (10 nM), or *(c)* estradiol plus 10% endometrial-conditioned media. After incubation, progesterone levels were determined in both media and tissue by RIA.

Preparation and Culture of Dissociated Luteal Cells. Corpora lutea were dissected from 4 rabbits on day 6 of pseudopregnancy, cut in quarters, and dissociated with 50-U/mL collagenase, 2.4-U/mL Dispase, and 100-ug/mL DNase in Hank's balanced salt solution containing 25-mM HEPES, 2% BSA, and antibiotics (pH 7.4). Tissue was incubated for 30 min at 37°C in a cell stirrer set at low speed. After allowing time for the intact cell clumps to settle, the dissociated cells were removed and washed. After 4 dispersal periods, the remaining tissue was incubated in sterile phosphate-buffered saline containing 0.2% EDTA and 2% BSA for an additional 15 min in the cell stirrer. After incubation, the tissue was centrifuged at 800 × g to complete the disruption of the tissue. The dispersed cells were combined, washed 3 times to completely remove EDTA and any remaining enzymes, and counted, and their viability was assessed using trypan blue exclusion. The dispersed luteal cells were plated in 24 well plates at a density of 40,000 cells/well in 1.5-mL Medium 199 containing 5% fetal calf serum (day 0) to ensure cell attachment. On day 2, media was replaced with media containing 0.1% BSA, with or without added LH (NIH-S14, 20 ng/mL), estradiol (10 nM), and endometrial-conditioned media (10%). Media was changed daily for 6 days, and progesterone concentrations were measured in the spent media by RIA.

Results

Progesterone secretion was not affected by the presence of endometrial-conditioned media alone in either luteal minces (Fig. 1) or in cultures of dissociated luteal cells (Fig. 2). However, when estradiol was included in the

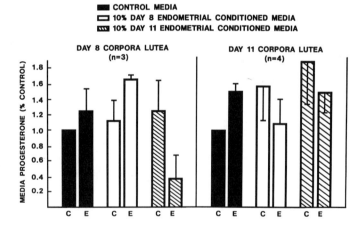

FIGURE 1. Corpora lutea, removed on either day 8 or day 11 of pseudopregnancy, were minced and incubated in control media (black bars) or in media containing 10% conditioned media from day-8 (open bars) or day-11 (hatched bars) endometrial incubates. Tissue was incubated in media alone (C) or in media containing 10-nM estradiol (E). After 4 h, the media was replenished, and the incubation continued for an additional 24 h. Results are calculated as media progesterone per mg tissue protein and expressed as a percentage of progesterone secreted in response to media alone.

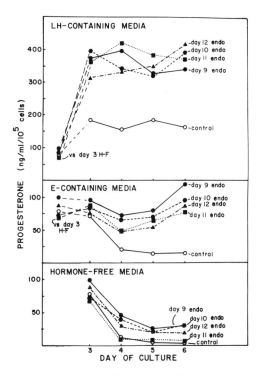

FIGURE 2. Day-6 corpora lutea were dispersed and incubated in Medium 199 containing 5% fetal calf serum to enhance attachment of cells. On day 2, media was replaced with Medium 199 containing 0.1% BSA alone (hormone-free media), with 10-nM estradiol (E), or with 100-ng/mL LH. In addition, cells were incubated in the presence of 10% conditioned media from day-9, -10, -11, or -12 endometrial incubates, which had been dialyzed against 10-mM Tris, pH 8.2. Control media contained 10% 10-mM Tris. Media was changed daily and serum progesterone concentrations were measured by RIA.

incubation media for 24 h (Fig. 1), progesterone secretion by day-8 luteal minces was increased in the presence of conditioned media from day-8 endometrium, while day-11 endometrial-conditioned media inhibited progesterone secretion in response to estradiol. Corpora lutea removed on day 11 of pseudopregnancy were not affected either by estradiol or endometrial-conditioned media under these same conditions. Similar results were observed after 48 h of incubation; however, no differences were detected after only 4 h of incubation.

When dissociated luteal cells were incubated in serum-free media, media progesterone secretion quickly fell, was slightly enhanced in the presence of estradiol (10 nM), and was stimulated approximately 2-fold in the presence of LH (Fig. 2). When endometrial-conditioned media (10%) was added to the culture media, estrogen responsiveness was restored so that progesterone secretion was maintained at a constant output. In addition, LH responsiveness was also augmented, so that progesterone levels averaged 3-5 fold compared to initial values in control cultures without conditioned media added. The addition of endometrial-conditioned media alone, in serum-free media, had no significant affect on luteal progesterone secretion.

Discussion

Results from luteal cell cultures, either using minced tissue or dissociated cells in culture, clearly demonstrate that products secreted by the rabbit endometrium modulate progesterone secretion by promoting responsiveness to estradiol and by augmenting responsiveness to LH. Since endometrial-conditioned media had been extensively dialyzed (12–14,000 M_r cutoff) and is ineffective after heating at 100°C for 1 h (data not shown), these results are consistent with the concept that some protein(s) of greater than 12,000 Da is (are) secreted by the endometrium and synergize(s) with estradiol (or LH) to stimulate luteal progesterone secretion. Since day-11 corpora lutea were not affected by this treatment, important changes must have occurred in vivo to alter luteal responsiveness to estradiol. We propose that these changes were initiated by some products secreted by the uterus during this critical period.

The identity of the endometrial secretory product(s) is not known. In recent years, however, the importance of growth factors, both as intermediates and regulators of hormone action in ovarian function, has become increasingly clear. In the case of IGF, its action may depend not only on its synergy with LH, FSH, or estradiol (6), but on the presence or absence of specific IFG binding proteins. Granulosa cells have been shown to secrete a low molecular weight IGF-I binding protein that is thought to adhere to the cell surface and amplify both IGF-I binding and hormone action (7). In addition, there is a larger binding protein that is synthesized by the liver in response to growth hormone. This binding protein, which forms a stable complex with IGF, is thought to prevent its action (8).

The uterus may prove to be a key player in the IGF story. In the rat uterus, the synthesis of IGF is second only to that in the liver (6). In addition, both the human and baboon endometria secrete an IGF-binding protein whose synthesis is regulated by progesterone (5, 9). Although it is clearly speculative at this time, it is interesting to propose that the rabbit endometrium may secrete a binding protein(s) to some growth factor, which could then enter the general circulation and alter the biological effect of estradiol on the corpus luteum. Since the ovarian and endometrial IGF-I binding proteins are 33–35,000 Da and thus within the size range of the rabbit endometrial protein targeted by our preliminary studies, it is possible that the rabbit protein may also be an IGF-binding protein. Clearly, there are multiple possibilities in this line of thinking. However, this pursuit could lead to significant and novel insight into how the ovary and uterus may interact to regulate hormone action in general and progesterone synthesis in particular. Thus, our results point to an important role for endometrial secretory products in regulating the action of estradiol on the rabbit corpus luteum and demonstrate their activity in vitro. The aim of future studies will be to identify these regulators of luteal function and to study the mechanisms through which these factors interact with estradiol to regulate luteal progesterone synthesis.

References

1. Miller JB, Keyes PL. A mechanism for regression of the rabbit corpus luteum: Uterine-induced loss of luteal responsiveness to 17-estradiol. Biol Reprod 1976; 15:511-8.
2. Bill CH, Keyes PL. 17-estradiol maintains normal function of corpora lutea throughout pseudopregnancy in hypophysectomized rabbits. Biol Reprod 1983; 28:608-17.
3. Miller JB, McLean MP. Evidence for multiple uterine modulators of rabbit luteal function: The effect of hysterectomy during pseudopregnancy in the estrogen-treated rabbit. Biol Reprod 1987;36:572-80.
4. Miller JB, Jarosik C, Staninic D, Wilson L, Jr. Alterations in plasma and tissue prostaglandin levels in rabbits during luteal regression. Biol Reprod 1983;29: 824-32.
5. Fazleabas AT, Verhage HG, Waites G, Bell SC. Characterization of an insulin-like growth factor binding protein, analogous to human pregnancy-associated secreted endometrial 1-globulin, in decidua of the baboon *(Papio anubis)* placenta. Biol Reprod 1989;40:873-85.
6. Adashi EY, Resnick C, Hernandez ER, et al. Rodent studies on the potential relevance of insulin-like growth factor (IGF-I) to ovarian physiology. In: Hirshfield AN, ed. Growth factors in the ovary. New York: Plenum Press, 1989: 95-105.
7. Hammond JM, Bamanao HLS, Skaleris D, Knight AB, Romanus JA, Rechler MM. Production of insulin-like growth factors by ovarian granulosa cells. Endocrinology 1985;117:2553-5.
8. Ui M, Shimonaka M, Shimasaki S, Ling N. An insulin-like growth factor-binding protein in ovarian follicular fluid blocks follicle stimulating hormone-stimulated steroid production by ovarian granulosa cells. Endocrinology 1989;125:912-6.
9. Bell SC. Secretory endometrial and decidual proteins: Studies and clinical significance of a maternally derived group of pregnancy-associated serum proteins. Hum Reprod 1986;1:129-43.

44

Baboon Corpus Luteum Oxytocin

FIRYAL S. KHAN-DAWOOD, M. YUSOFF DAWOOD,
AND RICHARD IVELL

The role of luteal oxytocin (OT) in the ruminant reproductive cycle has been examined extensively, and it appears to be the luteolytic factor, with the release of OT from the corpus luteum being controlled by prostaglandin $F_{2\alpha}$ produced by the uterine endometrium (1). However, the role of this peptide in the primate ovary is not clearly defined as yet. OT was first described in the human corpus luteum in 1982 (2). Our studies have confirmed the presence of this peptide in the human corpus luteum (3, 4) and have provided evidence for its presence in the cynomolgus monkey corpus luteum (5) and the baboon corpus luteum (6). The techniques used in these studies involved radioimmunoassay, immunocytochemistry, and high pressure liquid chromatography. Using immunocytochemical methodology, the carrier protein neurophysin has also been localized in the human and baboon luteal cells (7, 8).

The concentrations of OT within the primate corpus luteum are several-fold lower than in the ruminant corpus luteum (9). In the olive baboon *(Papio anubis)*, the concentrations vary through the luteal phase as in the human (4, 6). Thus, compared to the early luteal phase (2.1 ± 1.1 ng/gm), the concentrations rose to a peak in the mid-luteal phase (18.1 ± 4.3 ng/gm). Regressing corpora lutea and ovarian stroma had comparatively lower OT concentrations.

Since the concentrations of OT are low, it is unlikely that luteal OT acts in a similar way to that proposed for the ruminant corpus luteum, particularly since its secretion to distant sites outside the ovary is likely to end in significant dilution. Hysterectomy does not affect the life-span of the corpus luteum nor luteolysis. It is thus likely that OT may exert an intragonadal effect. Thus, OT in concentrations as low as 4 μU to as much as 800 μU (similar to concentrations found in baboon corpus luteum, 1 μU = 2 pg) significantly inhibited both basal and human chorionic gonadotropin (hCG)-stimulated luteal cell progesterone production in vitro (6). OT also inhibited basal estradiol production and, in low doses (4- to 40-μU OT), further stimulated hCG-stimulated 17α-hydroxyprogesterone production in luteal cells of the early luteal phase corpus luteum (10). This steroid-modulatory effect is dependent on the age of the corpus luteum; it is more pronounced in the early luteal phase and less marked in the corpus luteum of the late luteal phase when 200–400 μU are necessary to produce a significant inhibition of progesterone production. A similar effect is also seen in vivo (11). The major question these studies have posed is whether the primate corpus luteum has the capacity to synthesize OT de novo.

Thus, polymerase chain reaction (PCR) method was employed to examine the baboon corpus luteum for evidence of transcription of the genes for OT.

Materials and Methods

Adult female baboons with established breeding histories and weighing 14 to 17 kg, were used for this study (n = 8), as previously described (6). Luteectomy or ovariectomy was performed in 2 or 3 cycles in each animal, and all animals had at least one rest cycle between the cycles during which the operation was performed. Thirteen corpora lutea were obtained for the study, which was approved by the Institutional Review Board for Animal Experimentation. The baboon corpora lutea were combined together in one pool. Total RNA was extracted from individual tissues in a guanidinium isothiocyanate buffer and isolated by ultracentrifugation through a cesium chloride cushion, as previously described (12). Total RNA from grouped tissues was pooled prior to enriching for poly(A)-containing transcripts by oligo (αT)-cellulose chromatography. The extracted RNA was first converted into single-strand DNA, using reverse transcriptase, and this DNA was used as a template in the PCR reaction, together with pairs of oligonucleotide primers specific for sequences in the first or third exons of the vasopressin (VSP) and OT genes as indicated in Figure 1, panel A.

After 30 cycles of amplification, aliquots of the PCR products were electrophoresed on an agarose gel and visualized by ethidium bromide staining (Fig. 1, panel B). Evidence of that RNA is guaranteed only when a specific mRNA-derived template DNA, which reacts with both 5' (exon 1) and 3' (exon 3) primers to yield a PCR product of the correct size, is present. For VSP mRNA and OT mRNA, the resulting DNA should be 300 and 310 bp respectively, for the primers used (Fig. 1, Panel B).

Final confirmation was provided by blotting the electrophoresis products onto a nylon membrane and hybridizing this with a radiolabeled oligonucleotide probe specific for exon 2 of the VSP and OT genes (Fig. 1, panel C). Only the bands of the correct size, shown in panel B, are evident in the resulting autoradiogram, thus confirming that all 3 exons are encoded within the mRNA and implying that this mRNA is capable of producing the hormone precursor.

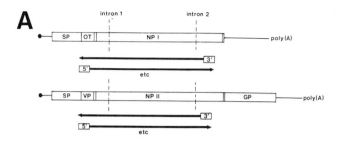

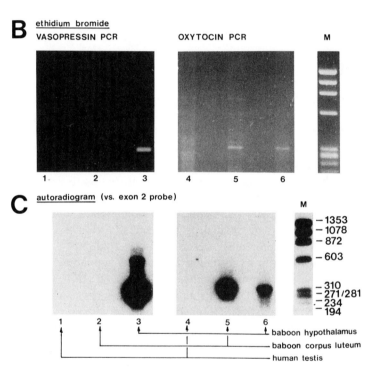

FIGURE 1. Examination of baboon corpus luteum for evidence of OT. Panel *A* shows the main features of the PCR assay used to detect VSP and OT mRNAs. Peptides encoded in the mRNA molecules are SP = signal peptide; OT = oxytocin; VP = vasopressin; NPI = oxytocin associated neurophysin; NP II = vasopressin-associated neurophysin; and GP = C-terminal glycopeptide. 5' and 3' represent the oligonucleotides used as primers for the Taq polymerase reaction shown for oxytocin ss-cDNA (upper structure) and vasopressin ss-cDNA (lower structure). Panel *B* shows autoradiograms of the radioactively probed PCR products derived from baboon corpus luteum. Positive signals for VSP are seen only in the baboon hypothalamus (lane 3); for OT, positive signals are seen in both the hypothalamus and corpus luteum (lanes 5 and 6, respectively). In panel *C*, hybridizing the bands (panel *B*) with radiolabeled oligonucleotide probe specific for exon 2 of the VSP and OT genes confirms the presence of the mRNA for OT in the corpus luteum (lane 5).

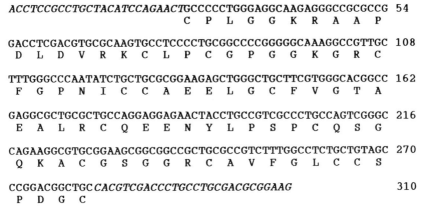

*ACCTCCGCCTGCTACATCCAGAAC*TGCCCCCTGGGAGGCAAGAGGGCCGCGCCG 54
                         C   P   L   G   G   K   R   A   A   P

GACCTCGACGTGCGCAAGTGCCTCCCCTGCGGCCCCGGGGGCAAAGGCCGTTGC 108
 D   L   D   V   R   K   C   L   P   C   G   P   G   G   K   G   R   C

TTTGGGCCCAATATCTGCTGCGCGGAAGAGCTGGGCTGCTTCGTGGGCACGGCC 162
 F   G   P   N   I   C   C   A   E   E   L   G   C   F   V   G   T   A

GAGGCGCTGCGCTGCCAGGAGGAGAACTACCTGCCGTCGCCCTGCCAGTCGGGC 216
 E   A   L   R   C   Q   E   E   N   Y   L   P   S   P   C   Q   S   G

CAGAAGGCGTGCGGAAGCGGCGGCCGCTGCGCCGTCTTTGGCCTCTGCTGTAGC 270
 Q   K   A   C   G   S   G   G   R   C   A   V   F   G   L   C   C   S

CCGGACGGCTGC *CACGTCGACCCTGCCTGCGACGCGGAAG*   310
 P   D   G   C

FIGURE 2. Sequence analysis of the cloned PCR product derived from baboon luteal RNA. The 5' and 3' primer sequences used are indicated in italics. The amino acid sequence for the encoded neurophysins is indicated below the nucleotide sequence.

Results

Positive results for both VSP and OT mRNA for baboon hypothalamus were obtained and used as a positive control. For luteal RNA extracted from a pool of corpora lutea gathered throughout the estrous cycle, only OT mRNA was evident; the PCR assay for VSP mRNA was negative. As negative controls in this assay, we used human testis RNA. The sizes (bp) of the marker DNA fragments (M) used in Figure 1, panels *B* and *C*, are indicated on the lower panel.

In a separate experiment, the OT-specific PCR product was eluted from the agarose gel, cloned into a plasmid vector, and sequenced. The resulting DNA sequence (Fig. 2) corresponded precisely with the expected region of the OT mRNA and differs from the human cDNA sequence in only 10 nucleotides, only one of which leads to an amino acid substitution in the neurophysin moiety.

Discussion

These results provide data to indicate that OT can be synthesized locally by baboon luteal tissue and, therefore, support the evidence previously obtained by immunological techniques for its presence in luteal extracts or in fluids derived from ovarian tissues or cells. However, the fact that OT mRNA can only be detected by PCR analysis of poly(A)-enriched RNA suggests a very low level of the specific RNA in the primate corpus luteum, sufficient only to supply a local intragonadal function.

Although the PCR method is not quantitative, the findings are consistent with OT gene transcription in the early to mid-luteal phase of the cycle, similar to the much more highly transcribed OT gene in the ruminant corpus luteum (13). This would fit with reports of OT peptide levels measured through the menstrual cycle in extracts (4, 6), where the hormone increases to a maximum in the mid-luteal phase.

If OT is a local paracrine factor in the primate ovary, what may be its role? When OT is applied to dispersed primate luteal cells, there appears to be a reduction in the hCG-stimulated production of progesterone (6, 14, 15), though in vivo this effect may be negligible (16), or OT may even be stimulatory to progesterone production when infused into whole, freshly excised human ovaries (17). It seems likely, therefore, that OT may be playing a modulatory role on ovarian steroidogenesis, acting in concert with other local factors.

References

1. McCracken JA, Schramm W, Okulicz WC. Hormone receptor control of pulsatile secretion of PG_{F22} from the bovine uterus during luteolysis and its abrogation in early pregnancy. Anim Reprod 1980;7:31-5.
2. Wathes DC, Swann RW, Pickering BT, et al. Neurohypophysial hormones in the human ovary. Lancet 1982;2:410-2.
3. Khan-Dawood FS, Dawood MY. Human ovaries contain immunoreactive oxytocin. J Clin Endocrinol Metab 1983;57:1129-32.
4. Dawood MY, Khan-Dawood FS. Human ovarian oxytocin: Its source and relationship to steroid hormones. Am J Obstet Gynecol 1986;154:756-63.
5. Khan-Dawood FS, Marut EL, Dawood MY. Oxytocin in the corpus luteum of the cynomolgus monkey *(Macaca fasicularis)*. Endocrinology 1984;115:570-4.
6. Khan-Dawood FS, Huang J-C, Dawood MY. Baboon corpus luteum oxytocin: An intragonadal peptide modulator of luteal function. Am J Obstet Gynecol 1988;158:882-9.
7. Khan-Dawood FS. Immunocytochemical localization of oxytocin and neurophysin in human corpora lutea. Am J Anat 1987;179:18-24.
8. Khan-Dawood FS. Localization of oxytocin and neurophysin in baboon *(Papio anubis)* corpus luteum by immunocytochemistry. Acta Endocrinol (Copenh) 1986;113:570-5.
9. Khan-Dawood FS, Dawood MY. Potential relevance of neurohypophysial hormones to ovarian physiology. Semin Reprod Endocrinol 1989;7:61-8.
10. Khan-Dawood FS, Huang J-C. Oxytocin (OT) a modulator of corpus luteum steroid production in the baboon [Abstract]. Biol Reprod 1987;36(suppl 1):136.
11. Khan-Dawood FS. Baboon corpus luteum: In vivo effect of oxytocin. Unpublished.

12. Ivell R, Hunt N, Khan-Dawood FS, Dawood MY. Expression of the human relaxin gene in the corpus luteum of the menstrual cycle and in the prostate. Mol Cell Endocrinol 1989;66:251-5.
13. Ivell R, Brackett KH, Fields MJ, Richter D. Ovulation triggers oxytocin gene expression in the bovine ovary. FEBS Lett 1985;190:263-7.
14. Bennegard B, Hahlin M, Dennefors B. Antigonadotropic effect of oxytocin on the isolated human corpus luteum. Fertil Steril 1987;47:431-5.
15. Tan GJS, Tweedale R, Biggs JSG. Oxytocin may play a role in the control of the human corpus luteum. J Endocrinol 1982;95:65-70.
16. Wilks JW. The effect of oxytocin on the corpus luteum of the monkey. Contraception 1983;28:267-72.
17. Maas S, Jarry H, Teichman A, Kuhn W, Wuttke W. PGF 2 alpha application into young human corpora lutea increases estradiol, oxytocin and progesterone release. Acta Endocrinol [Suppl I] (Copenh) 1990;122:120.

45

Inhibitory Effects of In Vivo and In Vitro Treatment of a LHRH Antagonist (Nal-Lys Antide) on Progesterone Levels During Early Pregnancy in the Rat

R.K. Srivastava, S. Harris-Hooker, and R. Sridaran

Endogenous gonadotropin releasing hormone (GnRH) maintains the normal reproductive function through its control of gonadotropin secretion from the pituitary. Hypophysis is essential for the maintenance of pregnancy for the first 12 days in rats (1). However, chronic administration of GnRH or its analogues exerts luteal suppression and an antifertility effect in pregnant and pseudopregnant rats (2). The abortifacient effect of GnRH is due to its ability to suppress plasma progesterone (PR) levels (3). GnRH or its analogs are known to act at several sites, including the pituitary, gonads, and reproductive tract (4). Several potent GnRH antagonists have been developed that bind to GnRH receptors in the pituitary (5), inhibit gonadotropin secretion, and thus exhibit an antifertility effect in animals (6). Therefore, the present investigation has been undertaken to determine the effect of a LHRH antagonist (Nal-Lys antide) on the serum PR level in vivo during early pregnancy or its direct effect on the luteal production of PR in vitro.

Materials and Methods

Timed-pregnant Sprague-Dawley rats were obtained from Holtzman Co. (Madison, WI) and housed at 23–25°C with a 14:10 light:dark photoperiod. The day of insemination was designated as day 1 of pregnancy.

On day 8 of pregnancy, laparotomy was performed under ether anesthesia in rats to observe the implantation sites. In one experiment, each group of rats received 10, 20, or 40 μg antide dissolved in 30% propylene glycol: water, sc, daily starting from day 8 through day 11 of pregnancy. The control group of rats received equal volume of vehicle (i.e., 30% propylene glycol:water). In another experiment, rats received either 80, 150, or 300 μg of antide once on day 8, and the control group received the same amount of vehicle. Rats were observed daily for vaginal bleeding. They were bled from the jugular vein daily from day 8 through day 12 of pregnancy under ether anesthesia. On day 12, rats were sacrificed with an overdose of ether.

On day 8 of pregnancy, the ovaries were dissected out, under ether anesthesia, and the corpora lutea were removed, cleaned carefully, transferred to Medium 199 containing 2.2 g/L $NaHCO_3$, and gassed with 95% O_2:5% CO_2. The basic procedure used here for enzymatic dissociation of corpora lutea for isolation of luteal cells was described earlier (7). Aliquots of approximately 5 × 10^5 viable luteal cells were suspended per mL of Medium 199 (containing 25-mM HEPES buffer, 10% fetal bovine serum, 100-IU penicillin and streptomycin, and 50-IU Gentacin/mL) and were preincubated for 90 min in 95% air:5% CO_2 in 24-well Falcon tissue culture plates. The medium was removed and fresh medium was added, after preincubation, and attached cells were treated with either 10^{-4} or 10^{-7}M of antide dissolved in 30% propylene glycol:water in a total volume of 10 μL. A control group of cells received only 10 μL of vehicle. These were incubated for 24 or 48 h in an atmosphere of 95% air:5% CO_2. After the incubation period, the media were removed, snap frozen, and stored at –20°C until assayed for PR. Luteal cells were treated with 0.5% trypsin, and viability was assessed by trypan blue. We found that viability was approximately 75% both before and after the incubation.

PR was measured in the serum or the medium after hexane extraction using the procedure described elsewhere (8). This assay employed a specific antibody (GDN-337) prepared against PR. The specificity of the antiserum is very high. The sensitivity of the assay was 0.10 ng/assay tube. Differences between the two groups were analyzed by Student's t-test. A P-value of less than 0.05 was considered significant.

Results

Administration of 3 different doses of antide (10, 20, or 40 μg) daily, sc, starting from day 8 of pregnancy was able to reduce the serum PR levels on day 10 by 33%, 42%, and 50%, respectively, and cause a further fall to 40%, 52%, and 72%, respectively, by day 12 of pregnancy as compared to controls (Fig. 1). One-time administration of 80- or 150-μg antide on day 8 was not able to reduce the serum PR level by day 12 of pregnancy; however, a single administration of 300-μg antide was able to reduce the serum PR levels to about 80% by day 12 of pregnancy (Fig. 2).

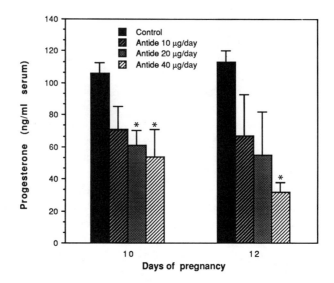

FIGURE 1. Effect of 3 different doses of antide (10, 20, or 40 μg/day) administered sc on days 8–11 of pregnancy on the serum PR levels in jugular vein blood on days 10 and 12 of pregnancy. (Values are mean ± SE; *P < 0.05 when compared to respective control.)

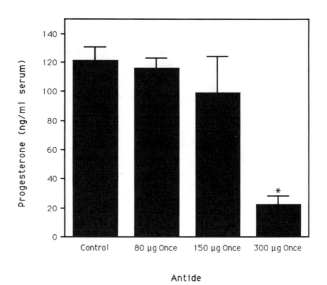

FIGURE 2. Effect of 3 different doses of antide (80, 150, or 300 μg) administered sc once on day 8 of pregnancy on the serum PR levels in jugular vein blood on day 12 of pregnancy. (Values are mean ± SE; *P < 0.05 when compared to control.)

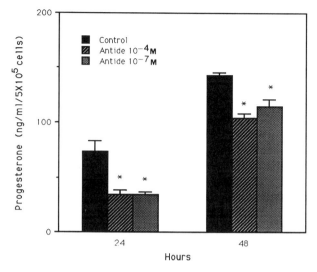

FIGURE 3. Mean (±SE) progesterone levels in medium containing luteal cells of day-8 pregnant rats after incubation with 2 different doses of antide for 24 or 48 h. (*P < 0.05 when compared to respective control.)

Treatment of 2 different doses of antide at 10^{-4} and 10^{-7}M in vitro to a population of approximately 5×10^5 luteal cells was able to reduce (P < 0.05) the PR release by these cells within 24 h after the treatment. PR levels in the media remain suppressed after 48 h (Fig. 3) of treatment.

Discussion

The results of this investigation have shown that a daily dose of 40 μg of antide was most effective in suppressing the serum PR level within 48 h of treatment to be incompatible for the maintenance of pregnancy in the rats, whereas a single administration of 300 μg of antide was able to reduce the serum PR level only after 96 h to be detrimental for the pregnancy. The antagonist analogs of GnRH are shown to bind the GnRH receptor (5) and inhibit the gonadotropin secretion, which, in turn, lowers the production of steroids to the incompatible level for maintenance of pregnancy. GnRH or its analogs are shown to act at several sites including the pituitary, gonads, and reproductive tract (4). The locus or loci at which GnRH acts directly upon ovarian function in vitro is much less clear. We are able to demonstrate here that antide is able to inhibit the PR release by the cultured luteal cells in the incubation medium within 24 or 48 h. Direct binding of a GnRH analog to isolated luteinized cells and the inhibition of steroidogenesis in vitro has been reported (9). Additionally, GnRH antagonists have been shown to compete with radiolabeled GnRH agonists for binding to gonadal membrane fractions (10) and thus antagonize the effects of GnRH on luteal cells in culture. The presence of a GnRH-like substance in the rat ovary (11) suggests a paracrine function for GnRH to regulate ovarian steroidogenesis. Ability of this potent LHRH antagonist to suppress the PR release by the luteal cells seems to be mediated by antagonizing the action of the endogenous LHRH present in the luteal cells.

Acknowledgments. We acknowledge the gift of Nal-Lys antide from Dr. Marvin Karten, Contraceptive Development Branch, NIH, and the gift of antisera to progesterone from Dr. G.D. Niswender, Colorado State University, Fort Collins, CO. We thank Sandra Milline for typing the manuscript. This work was supported by a grant from NIH, HD-17867 (RS) and a postdoctoral fellowship from Rockefeller Foundation (RKS).

References

1. Morishige WK, Pepe GJ, Rothchild I. Serum luteinizing hormone, prolactin and progesterone levels during pregnancy in the rat. Endocrinology 1973;92:1527-30.
2. Corbin A. Peptide contraception: Antifertility properties of LHRH analogues. Int J Gynaecol Obstet 1979;16:359-72.
3. Kledzik GS, Cusan L, Auclair C, Kelly PA, and Labrie F. Inhibitory effect of a luteinizing hormone (LH)-releasing hormone agonist on rat ovarian LH and follicle-stimulating hormone receptor levels during pregnancy. Fertil Steril 1978; 29:560-4.
4. Hsueh AJW, Jones PBC. Extrapituitary actions of gonadotropin-releasing hormone. Endocr Rev 1981;2:437-61.
5. Clayton RN, Catt KJ. Receptor binding affinity of gonadotropin releasing hormone analogs: Analysis by radioligand receptor assay. Endocrinology 1980; 106:1154-9.
6. Rivier C, Rivier J, Vale W. Antireproductive effect of a potent GnRH antagonist in the female rat. Endocrinology 1981;108:1425-30.
7. Smith CJ, Greer TB, Banks T, Sridaran R. The response of large and small luteal cells from the pregnant rat to substrates and secretagogues. Biol Reprod 1989; 41:1123-32.
8. Gibori G, Antczak E, Rothchild I. The role of estrogen in the regulation of luteal progesterone secretion in the rat after day 12 of pregnancy. Endocrinology 1977; 100:1483-95.
9. Clayton RN, Harwood JP, Catt KJ. Gonadotropin-releasing hormone analogue binds to luteal cells and inhibits progesterone production. Nature 1979;282:90-2.
10. Perrin MH, Vaughan JM, Rivier JE, Vale WW. High affinity GnRH binding to testicular membrane homogenates. Life Sci 1980;26:2251-5.
11. Aten RF, Williams AT, Behrman HR. Ovarian gonadotropin releasing hormone-like protein(s): Demonstration and characterization. Endocrinology 1986;118: 961-7.

46

Suppression of Luteal Production of Progesterone In Vitro by a GnRH Agonist During Pregnancy

R. SRIDARAN, R.K. SRIVASTAVA, AND S. HARRIS-HOOKER

Previous studies from this laboratory have demonstrated that in vivo treatment with a gonadotropin-releasing hormone agonist (GnRH-Ag) suppresses luteal progesterone (PR) synthesis in pregnant rats within 24 h, with no effect on the ability of the luteal synthesis of testosterone or estradiol (1, 2). Although PR secretion is acutely stimulated by luteinizing hormone (LH) during early pregnancy, the constant high titers of PR necessary to maintain pregnancy in the rat appear to be the result of indirect LH action through testosterone that is aromatized to estradiol by the corpus luteum (3). Recently, we observed, in pregnant rats treated with GnRH-Ag at the level of luteal ultrastructure, an increase in the number of lipid droplets and a decrease in the number of tubular cristae within the mitochondria (4). In addition, the in vivo GnRH-Ag treatment decreased the luteal P-450 side-chain cleavage (P-450$_{SCC}$) enzyme and mRNA content (5). These observations suggest that the in vivo treatment of GnRH-Ag within the corpus luteum inhibits PR synthesis by decreasing the amount of P-450$_{SCC}$ mRNA and enzyme content, which may alter the mitochondrial cristae structure. Collectively, these data indicate that the effect of GnRH-Ag in the pregnant rat may be due to its direct inhibitory action on luteal steroidogenesis. However, this has not been tested yet. Therefore, the purpose of this study was to determine if the in vitro GnRH-Ag treatment during early pregnancy has any suppressive effect on luteal steroidogenesis by utilizing an in vitro model system.

Materials and Methods

Hank's balanced salt solution (HBSS) without Ca^{++} and Mg^{++}, trypan blue, collagenase type IV, ethylenediaminetetraacetic acid (EDTA), bovine serum albumin (BSA; endotoxin-tested), and $NaHCO_3$ were purchased from Sigma Chemical Co. (St. Louis, MO). DNase I and dispase (neutral protease) were purchased from Boehringer-Mannheim Biochemicals (Indianapolis, IN); Medium 199 from GiBCO (New York), and [^{3}H]progesterone from NEN Research Products, DuPont (Boston, MA). Progesterone antiserum (GDN-337) was provided by Dr. G. D. Niswender; rLH (NIDDK-rLH-7) was supplied from the National Institute of Diabetes and Digestive and Kidney Diseases, Baltimore, MD, and GnRH-Ag (Wyeth-40972) was a gift from Wyeth-Ayerst Laboratories.

Timed-pregnant Sprague-Dawley rats were obtained from the Holtzman Co. (Madison, WI) and housed at 23–25°C with a 14:10 light:dark photoperiod (lights on from 0600 to 2000 h). Purina rat chow (Ralston-Purina Co., St. Louis, MO) and water were available *ad libitum*. The day of insemination was designated as day 1 of pregnancy.

On day 8 of pregnancy, the ovaries were dissected out from the rats while they were under ether anesthesia. The corpora lutea that were removed and cleaned carefully under a dissecting microscope were pooled and enzyme digested to obtain a dissociated mixed population of luteal cells, as previously described (6). Cells were counted in a hemocytometer and viability was calculated after incubation in 0.4% trypan blue.

Aliquots of approximately 5×10^5 viable luteal cells were suspended per mL of Medium 199 (containing 25-mM HEPES buffer, 10% fetal bovine serum, 100-IU penicillin and streptomycin, and 50-IU Gentacin/mL) and were preincubated for 90 min in 95% air:5% CO_2 in 24-well Falcon tissue culture plates. After this period of preincubation, the medium was removed and fresh medium was replaced and then the attached cells were treated with LH at a dose of 100 ng/mL or 10^{-4} or 10^{-7}M of GnRH-Ag dissolved in saline in a total volume of 10 μL. A control group of cells received only 10 μl of saline. These were incubated for 12 or 24 h in an atmosphere of 95% air:5% CO_2. After the incubation period, the media were removed, snap frozen, and stored at –20°C until assayed for PR. Attached luteal cells were treated with 0.5% trypsin for the detachment of the cells. Viability was assessed by trypan blue exclusion test. In our studies, we found that viability was approximately 75% both before and after the incubation.

PR was measured in the medium after hexane extraction using the procedure described elsewhere (7). This assay employed a specific antibody (GDN-337) prepared against PR. The specificity of the antiserum is very high. The sensitivity of the assay was 0.10 ng/assay tube. Differences between 2 groups were analyzed by Student's t-test. A P-value of less than 0.05 was considered significant.

Results

Administration of both doses of GnRH-Ag (10^{-4} and 10^{-7}M) suppressed the luteal synthesis of PR by a population of approximately 5×10^5 cells in vitro at 23 ± 2 and 17 ± 1 ng/mL, respectively, when compared to 66 ± 2 ng/mL in controls after 12 h of treatment (Fig. 1). Similarly, both doses were suppressive on luteal PR synthesis after 24 h of treatment (Fig. 2). LH at a dose of 100 ng/mL stimulated PR synthesis by these cells at both time periods (Fig. 3).

Discussion

The results of this study provide conclusive evidence that the suppressive effect of GnRH-Ag on luteal PR production is due to its direct action on the corpus luteum during early pregnancy. The ability of LH to stimulate PR production approximately 5-fold and 3-fold after 12 and 24 h of treatment, respectively, by these mixed populations of luteal cells indicates that these cells respond to LH like the corpora lutea in situ. Further evidence for the direct action of GnRH-Ag on the corpus luteum is provided by the presence

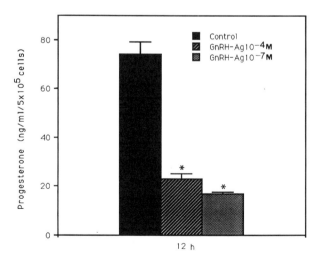

FIGURE 1. Mean (±SE) progesterone levels in medium containing mixed population of luteal cells after incubation with two different doses of GnRH-Ag for 12 h. (*P < 0.05 when compared to control.)

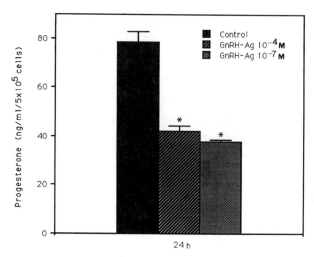

FIGURE 2. Mean (±SE) progesterone levels in medium containing a mixed population of luteal cells after incubation with 2 different doses of GnRH-Ag for 24 h. (*P < 0.05 when compared to control.)

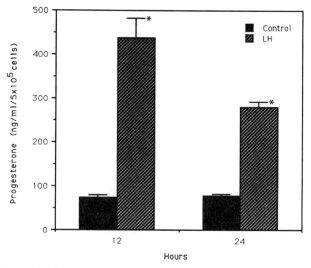

FIGURE 3. Mean (±SE) progesterone levels in medium containing a mixed population of luteal cells after incubation with LH at a dose of 100 ng/mL. (*P < 0.05 when compared to respective control.)

of high-affinity receptor sites for GnRH in the rat luteal cell membranes (8) and the fact that the number of these sites is not altered by in vivo treatment of GnRH-Ag during a 24-h time period (unpublished observations). Although previous studies (8) utilizing isolated luteinized cells obtained from immature rat ovaries treated with pregnant mare serum gonadotropin (PMSG) alone for 3 days have demonstrated the inhibitory effect of a GnRH-agonist on hCG-induced PR production, the results of the present study demonstrate, for the first time, the inhibitory effect of GnRH-Ag on the basal production of PR by luteal cells obtained from pregnant rats. Presently, studies are in progress to determine the minimum dose of GnRH-Ag and the minimum time period to be inhibitory on PR production by the mixed population of luteal cells. Other studies are focused on determining the inhibitory effect of in vitro GnRH-Ag on 2 populations of luteal cells, large and small, obtained by elutriation. Previous studies performed in this laboratory (6) appear to suggest that the major source of PR in the rat is large luteal cells during early pregnancy.

Recent observations in our laboratory indicate that in vivo GnRH-Ag treatment within 24 h decreased the luteal $P-450_{SCC}$ enzyme and mRNA content, while it increased the number of lipid droplets and decreased the number of tubular cristae within the mitochondria in the corpus luteum. Currently, studies are in progress to determine the in vitro GnRH-Ag effect on the $P-450_{SCC}$ enzyme and mRNA content in large and small luteal cells and on the production of pregnenolone, whose conversion from cholesterol is mediated by $P-450_{SCC}$ in the corpus luteum.

Acknowledgments. We thank Sandra Milline for typing the manuscript. This work was supported by grants from NIH, HD-17867 and RR-08248 (RS).

References

1. Sridaran R, Ghose M, Mahesh VB. Inhibitory effects of a gonadotropin-releasing hormone agonist on the luteal synthesis of progesterone, estradiol receptors and on prolactin surges during early pregnancy. Endocrinology 1988;123:1740-6.
2. Sridaran R, Mahesh VB. Suppression of luteal estradiol receptors and progesterone synthesis by a gonadotropin-releasing hormone agonist (WY-40972) during midgestation. Biol Reprod 1989;40:276-82.
3. Gibori G, Khan MI, Sridaran R, et al. Secretion and action of steroids in the luteal cell. In: McKerns KW, ed. Hormonal control of hypothalamo-pituitary-gonadal axis. New York: Plenum Press, 1984:289-307.
4. Smith CJ, Sridaran R. Effects of in vivo gonadotropin-releasing hormone agonist (GnRH-Ag) treatment on the ultrastructure of large luteal cells in the pregnant rat [Abstract]. Biol Reprod 1988;38:22A.

5. Sridaran R, Smith CJ. Effects of in vivo gonadotropin-releasing hormone treatment on luteal P450scc enzyme and mRNA content in the pregnant rat [Abstract]. Biol Reprod 1990;42:70A.

6. Smith CJ, Greer TB, Banks TW, Sridaran R. The response of large and small luteal cells from the pregnant rat to substrates and secretagogues. Biol Reprod 1989;41:1123-32.

7. Gibori G, Antczak E, Rothchild I. The role of estrogen in the regulation of luteal progesterone secretion in the rat after day 12 of pregnancy. Endocrinology 1977;100:1483-95.

8. Clayton RN, Harwood JP, Catt KJ. Gonadotropin-releasing hormone analogue binds to luteal cells and inhibits progesterone production. Nature 1979;282:90-2.

47

Effects of Long-Term Treatment of a GnRH Agonist on Ovarian Function in the Rat

R. SRIDARAN, A. KRISHNA, AND R.K. SRIVASTAVA

Gonadotropin-releasing hormone (GnRH) analogs are associated with the inhibition of a variety of female reproductive functions, such as ovarian steroidogenesis, ovulation, ovarian transport, ovarian implantation, pregnancy, and uterine growth (1). GnRH and its analogs are also shown to delay puberty, induce premature meiotic maturation of ova within preantral and preovulatory follicles and disrupt the normal ovarian cycle (1). Although the GnRH agonists are known to halt follicular development (2, 3), no studies quantified changes in follicle numbers and their size distribution following long-term treatment.

Materials and Methods

Sprague-Dawley (CD strain, Cobb variety) young adult female rats (160–175 g) were obtained from Charles River Laboratories (Wilmington, MA). Rats were exposed to a daily 14:10 light:dark photoperiod (lights on from 0600 to 2000 h) at 23–25°C. The estrous cyclicity of rats were monitored by taking vaginal smears daily. Only the rats that exhibited at least 2 regular estrous cycles were chosen for the experiment. Purina rat chow (Ralston-Purina Co., St. Louis, MO) was available *ad libitum.*

Each rat was implanted, sc, on the dorsal surface with a minipump (2002; Alza Corp., CA) containing a GnRH-agonist (GnRH-Ag; WY-40972, a gift from Wyeth-Ayerst Laboratories) starting on the day of estrus. Each minipump released continuously 0.2, 1, or 5 µg/day of GnRH-Ag for a period of 14 days. Therefore, on day 15, each minipump was replaced with a new pump containing identical drug treatment, with the rat under brief ether anesthesia. Sham surgery was performed in controls, but they received no treatment. Rats were weighed individually every week for the duration of the experiment. On day 29, the rats were dissected while they were under ether anesthesia. After obtaining the total ovarian weight, the ovaries were processed for light microscopy. Ovaries were sectioned serially 6–8 μ and stained with hematoxylin and eosin. Follicles were counted in every tenth section at 100× magnification according to the classification reported (4). At the end of the experiment, rats were exsanguinated by bleeding via the abdominal aorta. The blood was allowed to clot at room temperature and centrifused at 4°C, and the serum stored frozen at −20°C for the measurement of progesterone, testosterone, and estradiol by radioimmunoassay, as described by us previously (5). Differences between 2 groups were analyzed by Student's t-test. A P-value of less than 0.05 was considered significant.

Results

The ovarian histology revealed the inhibitory effect of GnRH-Ag on the follicular development (Table 1). The number of big antral follicles in 0.2 μg/day of the GnRH-Ag group was decreased when compared to controls. No big antral follicles were present in the remaining treated groups. The 2 high doses of GnRH-Ag suppressed the number of small antral follicles and also big and small atretic follicles when compared to controls (P < 0.001). However, GnRH-Ag at the dose of 0.2 μg/day was without any effect on these follicles.

The peripheral levels of serum progesterone in rats treated with all doses of GnRH-Ag were suppressed by the treatment (Table 2). Whereas the 2 high doses of GnRH-Ag suppressed the serum testosterone and estradiol levels, GnRH-Ag at the dose of 0.2 was ineffective.

The 2 high doses of GnRH-Ag increased the body weight of these rats (P < 0.05), as compared to controls (Table 3). The treatment at 0.2 μg/day had not

TABLE 1. Effect of GnRH agonist treatment on ovarian follicles.

GnRH-Ag Treatment	Big Antral Follicle	Small Antral Follicle	Big Atretic Follicle	Small Atretic Follicle
Control (none)	8.2 ± 1.5	14.3 ± 2.3	8.5 ± 2.0	10.0 ± 1.8
0.2 μg/day	4.1 ± 1.5	10.7 ± 1.3	7.5 ± 1.1	13.0 ± 1.9
1.0 μg/day	0.0	2.0 ± 1.2	0.0	4.8 ± 1.9
5.0 μg/day	0.0	1.6 ± 0.6	0.0	2.3 ± 0.9

Note: Values represent number of follicles counted in one ovary from treated rats, expressed as the mean ± SE.

TABLE 2. Effect of GnRH agonist treatment on serum levels of steroids.

GnRH-Ag Treatment	Progesterone (ng/mL)	Testosterone (pg/mL)	Estradiol (pg/mL)
Control (none)	32 ± 6	531 ± 76	53 ± 19
0.2 µg/day	17 ± 3	518 ± 77	20 ± 9
1.0 µg/day	18 ± 2	229 ± 15	16 ± 8
5.0 µg/day	18 ± 4	197 ± 22	11 ± 3

Note: Values are expressed as the mean ± SE.

shown such effect on the body weight gain, although an increasing trend was noticed. The ovarian weight was decreased by the treatment at all doses.

Discussion

The continuous administration of GnRH-Ag at the dose of 1.0 or 5.0 µg/day suppressed the number of small and big antral follicles following long-term treatment. The treatment also suppressed the number of big and small atretic follicles. The recruitment of new big follicles was totally absent, and the number of new small follicles was greatly reduced. This is indicative of the absence of a secondary FSH surge in these rats (6). The minimum dose of GnRH-Ag appears to be 1.0 µg/day to be inhibitory on the follicular development by the continuous mode of administration. The results also suggest that GnRH-Ag arrests the growth of antral and atretic follicles of both sizes, as reflected in the secretion of various steroid hormones. The reduction in the serum steroid hormonal milieu and associated changes in this follicular development are evidence of an interruption in the estrous cyclicity of these rats and thus an inhibition of ovulation. These inhibitory effects of GnRH-Ag could be due to its inhibition of the preovulatory proestrus gonadotropin surge (7) and/or to its direct effect on the ovary since rat ovaries are known to

TABLE 3. Effect of GnRH agonist treatment on body and ovarian weights.

GnRH-Ag Treatment	Body Weight Gain (gm)	Ovarian Weight (mg)
Control (none)	53.9 ± 6.6	137.1 ± 5.5
0.2 µg/day	62.8 ± 3.8	46.1 ± 5.7
1.0 µg/day	88.2 ± 7.7	78.7 ± 2.8
5.0 µg/day	96.5 ± 4.6	54.0 ± 3.1

Note: Values are expressed as the mean ± SE.

have receptors for GnRH (8) and the GnRH-agonists are known to halt follicular development in hypophysectomized rats (2).

The dose-dependent weight gain noticed in these rats is an interesting observation, and the mechanism by which this is triggered is presently under investigation in this laboratory. Neuropeptide Y (NPY), another neuropeptide like GnRH, is abundant in the rat brain and has been shown to play an important role in the neural regulation of feeding behavior (9). It has been speculated that NPY releases endogenous opioid peptide or catecholamines in critical brain areas, which may in turn activate feeding in the rats. Therefore, the weight gain triggered by the administration of GnRH-Ag in these rats may play a role in the stimulation of feeding in these rats, which may be associated with the secretion of NPY, endogenous opioid peptides, and/or catecholamines.

Acknowledgments. We thank Sandra Milline for typing the manuscript. The research reported in this chapter was supported by a grant from U.S. Agency for International Development (DAN-5053-G-SS08028).

References

1. Hsueh AJW, Jones PBC. Extrapituitary actions of gonadotrophin-releasing hormone. Endocr Rev 1981;2:437-61.
2. Ying S, Guillemin R. [D-Trp^6-Pro^9-Net]-luteinizing hormone releasing hormone factor inhibits follicular development in hypophysectomized rats. Nature 1979; 280:593-5.
3. Ataya K, McKanna J, Weintraub A, Clark M, LeMaire W. A luteinizing releasing hormone agonist for the prevention of chemotherapy-induced ovarian follicular loss in rats. Cancer Res 1985;45:3651-6.
4. Greenwald GS. Quantitation aspects of follicular development in the untreated and PMS-treated cyclic hamster. Anat Rec 1974;178:139-43.
5. Smith CJ, Greer TB, Banks TW, Sridaran R. The response of large and small luteal cells from the pregnant rat to substrates and secretagogues. Biol Reprod 1989;41:1123-32.
6. Hirshfield AN. Role of FSH in the secretion of ovulatory follicles. In: Schwartz NB, Hunzicker-Dunn M, eds. Dynamics of ovarian function. New York: Raven Press, 1981;79-82.
7. Corbin A, Beattie CW. Inhibition of the pre-ovulatory proestrus gonadotropin surge, ovulation and pregnancy with a peptide analogue of luteinizing hormone releasing hormone. Endocr Res Commun 1975;2:1-23.
8. Clayton RN, Harwood JP, Catt KJ. Gonadotropin-releasing hormone analogue binds to luteal cells and inhibits progesterone production. Nature 1979;282:90-2.
9. Clark JT, Kalra PS, Crowley WR, Kalra SP. Neuropeptide Y and human pancreatic polypeptide stimulate feeding behavior in rats. Endocrinology 1984; 115:427-9.

48

Modulation of the Steroidogenesis of Cultured Human Preovulatory Granulosa Cells by LHRH Analogs

I. Bussenot, C. Azoulay-Barjonet, and J. Parinaud

Luteinizing hormone-releasing hormone (LHRH) analogs are widely used in reproductive medicine in order to create a hypogonadotropic hypogonadism. Besides their well-documented pituitary actions, LHRH and its agonists seem to have extrapituitary effects particularly on the ovary, placenta, and breast (1). In animals, their activity on granulosa cells is different according to the maturation state of the cells. They display an antigonadotropic effect on small follicles and a gonadotropic action on preovulatory follicles and corpus luteum, both in vivo and in vitro (2–5). Moreover, high-affinity LHRH receptors have been characterized on the internal thecal, granulosa, and luteal cells (6, 7). Their action is mainly mediated by phosphatidyl inositol hydrolysis (2, 8, 9).

In humans, the results are contradictory: no modification (10, 11) or antigonadotropic action (12) of the LHRH agonists on the steroidogenesis. The description of high-affinity LHRH receptors in corpus luteum (13–15) and the evidence of LHRH-like activity in the follicular fluid (16) argue for a direct ovarian action of LHRH and its agonists.

LHRH analogs are commonly used for in vitro fertilization (IVF) protocols in association with human menopausal gonadotropin (hMG). The higher plasmatic E2 levels and increased pregnancy/transfer rate obtained with them (compared with hMG alone) could also suggest a direct ovarian effect.

The present study was undertaken to evaluate the effect of LHRH and triptorelin, buserelin, and leuprorelin (Gly^6- or Gly^6 + Gly^{10}-substituted agonists used for clinical purpose) on the steroidogenesis of human granulosa cells in culture.

Materials and Methods

Cell Collection. Granulosa cells were collected by aspiration of follicles during ovocyte retrieval for IVF. Follicular growth was stimulated by a combination of LHRH agonist and hMG. Ovulation was induced by an injection of 10,000-IU human chorionic gonadotropin (hCG) 36 h before the puncture, when serum E2 levels reached 300 pg/mL/growing follicle (>15 mm).

Culture Protocol. Modified INRA B2 Menezo culture medium was used (B2 supplemented with insulin [5 µg/mL] and transferrin [5µg/mL] and depleted in cholesterol and phenol red). Granulosa cells were separated from red blood cells by successsive centrifugations at 1500 g, washed with Dulbecco's phosphate buffer saline (DPBS), and incubated in a 5% CO_2 atmosphere at 37°C in 1 mL modified B2 containing 10% heat-inactivated human fetal cord serum to allow cell attachment. Twenty-four hours later, the attached cells were washed with DPBS and incubated in modified B2 alone. [^{14}C]androst-4-ene-3,17-dione ([^{14}C]D4A, Amersham France, Paris), a precursor of estrogen synthesis was added on day 3 and day 4. D4A concentration (5 nM; 200,000 dpm/mL) was previously determined to enable maximum E2 production (17). FSH (Metrodine, Serono, Levallois-Perret, France, 0.5 IU/mL) or LHRH (Biochem), buserelin (Hoechst, Paris), triptorelin (Ipsen, Paris), and leuprorelin (Abbott, Paris) at concentrations between 0.1 and 100 ng/mL were also added on day 4. Incubation media were collected daily.

Steroids Quantification. After extraction from incubation media with ethyl acetate, steroids were separated by high-performance liquid chromatography (HPLC) with a 5 µm spherical C18 resolve TM column (Waters, Millipore, Milford, MA). A 1-mL/mn flow rate of acetonitrile/H_2O (32/68%) allowed the separation of estrone (E1), 17β-estradiol (E2), estriol (E3), dihydrotestosterone (DHT), testosterone (T), and D4A. The reproductibility of the HPLC method was assessed daily by migration of pure standards. Their radioactivity was measured using an HPLC radioactivity monitor (LB 506D, Berthold, Elancourt, France) with automatic quenching correction, authorizing the detection of 50 dpm of [^{14}C] steroids.

Statistical Analysis. Results are expressed as the percentage of steroid production on day 4 compared to that of day 3 in the same culture sample. This representation of data is used to avoid variations due to different number of cells in the wells. Results are the mean ± SE from 10 individual experiments. Statistical comparisons used the nonparametric Wilcoxon paired test, each culture well being its own control.

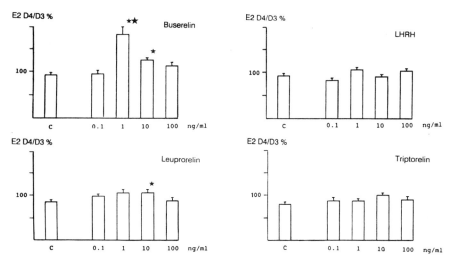

FIGURE 1. Effect of LHRH and three of its agonists on E2 secretion by human preovulatory granulosa cells in culture. Data are means $\pm$ SEM from 10 individual experiments. (*P < 0.05;**P < 0.01.)

Results

The steroid production in basal conditions was 0.18 $\pm$ 0.052 nM/mL/24 h for E2 and 0.44 $\pm$ 0.078 nM/mL/24 h for T, the 2 main D4A metabolites. The secretion of E1 and E3 was lower (0.044 $\pm$ 0.009 and 0.02 $\pm$ 0.008 nM/mL/24 h, respectively). DHT was not detectable.

The 2 Gly^6 + Gly^{10}-substituted agonists, buserelin (D-Ser(Bu^t)^6,Pro^9-N-Et)LHRH at concentrations of 1 and 10 ng/mL (+100%, P < 0.01; +35%, P < 0.05) and leuprorelin (D-Leu^6,Pro^9-N-Et)LHRH at 10 ng/mL, significantly increased E2 production (+24%, P < 0.05). LHRH and triptorelin, substituted only on Gly^6[(D-Trp^6)LHRH], had no effect on E2 secretion at any of the tested concentrations (Fig. 1). The secretion of other steroids was modified by none of the four molecules.

Discussion

These results suggest that buserelin and leuprorelin modulate steroidogenesis of human granulosa cells from preovulatory follicles. The effective concentrations are close to those observed in plasma during clinical use, since plasmatic buserelin and leuprorelin levels range from 1 to 10 ng/mL.

Results obtained with buserelin and leuprorelin are in good agreement with those of animal studies reporting the gonadotropic effect of LHRH agonists in the late follicular phase of hypophysectomized rats. LHRH analogs were shown to induce ovulation and germinal vesicle break down of oocyte and granulosa cells luteinization (2, 3, 5). Similar results were obtained with cultured preovulatory granulosa cells where LHRH agonists stimulated steroidogenesis (8, 9). This action is related to the presence of high-affinity receptors (Kd = 10^{-9}M) (6, 7). Human studies on the effect of LHRH agonists on steroidogenesis are few in number, and results are contradictory (10–12). This discrepancy could be explained by the different maturation stages of the cells (mid-follicular or luteal phase versus preovulatory stage in our study). Indeed, GnRH receptors have been described only in granulosa cells of preovulatory follicles and in corpus luteum (13, 17). Moreover, methodologic differences (presence or absence of serum and steroidogenic precursors) modify cell function (18) and thus make the comparison between studies difficult.

In our study, LHRH and the 3 tested agonists do not display the same ovarian effect despite a similar pituitary action. This discrepancy could be explained by the differences between pituitary and ovarian LHRH receptors described in humans and animals; in humans, Kd = 10^{-11}M and 10^{-9}M, respectively (13, 17). Moreover, their fate after binding of the ligand appears to be different. Indeed, after internalization, there is a recycling of receptors in the ovaries instead of degradation in the pituitary (19).

Of the 4 tested molecules, only the Gly^6 + Gly^{10}-substituted ones (buserelin and leuprorelin) have a gonadotropic effect on E2 secretion. The modification in position 10 of the native molecule could thus be involved in its ovarian biological activity and/or in its affinity for granulosa LHRH receptors.

In conclusion, it appears that the Gly^6 + Gly^{10}-substituted LHRH agonists modulate the steroidogenesis of cultured human preovulatory granula cells. This modulation occurs differently according to the agonist and the concentrations involved. The mean plasmatic level observed in their use in IVF protocols is about 1 ng/mL. The ovarian effects of buserelin and leuprorelin could thus be considered to optimize the therapeutic use of the LHRH analogs. This in vivo implication remains to be assessed by future therapeutic trials.

References

1. Fraser HM, Bramley TA, Miller WR, Sharpe RM. Extrapituitary actions of LHRH analogs in tissues of the human female and investigation of the existence and function of LHRH-like peptides. Prog Clin Biol Res 1986;225:29-54.
2. Naor Z, Zilberstein M, Zakut H, Linder HR, Dekel N. Dissociation between the direct stimulatory and inhibitory effects of a gonadotropin-realizing hormone analog on ovarian functions. Mol Cell Endocrinol 1983;31:261-70.

3. Ranta T, Knecht M, Baukal AJ, Korhonen M, Catt KJ. GnRH agonist-induced inhibitory and stimulatory effects during ovarian follicular maturation. Mol Cell Endocrinol 1984;35:55-63.
4. Maruo T, Otani T, Mochizuki M. Antigonadotropic actions of GnRH agonists on ovarian cells in vivo and in vitro. J Steroid Biochem 1985;23:765-70.
5. Malozowski S, Cassorla F, Gelato M, et al. Direct effect of the luteinizing releasing hormone analog D-Trp^6-Pro^9-Net-LHRH on rat ovarian steroidogenesis. Horm Metab Res 1985;17:321-2.
6. Seguin C, Pelletier G, Dube D, Labrie F. Distribution of luteinizing hormone realizing hormone receptors in the rat ovary. Regul Pept 1982;4:183-90.
7. Hazum E, Nimrod A. Photoaffinity-labeling and fluorescence-distribution studies of gonadotropin-releasing hormone receptors in ovarian granulosa cells. Proc Natl Acad Sci USA 1982;79:1747-50.
8. Kawai Y, Clark MR. Mechanism of action of gonadotropin releasing hormone on rat granulosa cells. Endocr Res 1986;12:195-209.
9. Eckstein N, Eshel A, Ayalon, Naor Z. Calcium dependent actions of gonadotropin-releasing hormone agonist and luteinizing hormone upon cyclic AMP and progesterone production in rat ovarian granulosa cells. Mol Cell Endocrinol 1986;47:91-8.
10. Casper RF, Erickson GF, Rebar RW, Yen SSC. The effect of luteinizing hormone-releasing factor and its agonist on cultured human granulosa cells. Fertil Steril 1982;37:406-9.
11. Casper RF, Erickson GF, Yen SSC. Studies on the effect of gonadotropin-realizing hormone and its agonist on human luteal steroidogenesis in vitro. Fertil Steril 1984;42:39-43.
12. Tureck RW, Mastroianni L, Blasco L, Strauss JF. Inhibition of human granulosa cell progesterone secretion by a gonadotropin-releasing hormone agonist. J Clin Endocrinol Metab 1982;54:1078-80.
13. Bramley TA, Menzies GS, Baird DT. Specific binding of gonadotropin-realizing hormone and an agonist to human corpus luteum homogenates: Characterization, properties, and luteal phase levels. J Clin Endocrinol Metab 1985;61:834-41.
14. Bramley TA, Menzies GS. Subcellular fractionation of the human corpus luteum: Distribution of GnRH agonist binding site. Mol Cell Endocrinol 1986;45:27-36.
15. Bramley TA, Menzies GS, Baird DT. Specificity of gonadotropin-releasing hormone binding sites of the human corpus luteum: Comparison with receptors of rat pituitary gland. J Endocrinol 1986;108:323-8.
16. Aten RF, Williams AT, Behrman HR. Ovarian gonadotropin-releasing hormone-like protein(s): Demonstration and characterization. Endocrinology 1986;118:961-7.
17. Latouche J, Crumeyrolle-Arias N, Jordan D, et al. GnRH receptors in human granulosa cells: Anatomical localization and characterization by autoradiographic study. Endocrinology 1989;125:1739-41.
18. Erickson GF. Primary cultures of ovarian cells in serum-free medium as models of hormone-dependent differentiation. Mol Cell Endocrinol 1983;29:21-6.
19. Childs GV, Hazum E, Amsterdam A, Limor R, Naor Z. Cytochemical evidence for different routes of gonadotropin-releasing hormone processing by large gonadotropes and granulosa cells. Endocrinology 1986;119:1329-38.

49

Regulation of Ovarian Steroidogenesis in the Little Skate *(Raja erinacea)*

LISA A. FILETI AND IAN P. CALLARD

Ovarian regulation in the most primitive jawed vertebrates, the elasmobranchs, is poorly understood (1). Most recently, we have investigated the little skate, *Raja erinacea*, and the spiny dogfish, *Squalus acanthias*, and have characterized endocrine aspects of the ovarian cycle (2, 3). These studies suggest pituitary regulation of the ovary.

In this vertebrate group, gonadotropic activity of the hypophysis is primarily confined to the ventral lobe, which is anatomically separated from the rest of the gland and which recieves its vascular supply from the internal carotid arteries (4). Since the presence of GnRH in the peripheral circulation has been demonstrated in several species (5, 6), elasmobranchs are ideal models for understanding potential physiological extrapituitary actions of GnRH and its interactions with GTH in ovarian regulation.

As a model for these studies, we have used the little skate, which ovulates pairs of eggs in a well-defined 8–10 day cycle (7). We have asked the following questions: *(a)* How does hypophysectomy influence the ovarian cycle and basal steroidogenesis; *(b)* what is the effect of ventral lobe extract (homologous gonadotropin) on ovarian steroidogenesis; and *(c)* what are the potential direct and indirect actions of GnRH on ovarian steroid synthesis?

Materials and Methods

Follicles ranging in diameter from 6–25 mm and corpora lutea (CL) were pooled from reproductively active females and placed in cold calcium/magnesium-free elasmobranch buffer. Follicles were punctured to remove yolk, and tissues were collected, rinsed, weighed, scissor minced, and triturated. The tissue fragments were washed twice in fresh buffer to remove excess yolk and red blood cells and were then resuspended in an appropriate volume of Eagles Basal Medium (BME) adusted to 350-mM urea, 280-mM NaCl, 10mM-HEPES (pH 7.4) to yield 80-mg wet weight tissue per mL of medium. Aliquots of 0.5 mL were distributed to glass culture tubes (12 × 75mm), and the volume made up to 1.0 mL with various additives and BME. As a membrane permeable substrate for steroidogenesis 1 µg of 25-hydroxy-cholesterol was added to the incubation medium where indicated. Incubations took place in a humidified chamber with an atmosphere of 95% oxygen/5% carbon dioxide for 8 h at room temperature. The incubations were stopped by spinning down at 2500 rpm for 15 min, and the medium was collected and frozen at −20°C until analysis by radioimmunoassay. The tissue pellets were frozen and used for protein assay by the method of Lowry. Results were expressed as picograms of steroid/mg protein/tube (±SE). Data were analyzed by ANOVA and Duncan's multiple comparison analysis. In the graphs, bars with different letters are significantly different (P < 0.05). The GnRH forms used were chicken II (His 5,Trp 7,Tyr 8-GnRH), a superagonist (Trp 6 GnRH), and an antagonist (Phe 2,Trp 6 GnRH).

Results

Hypophysectomy and ventral lobe extract in vitro showed the following influences to the ovarian cycle: Ovulation and oviposition continued normally in control and sham-operated animals, whereas after total hypophysectomy, only 2/12 animals ovulated, and after ventral lobectomy, 2/10 animals ovulated. In intact skates, testosterone (T) and estradiol (E) were produced by all follicular-size classes (Fig. 1), with T being the most abun-

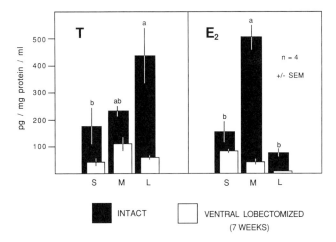

FIGURE 1. Steroid production by small, medium, and large follicles from intact and hypophysectomized skates. (S = <10 mm; M = 11–19 mm; and L = 20–25 mm.)

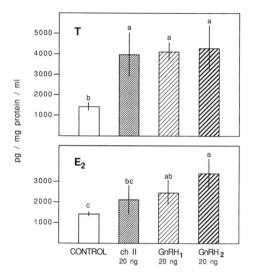

FIGURE 2. The effect of 3 forms of GnRH on follicular steroidogenesis in the presence of substrate.

dant product of large follicles and E being most abundant from medium follicles. Steroid production from follicles of ventral lobectomized animals was significantly lower than in controls. Increasing quantities of ventral lobe extract (homologous gonadotropin) did not stimulate steroidogenesis significantly in any follicular-size class from either intact or ventral lobectomized animals (data not shown).

The effects of GnRH on steroidogenesis in vitro are shown in Figures 2 and 3. All 3 GnRH forms acted directly on follicular tissue to stimulate T and E production and on luteal tissue to stimulate progesterone (P) and T (no E was found in luteal minces). Doses higher than 20 ng had the same effect.

Discussion

These results show that while the pituitary gland is important for cyclic ovarian follicular maturation and ovulation in the little skate, the effects of homologous ventral lobe extracts on steroidogenesis are not definitive under the conditions used here. In contrast, GnRHs have potent initial direct stimulatory effects on follicular and luteal steroidogenesis, while long-term administration in vivo depresses steroidogenesis (unpublished results). Local ovarian transduction of peptide signals is likely to be via known second messenger systems (8).

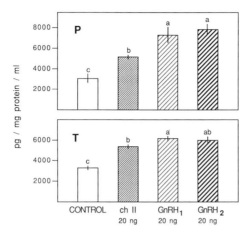

FIGURE 3. The effect of 3 forms of GnRH on luteal steroidogenesis in the presence of substrate.

Since GnRH is present in peripheral blood of some elasmobranch fishes, the results suggest that GnRH may be involved in the short-term regulation of steroid biosynthesis and secretion and that ventral lobe gonadotropic hormone(s) control ovarian growth through a gametogenic (i.e., FSH-like) action. Direct effects of the hypothalamic peptide in addition to indirect effects via control of ventral lobe gonadotropin secretion may be necessary for the full steroidogenic response at this phyletic level. These results provide a new perspective and background for observations on GnRH receptors in the mammalian ovary (11).

It is important to note that ovarian granulosa cells of the elasmobranch *(Squalus acanthias)* are capable of the complete steroidogenic pathway from cholesterol to estradiol without participation of thecal elements (2, 3, 9) and that theca cells have not been identified in elasmobranchs. Similarly, Sertoli cells are the primary steroidogenic element of the elasmobranch testis, whereas Leydig cells have not been definitively identified (10). It is thus possible that elasmobranch ovarian control mechanisms represent an intermediate stage in the evolution of definitive vertebrate-type gonadal control mechanisms in which peripheral GnRH has a dual function (ventral lobe regulation and direct control of steroidogenesis by granulosa elements). While ventral lobe gonadotropic activity is seen as primarily gametogenic, it provides the morphological substrate upon which GnRH can act to stimulate steroidogenesis and possibly ovulation through local paracrine effects of steroids such as progesterone.

It remains to be seen whether two putative gonadotropic moieties can be demonstrated in the elasmobranch pituitary and exactly how a second gonadotropic moiety (LH-like?) could be integrated to provide control over steroidogenesis in a second cell type.

Acknowledgment. The research reported in this chapter was supported by N.S.F. 8606344 (IPC).

References

1. Demski LS. Pathways for GnRH control of elasmobranch reproductive physiology and behavior. J Exp Zool 1989;(suppl 2):4-11.
2. Dodd JM, Sumpter JP. Fishes. In: Lamming GE, ed. Marshall's physiology of reproduction. 4th ed. Edinburgh, Churchill Livingstone.
3. Callard IP, Klosterman LL. Reproductive physiology: A, the female. In: Shuttleworth T, ed. The physiology of elasmobranch fishes. Springer-Verlag.
4. Callard IP, Klosterman LL, Sorbera LA, Fileti LA, Reese JC. Endocrine regulation of reproduction in elasmobranchs: Archetype for terrestrial vertebrates. J Exp Zool 1989;(suppl 2):12-21.
5. King JA, Millar RP.Comparative aspects of luteinizing hormone releasing hormone structure and function in vertebrate phylogeny. Endocrinology 1980;106:707-17.
6. Sherwood NM. The origin of the mammalian form of GnRH in primitive fishes. Fish Physiol Biochem (in press).
7. Koob TJ, Laffan J, Callard IP. Plasma estradiol, testosterone and progesterone levels during the ovulatory cycle of the skate (*Raja erinacea*). Biol Reprod, 35: 267-75.
8. Fileti LA, Callard IP. Regulation of ovarian steroidogenesis in the little skate, *Raja erinacea*. Biol Reprod 1990;42(suppl 1):115.
9. Tsang P. Endocrine correlates and regulation of the follicular development and luteal function during the reproductive cycle of the viviparous shark, *Squalus acanthias* [Dissertation]. Boston University, Boston, MA.
10. Pudney JP, Callard GV. Identification of Leydig-like cells in the interstitium of the shark testis *(Squalus acanthias)*. Anat Rec 1984;209:322-30.
11. Hsueh AJW, Jones PBC. Extrapituitary actions of gonadotropin-releasing hormone. Endocr Rev 1981;2:437-61.

50

Localization of Specific GnRH Receptors on Porcine Granulosa Cells and Mast Cells Within Ovarian Follicles

P. DeMent-Liebenow

Follicular atresia is most likely a process involving several molecules and, perhaps, the ratios between them. There is evidence that the process may be influenced by a receptor capable of binding gonadotropin releasing hormone (GnRH). It has been reported that GnRH has direct effects on the rat ovary (1–4). Together, these and other reports support the conclusion that receptors capable of binding and mediating a response to GnRH exist in the rat ovary and that a GnRH-like molecule might play a role as an atretogenic factor in the ovary.

While investigations into the role of GnRH in the rat ovary continue, others have sought to identify gonadotropin releasing hormone receptors (GnRH-R) in other species. Our laboratory reported in 1987 that a GnRH agonist mimics the inhibitory effects of follicular fluid from small porcine follicles (SFFl) but is not additive or synergistic with SFFl, while a GnRH antagonist does not antagonize the effects of SFFl (5), suggesting that these receptors are able to mediate specific physiological events in the sow. In 1988, we reported immunohistochemical evidence of the presence of specific GnRH receptors as well as further actions of GnRH in the porcine ovary (6). The present study seeks to identify the specific cell types that possess these GnRH receptors.

Materials and Methods

Porcine ovaries were obtained within 4 h of death from a local slaughter-house, cut into 0.5- to 1.0-cm slices, frozen on foil on dry ice, and mounted with OTC on microtome chucks. Approximately 8-μm sections were thaw-mounted to glass slides. Sections were fixed with acetone for 10 min at −20°C. Granulosa cells from a small (3 mm) porcine follicle were collected and washed with phosphate buffer. Cells were resuspended and distributed in 8-well slide chambers. After allowing 1 h for attachment of cells to slides, cells were fixed with acetone for 10 min at −20°C.

Fixed tissues were rehydrated with buffer and by buffer containing 1.0% bovine serum albumin. Tissues were then exposed to 10 μg/mL GnRH for 1 h at room temperature. Tissues were rinsed with buffer followed by exposure to a 1:200 concentration of rabbit anti-GnRH overnight at room temperature. After rinsing with buffer, tissues were finally exposed to anti-rabbit IgG Phycoerythrin (phycoprobe) for 1 h at 37°C, rinsed, mounted with Gel-Mount coverslip adhesive, and examined with a fluorescent microscope. To test for specificity, control sections were exposed to a GnRH antagonist [D-pGlu[1],D-phe[2];D-Trp[3,6]]LHRH (GnRHan), which does not bind the anti-GnRH as the receptor-binding ligand. Additional control sections were exposed to anti-GnRH, and phycoprobe in the absence of exogenous GnRH (antibody control), or phycoprobe alone (probe control). LH-receptors (LH-R) were demonstrated using 10 μg/mL LH and anti-LH in an analogous procedure. All histological specimens were examined for the bright yellow Phycoerythrin fluorescence with a Leitz Laborlux microscope fitted with a fluorescence light source using an IL-2 excitation filter and a 580-nm barrier filter.

The ability of anti-GnRH to bind GnRH and GnRH analogs was determined by ELISA, using an ABC staining kit. GnRH and GnRH analogs were bound to glutaraldehyde pretreated microtitre plates with an overnight incubation. After rinsing with buffer and blocking nonspecific binding with normal goat serum, 1:200 and 1:1000 anti-GnRH was added to wells for an overnight incubation. After rinsing with buffer, development was as suggested by the kit.

Routine histological examination with hematoxylin-eosin or Wright's-Giemsa staining was used to identify mast cells in ovarian sections.

Results

Pubertal and cycling porcine ovaries (n = 10) were examined. Sections incubated with GnRH, but not those incubated with the antagonist, exhibited bright yellow fluorescence (Figs. 1–4). Probe control and antibody control sections did not exhibit the yellow fluorescence. Examination of serial sections indicated that the only cells that fluoresced in the thecal layer were mast cells. Mast cells were found in only some follicles. Granulosa cells were also found to fluoresce in some follicles but not in all follicles within the same ovary. Examination of cell suspensions of fresh granulosa cells suggests the

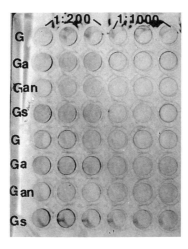

FIGURE 1. ELISA assay showing binding of anti-GnRH (Sigma L-8391) to GnRH analogs. GnRH (G), GnRH agonist [D-Lys^6]LHRH (Ga), and a GnRH acetate salt (Gs) exhibit binding as indicated by the slightly darker color in the wells, while the GnRH antagonist [D-PGlu^1,D-Phe^2,D-Trp^{3,6}]LHRH (Gan) shows little or no binding.

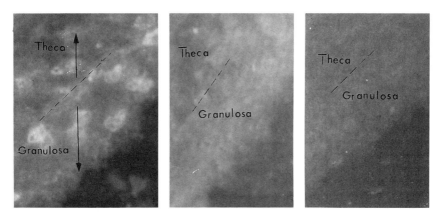

FIGURE 2. GnRH receptors on cells in a small follicle from an early pubertal porcine ovary containing small-to-medium (3–5 mm) follicles. The fluorescence suggests the presence of GnRH receptors on cells in both the theca and granulosa layers of the follicle. *Left*: Fluorescence view (×625). *Center*: Antibody control (no exogenous GnRH) of serial section of same follicle (×625). *Right*: Probe control (anti-rIgG phycoprobe only) of serial section of same follicle (×625).

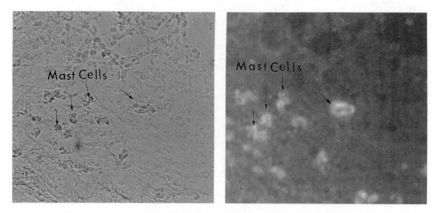

FIGURE 3. GnRH receptors on mast cells of frozen sections of a pubertal periovulatory porcine ovary. Cells exhibiting fluorescence appear to be mast cells in the light microscopic sections. Light and fluorescence views are of same sections. *Left*: Light microscopic view (×400). *Right*: Fluorescence view of same section (×400).

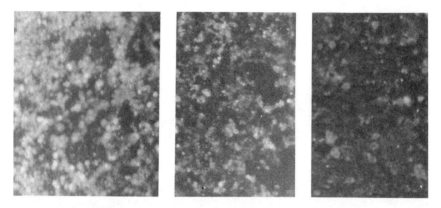

FIGURE 4. GnRH receptors on fresh granulosa cells from a small (3 mm) porcine follicle from a pubertal ovary with medium-to-large (5–7 mm) follicles. *Left*: Cells with GnRH as receptor ligand (×400). *Center*: Cells from same follicle with GnRHan as receptor ligand (×400). *Right*: Probe control (anti-rIgG phycoprobe only) of cells from same follicle (×400).

presence of GnRH receptors on many but not all granulosa cells of follicles that do exhibit fluoresence. We have not observed specific GnRH receptors on corpora lutea or interstitial tissue.

Discussion

The presence of receptors capable of binding GnRH in only specific follicles suggests that these receptors may have a role in follicular processes at only certain stages of development. Ovulation has been compared to an inflammatory event for the last ten years (7). The processes of ovulation and atresia involve a complex of events, all apparently initiated by a surge of luteinizing hormone (LH) from the pituitary. The events mimic, in many ways, those of inflammation subsequent to tissue injury: invasion of mast cells (8), macrophages (9), and platelets leading to collagen restructuring, vascularization, extravasation, and edema. Coincident with the LH surge, the mast cells in both atretic and periovulatory follicles can be seen to actively degranulate (10), presumably releasing histamine, serotonin, and bradykinin and mediating the collagenolytic processes of both atresia and ovulation. GnRH has been reported to cause mast cells to release histamine (11). These observations suggest that ovarian receptors capable of binding a GnRH-like molecule could have a role in the inflammatory events of atresia and ovulation.

Acknowledgments. This research was supported by NSF Graduate Fellowship RCD8758085, and Sigma Xi Grants-in-Aid of Research. The author wishes to thank Dr. F. Ledwitz-Rigby for her guidance and the use of laboratory space and equipment, Dr. P. Terranova for valuable advice, Dr. R. Toth for the use of the fluorescent microscope and M. Grzeszkowiak and R. Grey for assistance in preparation of prints.

References

1. Hsueh AJW, Wang C, Erickson GF. Direct inhibitory effect of gonadotropin-releasing hormone upon follicle stimulated hormone induction of luteinizing hormone receptor and aromatase activity in rat granulosa cells. Endocrinology 1980;106:1697-1705.
2. Harwood JP, Clayton RN, Catt KJ. Ovarian gonadotropin-releasing hormone receptors, I. Properties and inhibition of luteal cell function. Endocrinology 1980;107:407-13.
3. Harwood JP, Clayton RN, Chen TT, Knox G, Catt KJ. Ovarian gonadotropin-releasing hormone receptors, II. Regulation and effects on ovarian development. Endocrinology 1980;107:414-21.

4. Birnbaumer L, Shahabi N, Rivier J, Vale W. Evidence for a physiological role of gonadotropin releasing hormone (GnRH) or a GnRH-like material in the ovary. Endocrinology 1985;116:1367-1470.
5. Ledwitz-Rigby F. Local regulation of granulosa cell maturation. Steroid Biochem 1987;27:385-91.
6. Ledwitz-Rigby F, DeMent-Liebenow P. Direct action of gonadotropin releasing hormone and visualization of its receptors on porcine ovaries. In: Hirshfield A, ed. Growth factors and the ovary. New York: Serono Symposia, USA/Plenum Press, 1989:279-83.
7. Espey LL. Ovulation as an inflammatory reaction: A Hypothesis. Biol Reprod 1980;22:73.
8. Nakamura Y, Smith M, Krishna A, Terranova PF. Increased number of mast cells in the dominant follicle of the cow: Relationships among luteal, stromal, and hilar regions. Biol Reprod 1987;37:546.
9. Adashi EY. Editorial: Cytokine-mediated regulation of ovarian function: Encounters of a third kind. Endocrinology 1989;124:2043.
10. Krishna A, Terranova PF. Alterations in mast cell degranulation and ovarian histamine in the proestrous hamster. Biol Reprod 1985;32:1211.
11. Morgan JE, O'Neil CE, Coy DH, Hocart SJ, Nekola MV. Antagonistic analogs of luteinizing hormone-releasing hormone (LHRH) are mast cell secretagogues. Int Arch Allergy Appl Immunol 1986;80:70-75.

51

In Vitro Increase in Secretion of Oxytocin by Bovine Granulosa Cells After LH Surge

A.K. VOSS AND J.E. FORTUNE

Oxytocin (OT) mRNA has been detected in bovine granulosa cells (1). OT is secreted in vitro by bovine granulosa cells obtained at abattoirs (2, 3, 4), and OT secretion is enhanced in the presence of theca interna (3, 4). We observed previously that the addition of exogenous OT to granulosa cell cultures had a dose-dependent stimulatory effect on progesterone secretion by granulosa cells (5). Since the OT gene is expressed in ovarian follicles, and there is indirect evidence that OT secretion might change during the course of follicular development (6, 7), we have examined the ability of granulosa cells obtained at specific stages of development of the preovulatory follicle to secrete OT. Here we show that OT secretion is much greater when granulosa cells are isolated late in the follicular phase, as compared with follicles obtained earlier, but that OT secretion is enhanced by gonadotropins and co-culture with theca only when granulosa cells are obtained during early follicular phase.

Materials and Methods

Holstein heifers were injected with 25-mg $PGF_{2\alpha}$ on day 14 of the estrous cycle to induce luteal regression and initiate a follicular phase. Plasma progesterone was monitored to verify luteal regression. The preovulatory follicle was identified by daily ultrasonography (8), and its identity was confirmed by inspection under a dissecting microscope, as we have described previously (9). Beginning 44 h after the $PGF_{2\alpha}$ injection, blood samples were taken every 4 h to determine the time of the LH surge. Animals were checked for estrous behavior every 4 h to detect the onset of estrus.

Ovaries bearing the preovulatory follicle were removed either early (24 h after $PGF_{2\alpha}$ injection; n = 3) or late in the follicular phase (20 h after onset of estrus, i.e., after the LH surge; n = 4) and were transported to the laboratory in ice cold HEPES buffered Eagle's Minimum Essential Medium (MEM).

In Vitro Culture. Preovulatory follicles were dissected from the ovary and granulosa cells and theca interna isolated, as described previously (9). Granulosa cells (200,000 cells/well) and pieces of theca interna (3 pieces/culture = 5% or 2.5% of the total theca interna of follicles isolated at 24 h after $PGF_{2\alpha}$ or 20 h after the onset of estrus, respectively) were cultured separately or in combination in 24-well plates in MEM supplemented with 20-mM L-glutamine, 100-µM nonessential amino acids, 50-IU penicillin G/mL, 50-µg streptomycin sulfate/mL, 27.6-mIU insulin/mL, 5-µg transferrin/mL, and 40-ng cortisol/mL. Media were prepared with or without LH (300 ng/mL) or FSH (300 ng/mL). Treatments were applied to duplicate cultures from each of 3 or 4 animals ovariectomized early or late in the follicular phase, respectively. Cultures were maintained at 37°C, at 100% relative humidity in an atmosphere of 5% CO_2 in air. Media were collected and replaced with fresh medium every 24 h for 5 days.

Radioimmunoassay. LH concentrations in the plasma were assayed, as described before (10). OT was determined in nonextracted medium samples by the method of Shukovski et al. (11). OT antiserum was generously provided by Dr. Dieter Schams (Technical University, Munich, FRG). It did not cross-react with related peptides like vasopressin or other pituitary hormones (12). The sensitivity was 0.25 pg/tube, and intra- and inter-assay coefficients of variation were 7.3 and 11.0%, respectively.

Statistical Analysis. Differences in OT accumulation in vitro were tested by 4-factor, mixed-model analysis of variance (ANOVA) with gonadotropins, cell type(s) cultured, experiment (heifer), and time in culture as the 4 factors. If differences were observed, individual means were compared by Duncan's multiple range test. To simplify graphical presentation, some data are expressed as total OT secretion per follicle or depicted as sum of OT production per culture over 5 days. In the latter case, results were subjected to 3-factor ANOVA with gonadotropins, cell type, and experiment as the 3 factors.

Results

Granulosa cells isolated early or late in the follicular phase released substantial amounts of OT. However, granulosa cells obtained 20 h after the onset of estrus (14 ± 4 h after the peak of the LH surge) secreted 42-fold more OT over 120 h of culture as compared to granulosa cells isolated early in the

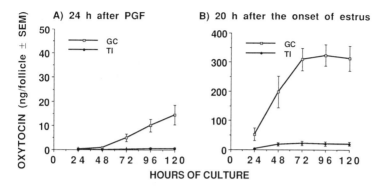

FIGURE 1. OT secretion by granulosa cells (GC) and theca interna (TI) isolated early (panel *A*; n = 6 cultures) and late (panel *B*; n = 8 cultures) in the follicular phase. Data are depicted as total OT secretion per follicle.

follicular phase (Fig. 1, *A* and *B*). OT secretion by granulosa cells isolated early in the follicular phase was low for the first 2 days of culture and then increased linearly (Fig. 1*A*), whereas OT secretion by granulosa cells isolated after the LH surge increased during the first 3 days of culture and then maintained a plateau (Fig. 1*B*). OT production by theca isolated early and late in the follicular phase was 5.0 and 7.4%, respectively, of the secretion by granulosa cells (Fig. 1, *A* and *B*).

Granulosa and theca cells cultured in combination secreted more OT than granulosa cells alone, when cells were isolated early in the follicular phase (P < 0.01, Fig. 2*A*). In contrast, co-culture had no effect on cells isolated after

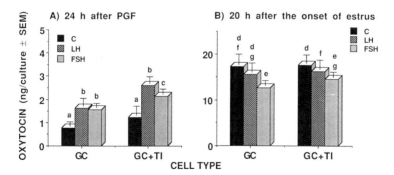

FIGURE 2. OT secretion by granulosa cells (GC) or granulosa cells in co-culture with theca interna (GC + TI) isolated early (panel *A*; n = 6 cultures) or late (panel *B*; n = 8 cultures) in the follicular phase. Data are depicted as total OT secretion per culture summed over 5 days; a < b:P < 0.01; b > c:P < 0.01; d > e:P < 0.01; and f > g:p < 0.05.

the LH surge (P > 0.05, Fig. 2*B*). The addition of LH or FSH to the culture medium stimulated OT secretion by granulosa cells alone or in co-culture with theca, when cells were obtained early in the follicular phase (P < 0.01, Fig. 2*A*). OT secretion by granulosa cells isolated after the LH surge could not be further stimulated by LH or FSH and/or co-culture with theca interna. On the contrary, the addition of FSH or LH to the medium slightly reduced OT secretion by granulosa cells obtained late in the follicular phase (P < 0.01 for FSH versus control and P < 0.05 for LH versus control, Fig. 2*B*).

Discussion

These results show that OT secretion by granulosa cells in vitro increases as the preovulatory follicle differentiates. Granulosa cells obtained after the LH surge secreted 42-fold more OT than granulosa cells isolated early in the follicular phase. These findings are consistent with studies showing that OT was detected in ovine follicle wall and secreted by caprine granulosa cells in vitro only when follicles were obtained after the LH surge (7, 13). Since the theca interna secreted only 5.0–7.4% of the amounts of OT secreted by granulosa cells, secretion by theca interna cultures may be due to contamination with granulosa cells. The finding that granulosa cells are the sole or primary site of OT production in the follicle is consistent with the finding that large luteal cells of the bovine corpus luteum, believed to be granulosa-derived, produce, store, and release OT, whereas small cells, which are thought to be theca interna-derived, do not contain OT (14, 15). Addition of theca interna to granulosa cell cultures resulted in an increase in OT secretion when cells were isolated early in the follicular phase. However, the specificity of the effect of co-culture on OT accumulation is questionable, since others have reported that the stimulatory effect of co-culture could be obtained not only with theca interna, but also with tissue pieces from liver, kidney, aorta, muscle, and adrenal cortex (3, 11). The lack of an effect of co-culture on OT secretion by granulosa cells isolated after the LH surge may be due to maximal stimulation of the granulosa cells by endogenous stimuli, loss of granulosa cell capacity to respond to the theca, or a change in thecal ability to further stimulate OT secretion by granulosa cells. The loss of responsiveness to LH and FSH may also be attributed to maximal stimulation in vivo by the LH/FSH surge and desensitization. Kiehm et al. (13) reported that caprine granulosa cells did not increase OT secretion in response to FSH or LH in vitro.

In conclusion, granulosa cells appear to secrete OT in increasing amounts as they differentiate during the follicular phase. This developmental pattern suggests a role for OT in periovulatory events and luteinization. Follicular OT may be an important stimulus for smooth muscle cells in the wall of the preovulatory follicle, and upon release from the follicle at ovulation, it could affect contractility of the fallopian tubes and the uterus to promote gamete transportation. Alternatively or in addition, OT may play a part in regulating the shift from estrogenic to gestagenic steroidogenesis in the preovulatory follicle, thus preparing the follicle cells for differentiation into luteal cells.

Acknowledgments. We are grateful to Dr. Dieter Shams for the OT antiserum and to Dr. Gordon Niswender for the LH antiserum. This work was supported by a grant from the NIH (HD-14584).

References

1. Holtorf A-P, Furuya K, Ivell R, McArdle CA. Oxytocin production and oxytocin messenger ribonucleic acid levels in bovine granulosa cells are regulated by insulin and insulin-like growth factor-I: Dependence on developmental status of the ovarian follicle. Endocrinology 1986;125:2612-20.
2. Geenen V, Legros JJ, Hazée-Hagelstein MT, et al. Release of immunoreactive oxytocin and neurophysin I by cultured luteinizing bovine granulosa cells. Acta Endocrinol 1985;110:263-70.
3. Jungclas B, Luck MR. Evidence for granulosa-theca interaction in the secretion of oxytocin by bovine ovarian tissue. J Endocrinol 1986;109:R1-4.
4. Schams D, Koll R, Li CH. Insulin-like growth factor-I stimulates oxytocin and progesterone production by bovine granulosa cells in culture. J Endocrinol 1988; 116:97-100.
5. Aladin Chandrasekher Y, Fortune JE. Effects of oxytocin on steroidogenesis by bovine theca and granulosa cells. Endocrinology 1990.
6. Schams D, Kruip TAM, Koll R. Oxytocin determination in steroid producing tissues and in vitro production in ovarian follicles. Acta Endocrinol 1985; 109:530-6.
7. Wathes DC, Guldenaar SEF, Swann RW, Webb R, Porter DG, Pickering BT. A combined radioimmunoassay and immunocytochemical study of ovarian oxytocin production during the periovulatory period in the ewe. J Reprod Fertil 1986;78:167-83.
8. Sirois J, Fortune JE. Ovarian follicular dynamics during the estrous cycle in heifers monitored by real-time ultrasonography. Biol Reprod 1988;39:308-17.
9. Fortune JE, Hansel W. The effects of 17ß-estradiol on progesterone secretion by bovine theca and granulosa cells. Endocrinology 1979;104:1834-8.
10. Niswender GD, Reichert LE, Jr, Midgley AR, Jr, Nalbandov AV. Radioimmunoassay for bovine and ovine luteinizing hormone. Endocrinology 1969;84:1166-73.
11. Shukovski L, Fortune JE, Findlay JK. Oxytocin and progesterone secretion by bovine granulosa cells of individual preovulatory follicles cultured in serum-free medium. Mol Cell Endocrinol 1989;69:17-24.
12. Schams D. Oxytocin determination by radioimmunoassay, III. Improvement to

subpicogramm sensitivity and application to blood levels in cyclic cattle. Acta Endocrinol 1983;103:180-3.

13. Kiehm DJ, Walters DL, Daniel SAJ, Armstrong DT. Preovulatory biosynthesis and granulosa cell secretion of immunoreactive oxytocin by goat ovaries. J Reprod Fertil 1989;87:485-93.

14. Hansel W, Alila HW, Dowd JP, Yang X. Control of steroidogenesis in small and large luteal cells. Aust J Biol Sci 1987;40:331-47.

15. Rodgers RJ, O'Shea JD, Findlay JK, Flint APF, Sheldrick EL. Large luteal cells the source of luteal oxytocin in sheep. Endocrinology 1983;113:230-4.

52

LH Stimulation of Ovarian Thecal-Interstitial Cell Differentiation: Sensitizing Effect of Angiotensin II

DENIS A. MAGOFFIN

There is substantial evidence indicating that angiotensin II is produced locally in the ovary and may play a role in regulating atresia (1) and ovulation (2). All of the components of the renin-angiotensin system have been localized in human and rat ovaries (3–7), including high concentrations of angiotensin II in human follicular fluid (4, 5). Immunoreactive angiotensin II has been demonstrated in human and rat thecal and luteal cells (2). Collectively, these data suggest a physiological role for angiotensin II in ovarian function. The present studies demonstrate that angiotensin II sensitizes thecal-interstitial cells (TIC) to the stimulatory actions of LH.

Materials and Methods

Sprague-Dawley rats (25 days of age) were killed 4 days after hypophysectomy by cervical dislocation, and the ovaries were dispersed into a cell suspension with collagenase/DNase solution (8). The TIC were isolated from contaminating granulosa cells by centrifugation through 1.055-g/mL Percoll (9). Purified TIC (2×10^5 viable cells/well) were cultured up to 6 days in 96-well microtest plates (10) containing 0- to 100-ng/mL LH (G3-330BR, provided by Dr. H. Papkoff) and 0- to 100-ng/mL angiotensin II (Sigma) in 0.2-mL serum-free medium (10). The medium was collected at 2-day intervals and assayed for androsterone by specific radioimmunoassay (11). The dose-response curves were analyzed using the Allfit program (12).

Results and Discussion

Recently, we performed a series of studies using phorbol esters that indicated protein kinase C is an important modulator of LH stimulation of androgen biosynthesis in ovarian TIC (13). Long-term treatment (4 days) with phorbol ester caused an inhibition of LH-stimulated androgen biosynthesis in the TIC. In many cell types, long-term treatment with phorbol esters causes a depletion of protein kinase C in the cells. Inhibition of the stimulatory actions of LH by depleting protein kinase C suggests that protein kinase C exerts a positive modulatory effect on LH stimulation of TIC androgen biosynthesis. In the present studies, we examined the effects of a physiological activator of the inositol polyphosphate/protein kinase C pathway, angiotensin II, on TIC androgen biosynthesis.

Figure 1 shows the time-course of LH and angiotensin II action on TIC androgen production. When TIC were treated with angiotensin II alone (100 ng/mL), there was no effect on basal androsterone production. Androsterone is the principal androgen produced by immature rat TIC and is a good measure of total androgen production (9, 10). LH (50 ng/mL) stimulated an approximately 100-fold increase in androsterone production at 2 days, which then decreased at 4 and 6 days. This is a typical pattern of LH stimulation of androsterone production in this model (10). Addition of angiotensin II (100 ng/mL) did not alter LH-stimulated androsterone production. These results demonstrated that

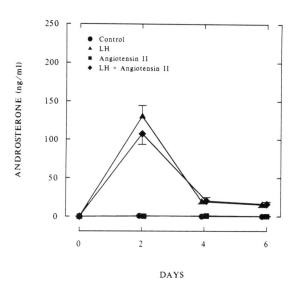

FIGURE 1. Time-course of LH and angiotensin II action on TIC androgen synthesis. Purified TIC were cultured for 6 days, with and without LH (50 ng/mL) and/or angiotensin II (100 ng/mL). The medium was collected and replaced every 2 days. The data are the mean ± SEM of 3 experiments with 4 replicates each.

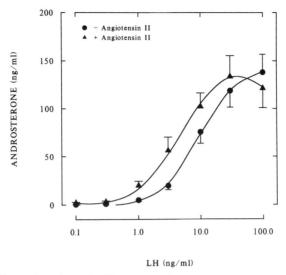

FIGURE 2. Effect of angiotensin II on LH-stimulated TIC androgen production. Purified TIC were cultured for 2 days with increasing concentrations of LH (0–100 ng/mL), with and without angiotensin II (100 ng/mL). The data are the mean ± SEM of 3 experiments with 4 replicates each.

angiotensin II did not affect TIC androgen production in the absence of LH or at a maximally stimulatory concentration of LH.

The effect of angiotensin II on the dose-response curve for LH stimulation of androgen production was examined next. As shown in Figure 2, LH stimulated a dose-related increase in androsterone production. The ED_{50} for LH stimulation was 9.3 ± 1.0 ng/mL. Treatment with angiotensin II (100 ng/mL) increased ($P < 0.01$) the sensitivity of the TIC to LH stimulation 2.5-fold. The ED_{50} for LH stimulation of androsterone production in the presence of angiotensin II was 3.7 ± 0.4 ng/mL. Basal androsterone production, maximum stimulated androsterone production, and the slope of the dose-response curve were unchanged by angiotensin II ($P = 0.205$).

To further characterize the interaction of angiotensin II with LH, dose-response studies were performed with angiotensin II. Figure 3 shows that in the absence of LH or in the presence of a saturating concentration of LH (50 ng/mL), there was no effect of angiotensin II on TIC androsterone production at any dose tested. In the presence of a submaximal stimulatory concentration of LH (3 ng/mL), angiotensin II caused a dose-related increase in androsterone production. The maximum amount of androsterone produced at 30 and 100 ng/mL of angiotensin II was equal to the androsterone production stimulated by a saturating concentration of LH alone. The ED_{50} for angiotensin II action was 10.1 ± 1.0 ng/mL.

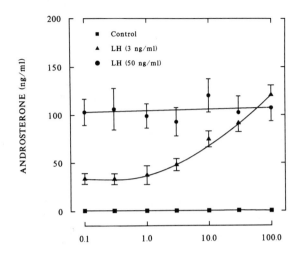

FIGURE 3. Effect of angiotensin II on LH-stimulated TIC androgen production. Purified TIC were cultured for 2 days with increasing concentrations of angiotensin II (0–100 ng/mL) in the presence of 0-, 3-, or 50-ng/mL LH. The data are the mean ± SEM of 3 experiments with 4 replicates each.

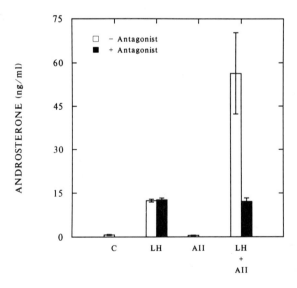

FIGURE 4. Effect of an angiotensin II antagonist on LH and angiotensin II stimulation of TIC androgen production. Purified TIC were cultured for 2 days with LH (50 ng/mL), angiotensin II (100 ng/mL), and/or [Sar^1,Ile^8]-angiotensin II (antagonist). The data are the mean ± SEM of 2 experiments with 4 replicates each.

These results indicate that in the absence of stimulation or in the presence of a saturating concentration of LH, angiotensin II does not affect TIC androgen production. Only at stimulatory but submaximal concentrations of LH is the effect of angiotensin II observed. This finding suggests that the protein kinase C pathway interacts in a positive manner with the LH-stimulated cAMP signaling system to increase the sensitivity of TIC to LH. It appears that the effects of angiotensin II are exerted through interaction with the cAMP pathway and not independently because angiotensin II does not stimulate androgen production in the absence of LH. Some degree of activation of the cAMP pathway appears to be required in order to observe the effects of angiotensin II. In light of the lack of synergism between LH and angiotensin II, it is probable that angiotensin II does not amplify the cAMP signal beyond the level stimulated by saturating concentrations of LH. These results are consistent with interaction of the two signaling pathways at the level of GTP-binding proteins. Perhaps angiotensin II causes inhibition of G_i activity as has been shown for protein kinase C in other systems (14, 15).

As shown in Figure 4, the effects of angiotensin II were blocked by a specific angiotensin II receptor antagonist [Sar^1,Ile^8]-angiotensin II. LH (3 ng/mL) stimulated a small increase in androsterone production. Addition of antagonist (10 µg/mL) did not alter LH action. As before angiotensin II alone (100 ng/mL) did not stimulate androsterone production. Angiotensin II, together with LH, stimulated approximately a 4-fold increase in androsterone production. Addition of approximately a 100-fold molar excess of antagonist (10 µg/mL) completely blocked the stimulatory effect of angiotensin II, suggesting that the effects of angiotensin II are receptor mediated. These results are consistent with the demonstration of specific angiotensin II binding sites in the ovary (6, 7).

The results of these experiments demonstrate a novel modulatory effect of angiotensin II on LH-stimulated androgen production in ovarian TIC. Although there are other stimulatory modulators of LH action, such as insulin/IGF-I (10) and lipoproteins (10), angiotensin II is the only modulator to date that causes a sensitization of the TIC to LH action. Interestingly, angiotensin II does not alter the maximum capacity of the TIC to produce androgens. These results are consistent with the conclusion that angiotensin II may be an important autocrine/paracrine regulator of ovarian function. These new data may provide a mechanism for the block of ovulation caused by administration of an angiotensin II antagonist to intact rats in vivo (2).

References

1. Balla T, Baukal AJ, Guillemette G, Catt KJ. Multiple pathways of inositol polyphosphate metabolism in angiotensin-stimulated adrenal glomerulosa cells. J Biol Chem 1988;263:4083-91.

2. Pellicer A, Palumbo A, DeCherney AH, Naftolin F. Blockage of ovulation by an angiotensin antagonist. Science 1988;240:1660-1.
3. Fernandez LA, Tarlatzis BC, Rzasa PJ, et al. Renin-like activity in ovarian follicular fluid. Fertil Steril 1985;44:219-23.
4. Culler MD, Tarlatzis BC, Lightman A, et al. Angiotensin II-like immunoreactivity in human ovarian follicular fluid. J Clin Endocrinol Metab 1986;62:613-5.
5. Glorioso N, Atlas SA, Laragh JH, Jewelewicz R, Sealey JE. Prorenin in high concentrations in human ovarian follicular fluid. Science 1986;233:1422-4.
6. Husain A, Bumpus FM, De Silva P, Speth R. Localization of angiotensin II receptors in ovarian follicles and the identification of angiotensin II in rat ovaries. Proc Natl Acad Sci USA 1987;84:2489-93.
7. Speth RC, Husain A. Distribution of angiotensin-converting enzyme and angiotensin II-receptor binding sites in the rat ovary . Biol Reprod 1988;38:695-702.
8. Magoffin DA, Erickson GF. Primary culture of differentiating ovarian androgen-producing cells in defined medium. J Biol Chem 1982;257:4507-13.
9. Magoffin DA, Erickson GF. Purification of ovarian theca-interstitial cells by density gradient centrifugation. Endocrinology 1988;122:2345-7.
10. Magoffin DA, Erickson GF. An improved method for primary culture of ovarian androgen-producing cells in serum-free medium: Effect of lipoproteins, insulin, and insulin-like growth factor-I. In Vitro Cell Dev Biol 1988;24:862-70.
11. Zamecnik J, Barbe G, Moger WH, Armstrong DT. Radioimmunoassays for androsterone, 5α-androstane-3α,17β-diol and 5α-androstane-3β,17β-diol. Steroids 1977;30:679-89.
12. De Lean A, Munson PJ, Rodbard D. Simultaneous analysis of families of sigmoidal curves: Application to bioassay, radioligand assay, and physiological dose-response curves. Am J Physiol 1978;235:E97-E102.
13. Hofeditz C, Magoffin DA, Erickson GF. Evidence for protein kinase C regulation of ovarian theca-interstitial cell androgen biosynthesis. Biol Reprod 1988; 39:873-81.
14. Bell JD, Brunton LL. Enhancement of adenylate cyclase activity in S49 lymphoma cells by phorbol esters. Withdrawal of GTP-dependent inhibition. J Biol Chem 1986;261:12036-41.

53

Influence of Lipoproteins on the Synthesis of Apo E by Rat Ovarian Granulosa Cells

L.M. OLSON, K.L. WYNE, V.M. SCHMIT, E.L. GONG, G.S. GETZ, AND J.R. SCHREIBER

Apo E, a protein of 35,000 Da, is found associated with chylomicron remnants, very low-density lipoproteins, and a subset of large high-density lipoproteins (HDL; 1, 2). It is a ligand on lipoproteins that is recognized by the B/E or LDL receptor, the apo E-specific hepatic receptors, and the immunoregulatory receptors on lymphocyte membranes (1, 2). One function of apo E appears to be the transport of excess cholesterol from peripheral tissues to the liver for excretion in a process called *reverse cholesterol transport* (1, 2). The major site of apo E synthesis is the liver, although apo E mRNA has been detected in significant quantities in other tissues, including steroidogenic tissues (3).

Primary rat ovarian granulosa cells (ROGC) are being used in our laboratory to investigate the regulation of apo E synthesis in steroid-producing tissues in response to hormonal stimulation. We have previously reported that apo E synthesis in ROGC is regulated by a complex interaction of gonadotropin stimulation and sterol synthesis (4, 5). The following experiments were designed to examine the influence of exogenous cholesterol provided in the form of lipoproteins on the synthesis of apo E by ROGC.

Materials and Methods

Cell Culture. Rat ovarian granulosa cells were isolated from ovaries obtained from 23-day-old, hypophysectomized diethylstilbesterol-treated Sprague-Dawley female rats (Johnson Laboratories, Chicago, IL). Cells were cultured for 32 h in serum-free McCoy's 5A medium containing 2-mM L-glutamine, 100-U/mL penicillin, 100-µg/mL streptomycin, and 10^{-7}M androstenedione supplemented with various treatments as noted in the text and figure legends. Following 28 h of culture a 200-µL aliquot of the medium was analyzed for DHP by radioimmunoassay (RIA). Each flask then received 100-µCi/mL medium [^{35}S]methionine for the remaining 4 h. The relative differences in the amounts of radioactive apo E in the medium was determined by immunoprecipitation using an anti-rat apo E antibody as described previously (4). Relative amounts of apo E mRNA were determined by slot-blot hybridization using a rat apo E cDNA probe, as previously described (4). Autoradiograms and fluorograms were quantitated using laser densitometry. Results are expressed as the ratio of the experimental sample to the non-stimulated control.

Synthetic Particles and Isolation of Lipoproteins. Lipoproteins were isolated from plasma by sequential ultracentrifugation. Human low-density lipoprotein (LDL) and HDL were isolated in the density ranges 1.019–1.063 g/mL and 1.063–1.21 g/mL, respectively. Two synthetic lipoprotein particles obtained as a gift from Dr. Elaine Gong, Lawrence Berkeley Laboratory (Berkeley, CA), were utilized in our studies. Particle one contained 4.11 mg/mL phosphatidylcholine and 1.41 mg/mL apolipoprotein A-I. Particle two contained 3.39 mg/mL phosphatidylcholine, 1.57 mg/mL apolipoprotein A-I, and 0.7 mg/mL unesterified cholesterol.

Statistics. All experiments were analyzed as complete randomized designs using analysis of variance. Specific treatment differences were tested by orthogonal comparisons following ANOVA, with a probability of 0.05 being accepted as a significant difference. In certain cases a paired t-test was performed. Statistical analyses were performed using the SYSTAT software program (6).

Results

To examine if exogenous cholesterol supplied in the form of lipoprotein influences apo E synthesis, rat ovarian granulosa cells were cultured with (stimulated) and without (nonstimulated) CT and increasing concentrations of HDL (Fig. 1, *left panels*). Increasing amounts of HDL resulted in higher levels of radioactive apo E protein in the media of nonstimulated cells. The addition of HDL to CT-treated cells resulted in a significant increase in the amount of apo E in the media relative to CT-treated cells (P < 0.05). Culturing granulosa cells with CT resulted in a significant increase in apo E mRNA levels (P < 0.005), but HDL had no independent effect. A second set of dose-response experiments were conducted using LDL as a sterol source to determine whether the lipoprotein effect was specific for HDL. The effect

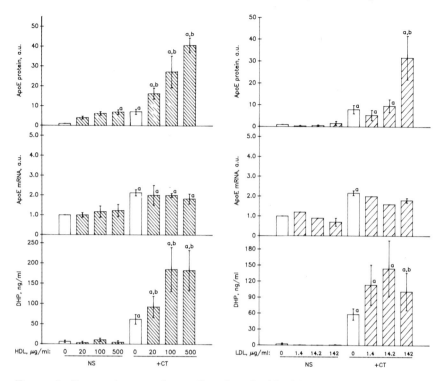

FIGURE 1. Rat ovarian granulosa cells cultured with either serum-free medium or serum-free medium supplemented with HDL (20, 100, or 500 µg/mL, *left panels*) or LDL (1.4, 14.2, or 142 µg/mL, *right panels*), with and without CT (1.25 µg/mL) for 32 h with 100-µCi [^{35}S]methionine/mL added for the last 4 h. DHP, apo E mRNA, and apo E protein levels were determined as described in text. (Data are expressed as means ± SEM. a, means are significantly different from nonstimulated, DHP, apo E protein: P < 0.001; apo E mRNA: P < 0.05. b, means are significantly different from CT-treated controls, DHP: P < 0.05; apo E protein: P < 0.01.)

of LDL on DHP synthesis, apo E mRNA, and protein levels was similar to that observed with HDL, although LDL was less effective (Fig. 1, *right panels*).

To determine whether the effect of the lipoproteins on apo E synthesis was due to the free-cholesterol component of the lipoproteins, the influence of 2 synthetic HDL-like particles on DHP and apo E synthesis were examined (Fig. 2). Granulosa cells were cultured with either HDL (100-µg protein/mL; 4.1-µg unesterified cholesterol/mL; 29.3-µg esterified cholesterol/mL), particle 2 (10.4-µg protein/mL; 4.1-µg cholesterol), or particle 1 (10.4-µg protein/mL; no cholesterol). In the presence of CT, HDL had the usual stimulatory effect on DHP synthesis, while both synthetic lipoprotein par-

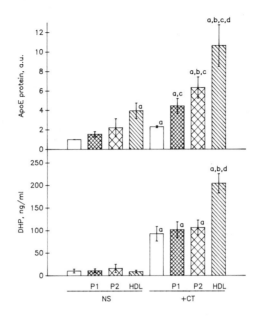

FIGURE 2. Rat ovarian granulosa cells cultured with either serum-free medium, particle 1 (10.4 μg protein/mL, no cholesterol), particle 2 (10.4 μg protein/mL, 4.1-μg unesterified cholesterol/mL) or HDL (100 μg protein/mL, 4.1-μg unesterified cholesterol/mL, and 29.3-μg esterified cholesterol/mL), with and without CT (1, 25 μg/mL) for 32 h with 100-μCi [^{35}S]methionine/mL added for the last 4 h. DHP, apo E mRNA, and apo E protein levels were determined as described in text. (Data are expressed as means ± SEM. a, means are significantly different from nonstimulated, P < 0.05. b, means are significantly different from CT-treated controls, P < 0.05. c, means are significantly different from each other using a paired t-test, P < 0.02. d, mean apo E protein level was significantly different from that determined for cells cultured with CT and either particle 1 or 2, DHP: P < 0.05; apo E: P < 0.01.)

ticles were without effect. In combination with CT, both particles raised apo E levels significantly above those measured from cells cultured with CT alone. Particle 2 was significantly more effective in raising apo E protein levels than particle 1, although neither particle increased apo E protein levels as effectively as HDL.

Discussion

These studies were designed to examine whether lipoproteins as sources of exogenous cholesterol, would replace the intracellular requirement for cholesterol for apo E production in hormone stimulated ROGC. The results of these experiments indicate that the increase in apo E observed with hormone stimulation of cells can be augmented when donors of exogenous cholesterol are also present. The mediator for this increase may be unesterified cholesterol since a synthetic particle containing unesterified cholesterol raised apo E levels to a greater extent than one with no cholesterol. The level of cholesterol is probably not the only mediator, however, for two reasons. Firstly, both synthetic lipoprotein particles raised apo E levels significantly over control levels despite their differences in cholesterol content, and secondly, HDL raised apo E levels in nonstimulated cells, a result not shared by LDL or either synthetic particle.

The lipoprotein effects on apo E production operate post-transcriptionally. A number of possible mechanisms could be envisaged. The translation of the apo E mRNA could be more efficient in the presence of lipoprotein. The lipoprotein could promote the secretion of apo E that might otherwise be degraded intracellularly. Alternatively, the secreted apo E might be recycled rapidly into the cell, perhaps employing the LDL receptor, after which it could be degraded. The lipoprotein would stabilize the extracellular apo E by association with the added lipoprotein. If the lipoprotein addition acts on some intracellular phase of apo E production (translation, secretion, or stabilization), it is not clear what might be involved. Effecting a redistribution of intracellular lipids (sterol or phospholipid) or an alteration of intracellular membrane properties (e.g., fluidity) are possible candidates. We are currently performing experiments to examine these possibilities.

Acknowledgments. The authors acknowledge Dr. M. Beckman for his assistance with the rats and Ms. Sarah Frazier for her help with the quantitation of the fluorographs.

References

1. Getz GS, Mazzone R, Soltys P, Bates, SR. Atherosclerosis and apoprotein E. Arch Path Lab Med 1988;112:1048-55.
2. Mahley RW. Apoprotein E. Science 1988;240:622-30.
3. Driscoll DM, Getz GS. Extrahepatic synthesis of apolipoprotein E. JLR 1984;25:1368-79.
4. Wyne KL, Schreiber JR, Larsen AL, Getz GS. Regulation of apolipoprotein E by cAMP and phorbol ester in rat ovarian granulosa cells. J Biol Chem 1989;264:981-9.
5. Wyne KL, Schreiber JR, Larsen AL, Getz GS. Rat granulosa cell apolipoprotein E secretion. J Biol Chem 1989;264:16530-6.
6. Wilkinson L. SYSTAT: The system for statistics. Evanston, IL: SYSTAT Inc, 1989.

54

Bovine Granulosa Cells
Steroidogenesis In Vitro, I:
Response to Androgens and Estrogens

M.-A. SIRARD, S. BILODEAU, M.A. FORTIER,
AND A. BÉLANGER

Granulosa cells steroidogenesis has been characterized at the cellular and molecular levels in the rat (1), but information gained with this species cannot be easily applied to the bovine. Therefore, specific tools must be developed to learn more about follicular growth in the cow in order to control superovulation. Attempts were made to culture bovine granulosa cells in vitro, but the capacity to aromatize androgens to estradiol was always rapidly lost (2, 3). Since estradiol is one of the most accurate means to evaluate follicular health in vivo (4), its production in vitro has been used as an indication of normal follicular behavior (2). It is also well reported that estradiol may be an important cofactor in its own synthesis through induction of FSH or other receptors. The suppressive effect of estradiol on the in vitro progesterone production was noticed with different classes of follicles (5–8). The study of Henderson and coauthors (2) and the preceding ones (4, 9) indicate that a suppression of progesterone production could be regarded as a nonatretic sign. Different approaches aimed at maintaining a high estradiol to progesterone ratio with serum or FSH supplementation, growth factors or co-culture with theca cells were not successful (10–13). The effect of serum has been described as suppressive towards the hormonal response (FSH), both in the bovine and the rat (10, 14) but serum-free culture requires additional growth factors and an extracellular matrix especially if small follicles are used (15, 16).

The objective of this study was to evaluate the steroidogenesis potential of bovine granulosa cells obtained at an early stage of differentiation and by a method that could be easily reproduced. We analyzed the effect of 3 culture media supplements: fetal calf serum (FCS), bovine follicular fluid (BFF) from small follicles, and bovine serum albumin (BSA) after coating the culture dishes with BFF. Secondly, we analyzed the effect of time in culture by looking at secretion of estradiol and progesterone, with and without androgenic or estrogenic supplementation after 1, 7, and 8 days of culture.

Materials and Methods

Granulosa Cells Preparation. Granulosa cells were collected by aspiration of follicles (1–5 mm) from ovaries of cows obtained at a slaughterhouse. Ovaries were transported (1 h) to the laboratory in a saline solution maintained between 30°C and 35°C (additives: 100,000-IU penicillin, 100-mg streptomycin, and 250-µg amphotericin B/L; Sigma Chemical Co., St. Louis, MO). The follicles were aspirated with a 10-mL syringe and an 18-G needle. Cumulus oocyte complexes were removed prior to centrifugation (450 g, 4°C, 10 min), and the supernatant was kept as bovine follicular fluid. The cells were washed twice in 30-mL calcium/magnesium-free Hank's balanced salt solution with antibiotics (450 g, 10 min, 4°C). The cells were resuspended in 1-mL TCM-199, and 1×10^6 cells were transferred into 24-well plates (Corning, NY) containing medium TCM-199 (1 mL/well), with Hank's salts, glutamine, and bicarbonate, supplemented with 1-µg/mL of insulin, 2.2-µg/mL pyruvate, and 50 µg/mL gentamicin sulphate (all from Sigma). Three protein supplements were used: 10% FCS (Flow Laboratories, McLean, VA), 10% BFF obtained from small follicles (FCs and BFF were treated with dextran charcoal for 24 h at 4°C), and BSA (5 mg/mL; Sigma). When BSA was used, the wells were coated with 200-µL BFF for 1 h at 38.5°C, then BFF was removed. The cells were cultured at 38.5°C in a humidified incubator with 5% CO_2 in air.

Experimental Design. The effects of testosterone (10^{-9}, 10^{-8}, and 10^{-7}M), clomiphene citrate (10^{-7}M), diethylstilbestrol (10^{-7}M) (all from Sigma), and EM-139 (10^{-7}), a potent anti-estrogen, were evaluated following 24-h of culture. The cells were used for a second and a third incubation of 144 h and 24 h, respectively, with the same treatments. All supernatants were centrifuged before freezing. Each treatment was replicated 3 times.

Steroids Measurements. Steroids were measured by standard radioimmunoassay following ether extraction. For estradiol, 500 µL of culture supernatant were extracted with 5 mL of solvent; for progesterone, 10 µL were diluted 1:100 in TCM-199 before extraction. The antibody specificity has been described before (18). Statistical analyses were performed with a SAS system using a Waller-Dunkan variance analysis.

Results

Media with FCS and BFF were analyzed for steroid concentration in order to evaluate the effectiveness of the dextran charcoal treatment. Medium with FCS contained 35.3 ± 7.7 pM/L of estradiol; the one with BFF contained 26.6 ± 2.3 pM/L. These levels were near the sensibility limit of the assay. Progesterone concentrations were below the sensibility limit of the assay (24 nM/L).

Figure 1 shows the steroid content after 24 h, 24 + 144 h, and 24 + 144 + 24 h of incubation in the medium with 10% FCS and testosterone. For the 3 periods of time, there is a positive correlation between the amount of testosterone and the amount of estradiol produced and a negative correlation with the amount of progesterone. These results indicate a sustained capacity of cultured granulosa cells to aromatize testosterone over 8 days.

During the first 24 h, the 3 media were able to sustain estradiol synthesis at a similar level, but after 7 or 8 days, there was a marked decrease in aromatase activity in the media containing BFF or BSA (Fig. 2). The amount of progesterone measured depended also on the medium as illustrated in Figure 3.

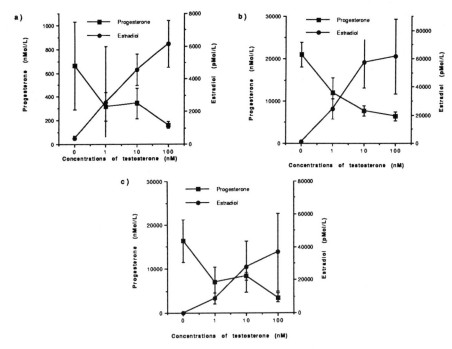

FIGURE 1. The effects of 3 concentrations of testosterone (10^{-9}, 10^{-8}, and 10^{-7}M) on the estradiol and progesterone secretion of cells cultured in the medium containing 10% FCS after 24 h *(a)*, 24 + 144 h *(b)*, and 24 + 144 + 24 h *(c)*.

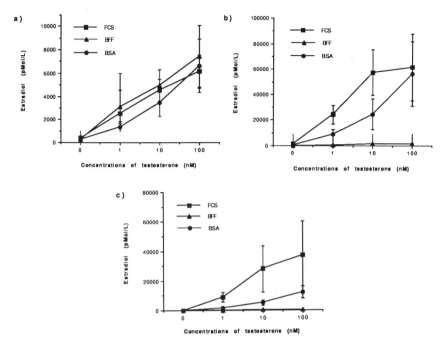

FIGURE 2. The effects of 10% FCS, 10% BFF, and 5-mg/mL BSA in TCM-199 on the production of estradiol in response to testosterone after 24 h *(a)*, 24 + 144 h *(b)*, and 24 + 144 + 24 h *(c)*.

Figure 4*a* shows that diethylstilbestrol inhibits progesterone synthesis. Clomiphen citrate also results in an inhibition, but the addition of testosterone does not seem to synergize with CC to reduce the amount of progesterone produced. The addition of EM-139 resulted in a small increase in progesterone synthesis. The estradiol production in the presence of these

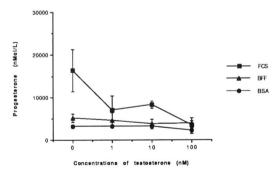

FIGURE 3. The effects of 10% FCS, 10% BFF, and 5-mg/mL BSA on the production of progesterone in response to testosterone after 24 + 144 + 24 h of culture.

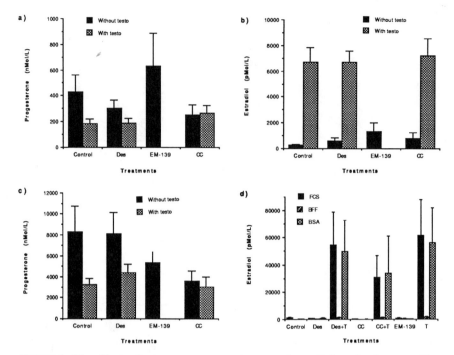

FIGURE 4. The effects of estrogens on progesterone and estradiol production. *a* and *b*: After 24 h of culture; *c*: after 24 + 144 + 24 h of culture; and *d*: after 24 + 144 h in the 3 media. In *a–c*, the results for the 3 media were pooled. (Des = diethylstilbestrol; EM-139 = anti-estrogen; and CC = clomiphen citrate.)

products is represented in Figure 4*b*, and no stimulation of estradiol synthesis is seen.

The effects of estrogens after 24 + 144 + 24 h are shown in Figure 4*c*. DES does not inhibit progesterone production; CC has an inhibitory effect, but does not seem to synergize with testosterone. The effect of EM-139 was between the one of DES and the one of CC. The results presented in Figure 4 were computed using the 3 media. The effects of estrogens on estradiol production after 24 + 144 h are shown in Figure 4*d*; these effects are the same as after 24 h except for the medium with BFF.

Discussion

Using successive incubations of bovine granulosa cells, the results presented here support the principal objective of this study, namely, the maintenance of modulated aromatase activity. The protocol used to harvest the granulosa cells resulted in an estradiol-to-progesterone ratio superior than previously published reports (2, 10). The use of a supplemented medium may not be the ideal solution, but to study aromatase regulation, a minimal activity has to be maintained.

The inhibition of aromatase capacity in the media containing either BFF or BSA cannot be explained by a reduced steroid-synthesizing ability since the progesterone production in the 3 media is comparable at least for the first 2 incubation periods (24 h and 24 + 144 h; results not shown). The BFF used in the medium originated from small follicles and could contain aromatase inhibitors since those follicles have a reduced capacity of aromatization in vivo. Finally, estrogens do influence the ability of granulosa cells to produce progesterone and could complement the androgen control of aromatase.

References

1. Hsueh AJW, Adashi EY, Jones PB, Welsh TH, Jr. Hormonal regulation of the differentiation of cultured ovarian granulosa cells. Endocr Rev 1984;5:76-127.
2. Henderson KM, McNatty KP, Smith P, et al. Influence of follicular health on the steroidogenic and morphological characteristics of bovine granulosa cells in vitro. J Reprod Fertil 1987;79:185-93.
3. Skinner MK, Osteen KG. Developmental and hormonal regulation of bovine granulosa cell function in the preovulatory follicle. Endocrinology 1988;123: 1668-75.
4. McNatty KP, Heat DA, Henderson KM, et al. Some aspects of thecal and granulosa cell function during follicular development in the bovine ovary. J Reprod Fertil 1984;72:39-53.
5. Fortune JE. Bovine theca and granulosa cells interact to promote androgen production. Biol Reprod 1986;35:292-9.
6. Fortune JE, Hansel W. The effects of 17β-Estradiol on progesterone secretion by bovine theca and granulosa cells. Endocrinology. 1979;104:1834-8.
7. Henderson KM, Franchimont P. Inhibin production by bovine ovarian tissues in vitro and its regulation by androgens. J Reprod Fertil 1983;67:291-8.
8. Kaplanski O, Shemesh M, Berman A. Effects of phyto estrogens on progesterone synthesis by isolated bovine granulosa cells. J Endocrinol 1981;89:343-8.
9. Henderson KM, Franchimont P, Charlet-Renard C, McNatty KP. Effect of follicular atresia on inhibin production by bovine granulosa cells in vitro and inhibin concentrations in the follicular fluid. J Reprod Fertil 1984;72:1-8.
10. Fortune JE. Effects of LH and FSH on steroidogenesis by bovine granulosa cells from proestrus follicles cultured with and without serum. In: Development and function of the reproductive organs. New York: Raven Press, 1987.
11. Gospodarowicz D, Bialecki H. The effects of the epidermal and fibroblast growth factors on the replicative lifespan of cultured bovine granulosa cells. Endocrinology 1978;103:854-65.
12. Adashi EY, Resnick CE, Brodie AMH, Svoboda ME, Van Wyk JJ. Somatomedin-C mediated potentiation of FSH-induced aromatase activity of cultured rat granulosa cells. Endocrinology 1985;117:2313-9.

13. Liu XY, Hsueh AJW. Synergism between granulosa and theca-interstitial cells in estrogen biosynthesis by gonadotropin-treated rat ovaries: Studies on the two-cell, two-gonadotropin hypothesis using steroid antisera. Biol Reprod 1986;35:27-36.
14. Orly J, Sato G, Erickson GF. Serum suppresses the expression of hormonally induced functions in cultured granulosa cells. Cell 1980;20:817-27.
15. Savion N, Laherty R, Lui G-M, Gospodarowicz D. Modulation of low density lipo protein metabolism in bovine granulosa cells as a function of their steroidogenic activity. J Biol Chem 1981;256:12817-22.
16. Luck MR. Greatly elevated and sustained secretion of oxytocin by bovine granulosa cells in serum-free culture. J Experi Zool 1989;251:361-6.
17. Dufour JJ, Cahill LP, Mauléon P. Short- and long-term effects of hypophysectomy and unilateral ovariectomy on ovarian follicular populations in sheep. J Reprod Fertil 1979;57:301-9.
18. Bélanger A, Caron S, Picard V. Simultaneous radioimmunoassay of progestins, androgens and estrogens in the rat testis. J Steroid Biochem 1980;13:185-90.

55

Bovine Granulosa Cells Steroidogenesis In Vitro, II: Response to FSH, Forskolin, and IBMX

M.-A. SIRARD, S. BILODEAU, MA. FORTIER,
AND A. BÉLANGER

There is a follicular population in the bovine that does not change upon sexual status of the animal: the small follicles (<5 mm) (1). This population is present in fetal life, and in sheep is partially independant of pituitary support since hypophysectomy does not prevent follicular growth up to 2–3 mm (2). The granulosa cells from those follicles are, therefore, available at the slaughterhouse and provide access to a large amount of research material. These follicles are further away from luteinization or final differentiation since they would require from 4–10 days in vivo to reach ovulation (3). This early stage of follicular growth represents the beginning of estradiol dominancy, and therefore, the granulosa cells possess aromatase capacity (4). The factors inducing differentiation and the apparition of FSH response are not precisely known in bovine, but they are well characterized in other species, such as the rat, and involve estradiol, androgens, and adenylate cyclase activity (5).

In this second study, we analyzed the effects of factors known to increase cAMP content—follicle stimulating hormone (FSH), forskolin (FSK), and Isobutyl-1-methylxanthine (IBMX)—with or without androgen supplementation on the steroid secretion (estradiol and progesterone) after 1, 7, and 8 days of culture in 3 different media: TCM-199 with fetal calf serum (FCS), bovine follicular fluid (BFF) from small follicles, and bovine serum albumin (BSA) after coating the culture dishes with BFF.

Materials and Methods

Granulosa Cells Preparation. Granulosa cells were obtained by aspiration of follicles from ovaries collected at the slaughterhouse from cows at different stages of their reproductive cycle. Ovaries were collected in the morning (1 h) and transported (1 h) to the laboratory in a saline solution 0.9% (w/v) NaCl maintained between 30°C and 35°C (additives: 100,000-IU penicillin, 100-mg streptomycin, and 250-µg amphotericin B/L; Sigma Chemical Co., St. Louis, MO). Follicles between 1 and 5 mm in diameter were aspirated using a 10-mL syringe and an 18-G needle. Cumulus oocyte complexes were removed prior to centrifugation (450 g, 4°C, 10 min), and the supernatant was kept as bovine follicular fluid. Subsequently, the cells were washed twice in 30 mL calcium/magnesium-free Hank's balanced salt solution containing antibiotics (450 g, 10 min, 4°C). The final pellet was resuspended in 1-mL TCM-199. A total of 1×10^6 cells were transferred into 24-well plates (Corning, NY) containing TCM-199 (1 mL/well) with Hank's salts, glutamine, bicarbonate, supplemented with insulin (1 µg/mL), pyruvate (2.2 µg/mL), and gentamicin sulphate (50 µg/mL) (all from Sigma) Three protein supplements were used: 10% FCS (Flow Laboratories, McLean, VA), 10% BFF obtained from small (1–5mm) follicles (FCS and BFF were treated with dextran charcoal for 24 h at 4°C), and BSA (5 mg/mL; Sigma). When BSA was used, the wells were coated with 200-µL BFF (cd) for 1 h at 38.5°C, then BFF was removed. The cells were cultured at 38.5°C in a humidified incubator with 5% CO_2 in air.

Experimental Design. The effects on steroid synthesis of 3 concentrations $10^{-9}, 10^{-8}$, and 10^{-7}M of testosterone (Sigma), FSH (100 ng/mL NIADDK), forskolin (1 µM), and IBMX (0.1 mM) (both from Sigma) were measured following a 24-h incubation. The same cells were used for a second and a third incubation of 144 h and 24 h, respectively, with the same treatments except that FSH was added every 24 h during the first 3 days of the second culture period. All supernatants were centrifuged before freezing. Each treatment was replicated 3 times.

Steroids Measurements. Steroids were measured by standard radioimmunoassay following ether extraction. For estradiol, 500 µL of culture supernatant were extracted with 5 mL of solvent; for progesterone, 10 µL were diluted in 990-µL TCM-199, then extracted. The antibody specificity has been described before (6). Statistical analyses were performed with a SAS system using a Waller-Dunkan variance analysis.

Results

Media with FCS and BFF were analyzed for steroid concentration in order to evaluate the effectiveness of the dextran charcoal treatment. The medium with FCS contained 35.3 + 7.7 pM/L of estradiol; the one with BFF contained 26.6 + 2.3 pM/L. These levels were near the sensibility limit of the assay. Progesterone concentrations were below the sensibility limit of the assay (24 nM/L).

The first set of figures (Fig. 1) illustrates the effects of FSH (100 ng/mL)

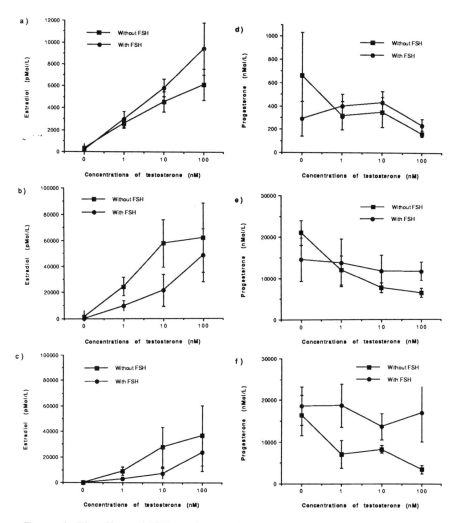

FIGURE 1. The effects of FSH supplementation, with or without testosterone in TCM-199 + 10% FCS on the estradiol synthesis after 24 h *(a)*, 24 + 144 h *(b)*, and 24 + 144 + 24 h *(c)* and progesterone synthesis after the same periods of time *(d, e,* and *f).*

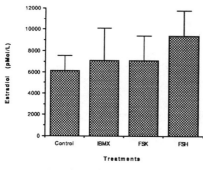 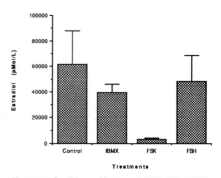

FIGURE 2. The effects of IBMX, FSK, and FSH on estradiol synthesis after 24 h in the medium containing 10% FCS with testosterone (10^{-7}M).

FIGURE 3. The effects of IBMX, FSK, and FSH on estradiol synthesis after 24 + 144 h in TCM-199 + 10% FCS with testosterone (10^{-7}M).

supplementation on the amount of estradiol and progesterone synthesized after 24 h, 24 + 144 h, and 24 + 144 + 24 h in the medium which was supplemented with FBS, since an effect of the medium was detected in the estradiol synthesis. FSH clearly enhanced progesterone production in the presence of a large amount of testosterone at the third incubation period and decreased estradiol production in all 3 media. Without testosterone, FSH had no effect.

During the first 24 h of incubation, in the presence of testosterone (10^{-7}), estradiol production can be enhanced by FSH, but not by IBMX or FSK (Figs. 1a and 2). Following the subsequent 144-h incubation period (Fig. 3), the effects of FSH, forskolin, and IBMX are different, since FSH had no more stimulatory effect, IBMX was partially inhibitory, and forskolin really suppressed aromatization in the presence of testosterone (10^{-7}M).

The progesterone production after the first 24 h of incubation (with testosterone, 10^{-7}M) was not affected by the media, so results were pooled and are presented in Figure 4. The 3 stimulants of cAMP accumulation resulted in an increase in progesterone synthesis after 24 h, and forskolin was the most

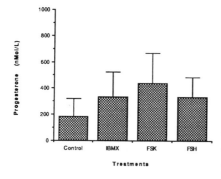

FIGURE 4. The effects of IBMX, FSK, and FSH on progesterone synthesis after 24 h. The results obtained with the 3 media in the presence of testosterone (10^{-7}M) were pooled.

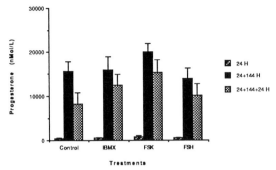

FIGURE 5. The amount of progesterone produced following 24 h, 24 + 144 h, and 24 + 144 + 24 h of incubation in the absence of testosterone. Media was supplemented with FSH, IBMX, FSK or was not supplemented as described in text.

potent stimulator. The same picture can be observed following a subsequent 144 h of incubation.

Without testosterone, the production of estradiol following treatments with either FSH, FSK, or IBMX was always lower than in the control media (results not shown). The progesterone production in the same conditions (without testosterone) is shown in Figure 5 and was much higher than with the androgen (Fig. 4, for example), but the substrate did not significantly influence the relative response to FSH, forskolin, and IBMX.

Conclusion

Previous reports using later stage follicles resulted in a rapid loss of aromatase activity even in presence of FSH (7, 8). In our study, after the first 24 h, FSH ceased to stimulate aromatization of androgens and increased progesterone production. This effect is supportive of previous observations using in vitro culture of bovine granulosa cells (9), but is contradictory to the in vivo effect of FSH and cannot be explained by a rapid desensitization of the receptor in vitro since the effect is still present after 7 days of culture. Gonadotropins are strong stimulators of cAMP accumulation in laboratory animals (5), and it is possible that the progesterone stimulation is a direct effect of this second messenger accumulation. In other species, products that stimulate cAMP accumulation by a direct action on the catalytic unit of the adenylate cyclase normally result in progesterone production by granulosa cells (10). Therefore, our results support a difference between the cAMP accumulation produced by FSH and the estradiol synthesis also stimulated in vivo by FSH. A second explanation comes from the capacity of FSH to induce differentiation of granulosa cells. In the bovine, the dominant follicle rapidly produces inhibin, creating a shortage of FSH to which it becomes independant by synthesizing LH receptors. The same mechanism could possibly explain the in vitro results. No LH stimulation was done in this study since this gonadotropin should induce luteinization; therefore, it is not known if LH would have stimulated estradiol production at a very low and pulsative level. A third explanation comes from the nature of FSH stimulation used in vitro: In our case, we used repeated doses of FSH at every 24 h over a 4-day period, but even if this protocol produces a small cyclicity in FSH, it does not mimic the natural pulsative release of this product in vivo.

References

1. Erickson BH. Development and senescence of the postnatal bovine ovary. J Anim Sci 1966;25:800-5.
2. Dufour JJ, Cahill LP, Mauléon P. Short- and long-term effects of hypophysectomy and unilateral ovariectomy on ovarian follicular populations in sheep. J Reprod Fertil 1979;57:301-9.
3. Pierson RA, Ginther OJ. Ultrasonic imaging of the ovaries and uterus in cattle. Theriogenology 1988;29:21-38.
4. Carson RS, Zhang Z, Hutchinson LA, Herington AC, Findlay JK. Growth factors in ovarian function. J Reprod Fertil 1989;85:735-46.
5. Hsueh AJW, Adashi EY, Jones PB, Welsh TH, Jr. Hormonal regulation of the differentiation of cultured ovarian granulosa cells. Endocr Rev 1984;5:76-127.
6. Bélanger A, Caron S, Picard V. Simultaneous radioimmunoassay of progestins, androgens and estrogens in the rat testis. J Steroid Biochem 1980;13:185-90.
7. Henderson KM, McNatty KP, Smith P, et al. Influence of follicular health on the steroidogenic and morphological characteristics of bovine granulosa cells in vitro. J Reprod Fertil 1987;79:185-93.
8. Skinner MK, Osteen KG. Developmental and hormonal regulation of bovine granulosa cell function in the preovulatory follicle. Endocrinology 1988; 123:1668-75.
9. Fortune JE. Effects of LH and FSH on steroidogenesis by bovine granulosa cells from proestrus follicles cultured with and without serum. In: Development and function of the reproductive organs. New York: Raven Press, 1987.
10. Goff AK, Armstrong DT. Changes in responsiveness of rat granulosa cells to PGE_2 and FSH during culture. Can J Physiol 1983;61:608-13.

56

Sustained Estradiol Production by Porcine Granulosa Cells In Vitro

J. JOE FORD

As ovarian follicles grow and develop to ovulatory size, granulosa cells (GCs) proliferate and secrete estrogens and progesterone. Estrogens play a central role in follicular development both directly and through amplification of responses to follicle stimulating hormone (FSH; 1, 2). Use of GC cultures has greatly expanded current understanding of regulation of steroidogenesis in these cells, but species differences exist in the ability of GCs to maintain estrogen secretion in culture when provided with aromatizable androgen. Rat GCs maintain FSH-stimulated estrogen production in culture (3); the response is sufficient to provide a sensitive bioassay (4). Human GCs also secrete estrogen during FSH stimulation in vitro, and this responsiveness continues in GCs obtained after in vivo stimulation with an ovulatory dosage of human chorionic gonadotropin (5, 6). In contrast to these rather consistent findings with rat and human GCs, less predictable observations occur with porcine GCs. In general, porcine GCs possess appreciable aromatase activity during the first 48 h in culture, after which this activity decreases (7, 8). Only two reports of prolonged FSH-stimulated estrogen synthesis by porcine GCs were identified (9, 10); thus, in most studies, in vitro differentiation progresses, and by day 4 in culture a majority of porcine GCs lose their ability to aromatize androgens to estrogens. The objective of the present studies was to overcome this limitation and identify conditions that extend estrogen production by porcine GCs on a reliable basis.

Methods

Porcine ovaries were obtained at slaughter and placed into cold saline that contained penicillin G (100 U/mL), streptomycin sulfate (100 µg/mL), and amphotericin B (0.25 µg/mL). Ovaries were transported to the laboratory and rinsed once with saline supplemented with antibiotics. Follicles (1–3 mm in diameter) were punctured with 25-G needles, and GCs were collected by aspiration. The GCs were washed twice with Dulbecco's Minimum Essential Medium without calcium and magnesium (MEM), were resuspended in MEM, and filtered through a 70-μm nylon filter (Spectrum, Los Angeles, CA). Cells that passed through the filter were designated as weakly associated (WAGCs).

Preliminary studies identified cells retained by the filter as candidates to maintain estrogen production in vitro. Retained material, which included oocytes and aggregates of tightly bound GCs (TBGCs), was rinsed from the filter with MEM, centrifuged (300 × g for 5 min) and resuspended in 2-mL MEM (0.5% BSA) that contained collagenase (Type II, 590 U/mL), hyaluronidase (1000 U/mL), and DNase (20 U/mL). During incubation at 39°C, cells were passed gently through a 1-mL disposable pipette tip on repeated occasions at 10 min intervals. After 30-40 min, cells were diluted in 20-mL MEM (1% BSA), centrifuged, washed with MEM (1% BSA), and passed through a 70-μm filter. Both WAGCs and TBGCs were resuspended in Hams F-12:DMEM (1:1; Gibco, Grand Island, NY) supplemented with 10% fetal bovine serum (FBS), antibiotics (100-U/mL penicillin G and 100-μg/mL streptomycin sulfate), antimycotic (0.25-μg/mL amphotericin B), and insulin (1 μg/mL). Cell viability was determined by trypan blue exclusion and cells were dispensed into 24-well culture plates (2 cm^2/well) at designated number of viable cells/well. Media were removed at 48-h intervals and replaced with fresh media (1 mL) formulated as indicated above, except that it contained 10^{-6}M androstenedione and the concentration of FBS varied as indicated. At termination of each study, each well was rinsed with 0.5 mL cold MEM. Cells were disrupted with 0.1 mL of 1% cholic acid, sodium salt, and 0.1% lauryl sulfate and were assayed for protein (Bio-Rad, Richmond, CA), or DNA concentration (11). Estradiol and progesterone concentrations were determined by direct assay of culture media (12). Steroid radioimmunoassays were modified to utilize ^{125}I-labeled hormones.

Results

Estradiol concentrations were 35 times greater ($P < 0.05$) in media of TBGCs that received FSH than in control cultures (Fig. 1). In contrast, FSH stimulation of WAGCs produced only a 1.6-fold increase in estradiol. For both populations of GCs, progesterone production increased ($P < 0.01$) with FSH stimulation (6.4- and 7.3-fold for WAGCs and TBGCs).

When cells were plated at 0.28, 0.84, 2.5, and 7.5 × 10^5 viable TBGCs/cm^2 and cultured in 10% FBS for 8 days (n = 3 pools), FSH-stimulated estradiol production per μg DNA was greater at the two intermediate plating densities.

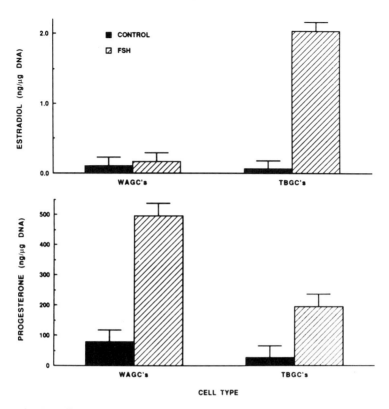

FIGURE 1. Estradiol and progesterone concentrations on day 8 of culture of porcine GCs plated at 2.5×10^5 viable cells/cm^2 and maintained in 10% FBS (n = 2 independent pools of WAGCs and TBGCs). Treatment with FSH (200 ng/mL; NIH-P1) was initiated on day 2.

Estradiol production continued for 14 days when TBGCs (1×10^5 cells/cm^2) were stimulated with FSH (200 ng/mL, NIH-P1) and cultured in 2.5, 5, or 10% FBS (n = 2 pools): 13.3 ± 3.0, 17.7 ± 3.9, and 13.9 ± 2.9 ng/mL on day 8 of culture and 7.2 ± 2.3, 20.5 ± 4.9, and 11.5 ± 3.8 ng/mL on day 14. For cells cultured in 2.5% FBS for 8 days (n = 2 pools), FSH-stimulated estradiol production was nonsignificantly greater at 1×10^5 TBGCs/cm^2 than at 0.34 or 3×10^5 cells/cm^2.

The response to increasing dosages of highly purified porcine FSH was maximal at 5 ng/mL for estradiol production (Fig. 2). Estradiol production in response to luteinizing hormone (LH) and forskolin stimulation was curvilinear, whereas progesterone production continued to increase with dosage. With forskolin (Fig. 3), estradiol concentration was greatest with a dosage of 0.2–1 µM. The situation differed for LH because on day 8 of culture maximal

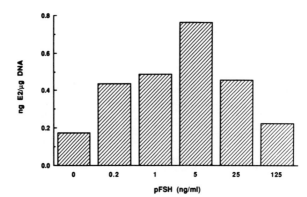

FIGURE 2. Estradiol concentrations on day 8 of culture (1×10^5 TBGCs/cm² in 2.5% FBS; n = 2 pools) in response to porcine FSH (LER-1419-3).

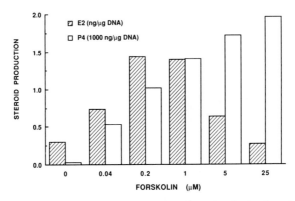

FIGURE 3. Estradiol and progesterone concentrations on day 8 of culture in response to forskolin treatment (1×10^5 TBGCs/cm² in 2.5% FBS; n = 2 pools). Similar results were observed with another pool of cells (2.5×10^5 TBGCs/cm²) cultured in 10% FBS.

estradiol production by the 3 pools of TBGCs occurred at different dosages of LH. When cultures with LH were continued through day 14, the dose-response relationship between LH and estradiol continued with 2 of 3 pools of cells, but was not evident after day 8 with the other pool.

Discussion

These studies identified a population of porcine GCs that consistently maintained FSH-stimulated estradiol secretion for 8 days in culture. Due to the tight affinity of these GCs to one another, isolation from the majority of the

GCs involved retention on filters with 70 µm openings followed by enzymatic dissociation. The TBGCs accounted for approximately 10% of the GCs isolated from small follicles, and in 3 of 4 pools, FSH-stimulated estradiol secretion continued through day 14 in culture. These TBGCs provide an in vitro system that more closely resembles the in vivo situation (i.e., synthesis of both estradiol and progesterone) and will be useful for further investigations into GC activity that is associated with follicular development. Such studies are needed because estradiol is assigned a central role in intraovarian regulation of follicular activity (1), but this is based primarily on studies conducted with rats. The contribution of estradiol to intraovarian regulation in other species remains less certain (2).

At present, an explanation for the success of Maruo et al. (9, 10) at stimulation of estrogen synthesis by porcine GCs for 6 days in culture is not apparent relative to the difficulties encountered by other investigators. In the present studies, estradiol synthesis occurred in culture medium that contained FBS (2.5–10%) and insulin (1 µg/mL); whereas Maruo et al. used 4% FBS plus thyroxin (10^{-7}M) or serum-free medium supplemented with insulin-like growth factor I (IGF-I, 100 ng/mL). With serum-free medium they determined that insulin would not substitute for IGF-I for maintenance of estrogen production although insulin and IGF-I were interchangeable for maintenance of progesterone synthesis. The FBS used in the current studies contained 55 ng IGF-I/mL; thus, this appears inadequate to support estrogen synthesis in view of the earlier report (10). This question requires further studies with TBGCs cultured in serum-free medium.

Summary

In summary, porcine GCs were separated into two populations: WAGCs and TBGCs. Progressive differentiation with time in culture appears to occur with WAGCs; their ability to secrete estrogen decreases concurrent with increased progesterone secretion. On the other hand, TBGCs continued to synthesize estrogen and progesterone when stimulated with FSH in culture. This heterogeneity for sustained estradiol synthesis emphasizes previously identified heterogeneity of GCs for other cellular activities (13, 14). If TBGCs were cultured with LH or forskolin (an intracellular stimulator of cyclic adenosine monophosphate production), lower dosages stimulated estradiol secretion while higher dosages were less stimulatory concurrent with further increases in progesterone secretion.

Acknowledgments. The author thanks S. Hassler and D. Griess for their excellent technical assistance, Dr. L E. Reichert, Jr., for purified porcine FSH and USDA-NIDDK for porcine FSH and LH.

References

1. Hsueh AJW, Adashi EY, Jones PBC, Welsh TH. Hormonal regulation of the differentiation of cultured ovarian granulosa cells. Endocr Rev 1984;5:76-127.
2. Hutz RJ. Disparate effects of estrogens on in vitro steroidogenesis by mammalian and avian granulosa cells. Biol Reprod 1989;40:709-13.
3. Leung PCK, Armstrong DT. Interactions of steroids and gonadotropins in the control of steroidogenesis in the ovarian follicle. Annu Rev Physiol 1980;71-82.
4. Wang C. Bioassays of follicle stimulating hormone. Endocr Rev 1988;9:374-7.
5. Steinkampf MP, Mendelson CR, Simpson ER. Regulation by follicle-stimulating hormone of the synthesis of aromatase cytochrome P-450 in human granulosa cells. Mol Endocrinol 1987;1:465-71.
6. Erickson GF, Garzo VG, Magoffin DA. Insulin-like growth factor-I regulates aromatase activity in human granulosa and granulosa lutea cells. J Clin Endocrinol Metab 1989;69:716-24.
7. May JV, Schomberg DW. Granulosa cell differentiation in vitro: Effect of insulin on growth and functional integrity. Biol Reprod 1981;25:421-31.
8. Stoklosowa S, Gregoraszczuk E, Channing CP. Estrogen and progesterone secretion by isolated cultured porcine thecal and granulosa cells. Biol Reprod 1982; 26:943-52.
9. Maruo T, Hayashi M, Matsuo H, Yamamoto T, Okada H, Mochizuki M. The role of thyroid hormone as a biological amplifier of the actions of follicle-stimulating hormone in the functional differentiation of cultured porcine granulosa cells. Endocrinology 1987;121:1233-41.
10. Maruo T, Hayashi M, Matsuo H, Ueda Y, Morikawa H, Mochizuki M. Comparison of the facilitative roles of insulin and insulin-like growth factor I in the functional differentiation of granulosa cells: In vitro studies with the porcine model. Acta Endocrinol (Copenh) 1988;117:230-40.
11. Labarca C, Paigen K. A simple, rapid, and sensitive DNA assay procedure. Anal Biochem 1980;102:344-52.
12. Christenson RK, Ford JJ, Redmer DA. Metabolic clearance and production rates of oestradiol and progesterone during pubertal and postpubertal development in gilts. J Reprod Fertil 1985;75:247-53.
13. Amsterdam A, Rotmensch S, Ben-Ze'ev A. Coordinated regulation of morphological and biochemical differentiation in a steroidogenic cell: The granulosa cell model. TIBS 1989;14:377-82.
14. Oliver JE, Aitman TJ, Powell JF, Wilson CA, Clayton RN. Insulin-like growth factor I gene expression in the rat ovary is confined to the granulosa cells of developing follicles. Endocrinology 1989;124:2671-9.

57

Initiation of Oocyte Maturation by Multiple Kinase Pathways

C.J. HUBBARD AND M. ROMANI

Numerous studies have indicated that LH provides the primary stimulus for oocyte maturation in mammals (1). An LH-initiated pulse of cAMP may be required to initiate meiosis; however, the mechanisms behind this event are not clear. LH can also activate protein kinase C (PKC; 2), and stimulation of PKC by phorbol esters will initiate maturation in follicle-enclosed oocytes (3). It is possible, therefore, that stimulation of maturation by LH may involve both protein kinase A (PKA) and PKC.

Meiosis in follicle-enclosed oocytes is triggered by epidermal growth factor (EGF; 4). While it is not clear that EGF is required during normal maturation, it may activate metabolic paths that have elements in common with those of both PKA and PKC.

The purpose of this study was to examine the mechanism by which different metabolic pathways involving cAMP, PKC, or tyrosine kinase can initiate oocyte maturation.

Materials and Methods

Mature female hamsters, 30 days of age, were injected ip with 25 IU of pregnant mare's serum gonadotropin (PMSG; Sigma) on day 1 of the estrous cycle. Graafian follicles were dissected from the ovaries of animals killed on day 4 of the cycle and incubated, as described previously (5). Follicle-enclosed oocytes were analyzed for percent maturation, and the data were transformed prior to statistical analysis (6).

The time during which oocytes from incubated follicles became committed to mature was determined by modifying the procedure used for analysis of spontaneously maturing oocytes in mice (7). Follicles were preincubated in control medium or experimental additive for various lengths of time, after which they were punctured and the COCs from each follicle were incubated for an additional 3 h in medium containing 0.2-mM IBMX. The oocytes were then evaluated for percent maturation.

Bound and total cAMP levels were measured in the granulosa cells and COCs, which were extracted from follicles following incubation. The separated cells were sonicated in cyclic nucleotide grind buffer (50-mM potassium phosphate, 2-M NaCl and 1-mM IBMX, pH 6.7). An aliquot of supernatant was added to 0.5-N HCl, which was dried and reconstituted with acetate buffer for assay of total cAMP by RIA. Bound cAMP was measured following filtration through nitrocellulose. The filters were washed and boiled in HCl to extract cAMP, after which the HCl was dried and assayed for cAMP by RIA.

Phosphoproteins were analyzed in follicle cells after a 1-h equilibration period followed by a 2-h incubation with various additives in phosphate-free medium containing [^{32}P]orthophosphate (1 mCi/well). After each incubation, the follicles were washed, and the granulosa cells and COCs were separated. Samples were processed and run on two dimensional SDS-PAGE gels (8). The dried gels were exposed to Kodak X-OMAT AR film to detect phosphoproteins.

Results

Maturation was initiated by 4 h in whole follicles incubated continuously with LH, EGF, or TPA, while exposure to forskolin for 30 min followed by 3.5 h in plain medium stimulated maturation (Table 1). To examine the role of different protein kinases in oocyte maturation, follicles were incubated with protein kinase inhibitors. Inhibitor H-8 is reported to inhibit both PKC and PKA at 15-μM concentration or PKA alone at 1.2 μM (9). Maturation was stimulated by 1.2-μM H-8 alone while groups incubated with higher (15 μM) and lower concentrations (0.48 μM) of H-8 were not different from controls (Table 1). Combining LH (1 μg/mL) with 1.2-μM H-8 significantly reduced the percent maturation compared with groups exposed to LH alone; however, these values were still statistically higher than controls. Groups exposed for 30 min to forskolin plus 1.2-μM H-8 were not different from controls.

LH plus acridine orange, an inhibitor of PKC (10), significantly reduced maturation compared with groups exposed to LH alone, but the values remained significantly higher than controls (Table 1). Acridine orange inhibited EGF-stimulated maturation as did genistine, a tyrosine kinase inhibitor (11). Genistine had no effect on stimulation of maturation by LH.

Studies were conducted to determine when follicle-enclosed oocytes from hamsters were committed to mature (Table 2). Most treatments did not

TABLE 1. Percent maturation in follicle-enclosed oocytes following 4-h continuous incubations.

Treatment	% Mature	Treatment	% Mature
Control	25.2	Acridine orange (100 µM)	15.7
LH (1 µg/mL)	51.4*	LH + acridine orange	42.0*†
EGF (50 ng/mL)	52.6*	EGF + acridine orange	20.1
TPA (20 µM)	52.6*	Genistine (30 µg/mL)	19.8
Forskolin (60 µM)	57.7*	EGF + genistine	38.4
		LH + genistine	50.7*
H-8 (15 µM)	34.7	LH + 15-µM H-8	28.0†
H-8 (1.2 µM)	54.6*	LH + 1.2-µM H-8	40.2*†
H-8 (0.48 µM)	24.6	LH + 0.48-µM H-8	53.9*
Forskolin + 1.2 µM H-8	34.7		

* = significantly different from controls ($P < 0.05$); † = significantly different from LH groups alone ($P < 0.05$).

stimulate maturation by 1 h (not shown); however LH, TPA, and EGF all triggered maturation by 2 h. Oocytes from follicles preincubated for 30 min with forskolin (60 µM) matured. H-8 inhibited LH-initiated commitment following a 2-h preincubation (Table 2).

Because cAMP and PKA are reported to play a role in oocyte maturation, total and bound cAMP were measured at various times in granulosa cells and COCs.

LH stimulated a significant rise in total cAMP (control = 55 ± 7; LH = 245 ± 42 fM/fol) and bound cAMP (control = 14 ± 1; LH = 21 ± 3 fM/fol) after 5 min in the granulosa cells. This pattern persisted throughout a 120-min incubation period (data not shown). No significant change in total or bound cAMP in the COCs was seen at any time (data not shown). EGF

TABLE 2. Maturation commitment in follicle-enclosed oocytes exposed to various additives.

Treatment	% Maturation	Treatment	% Maturation
Control	11.8	LH + 15 µM H-8	7.2†
LH (1 µg/mL)	43.9*	LH + 1.2 µM H-8	22.5*†
EGF (50 ng/mL)	51.9*	LH + 0.48 µM H-8	44.5*
TPA (20 µM)	54.0*		
Forskolin	50.0*		

* = significantly different from controls ($P < 0.05$); † = significantly different from LH groups alone ($P < 0.05$).

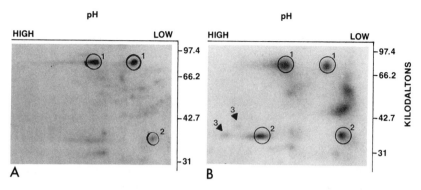

FIGURE 1. Phosphoproteins synthesized by control *(A)* and LH-stimulated granulosa cells *(B)*. 92-kDa proteins (1) showed constant intensity in all groups. The 39-kDa proteins (2, 3) were darkest in LH, EGF, TPA, and forskolin groups.

stimulated a small but significant rise in granulosa cell total cAMP at 1 h (EGF = 61.5 ± 1.3 fM/fol; controls = 41.8 ± 5 fM/fol), but it had no effect on COC cAMP. TPA had no effect on cAMP levels. The effects of forskolin on cAMP in hamster follicles have been reported previously (12).

LH stimulated phosphorylation of a 39-kDa group of proteins in granulosa cells, which was either absent or faint in the control groups (Fig. 1). No detectable phosphoproteins were seen in gels of COCs from the controls or LH groups. However, a full complement of phosphoproteins was present when COCs were stimulated by forskolin, TPA, or EGF (data not shown).

Discussion

Inhibiting LH-stimulated maturation with H-8 (1.2 μM) or acridine orange caused a reduction in percent maturation in continuous incubations and commitment experiments; however, the values remained above control levels. If, as proposed, LH initiates maturation by activating both PKC and PKA, then inhibiting one kinase while the other remains active may cause only half of the oocytes to mature. Interestingly, 1.2-μM H-8 alone initiated maturation, thus supporting the concept that a drop in cAMP (or PKA activity in this case) is required to initiate maturation. However, a large change in cAMP (either up or down) may be all that is necessary to induce maturation. Thus, forskolin causes a large increase in cAMP (12) while H-8 (1.2 μM) inhibits PKA activity. However, unlike LH, both additives are membrane permeable and act on all cell groups within the follicle. EGF-stimulated maturation was inhibited by genistine and acridine orange; however, LH-stimulated maturation was not affected by genistine, indicating that its effect was specific and not toxic. Inhibition of EGF-stimulated maturation by acridine orange indicates that EGF may trigger meiosis via PKC. EGF has been reported to indirectly stimulate PKC in other systems (13).

LH, EGF, and TPA all induced commitment to mature in follicle-enclosed oocytes by 2 h. Previous studies of spontaneously maturing mouse oocytes reported commitment after 60 min (7). It is probable that commitment time in follicle-enclosed oocytes is dependent on diffusion factors and may also involve a different mechanism of action.

LH significantly increased both total and bound cAMP in granulosa cells at 5 min compared with controls. This time, as expected, is well before maturation commitment at 2 h. That significant changes in cAMP occurred only in the granulosa cells and not the COCs suggests that the signal for oocyte maturation originates in the granulosa compartment.

LH initiated the phosphorylation of 39-kDa proteins in granulosa cells, which were faint or absent in the control groups. A similar group of proteins appeared in both the granulosa cells and COCs of groups incubated with either EGF, TPA, or forskolin. These results suggest that PKA, PKC, and tyrosine kinase may utilize a similar substrate(s). LH did not change cAMP in the COCs, and this correlates with the lack of detectable phosphoproteins in COCs from follicles incubated with LH. By contrast, membrane-permeable additives (TPA and forskolin) and EGF did stimulate detectable protein phosphorylation in COCs. Previous studies have demonstrated EGF receptors on hamster COCs while they contain few LH receptors (14).

References

1. Tsafriri A. Mammalian oocyte maturation: Model systems and their physiological relevance. Adv Exp Med Biol 1979;112:269-81.
2. Davis JS, Weakland LL, Farese RV, West LA. Luteinizing hormone increase inositol triphosphate and cytosolic free Ca^{2+} in isolated bovine luteal cells. J Biol Chem 1987;262:8515-21.
3. Aberdam E, Dekel N. Activators of protein kinase C stimulate meiotic maturation of rat oocytes. Biochem Biophys Res Commun 1985;132:570-4.
4. Dekel N, Sherizly I. Epidermal growth factor induces maturation of rat follicle-enclosed oocytes. Endocrinology 1985;116:406-9.
5. Hubbard CJ. Cyclic AMP changes in the component cells of Graafian follicles: Possible influences on maturation in the follicle-enclosed oocytes of hamsters. Dev Biol 1986;118:343-51.
6. Zar JH. Biostatistical Analysis. Englewood Cliffs, NJ: Prentice-Hall, 1974.
7. Schultz RM, Montgomery RR, Belanoff JR. Regulation of mouse oocyte meiotic maturation: Implication of a decrease in oocyte cAMP and protein dephosphorylation in commitment to resume meiosis. Dev Biol 1983;97:264-73.
8. O'Farrell PH. High resolution two-dimensional electrophoresis of proteins. J Biol Chem 1975;230:4007-21.

9. Hidaka H, Inagaki M, Kawamoto S, Sasaki Y. Isoquinolinesulfonamides, novel and potent inhibitors of cyclic nucleotide dependent kinase and protein kinase C. Biochemistry 1984;23:5036-40.
10. Hannun YA, Bell RM. Aminoacridines, potent inhibitors of protein kinase C. J Biol Chem 1988;263:5124-31.
11. Akiyama T, Ishida J, Nakagawa S, et al. Genestein, a specific inhibitor of tyrosine-specific protein kinases. J Biol Chem 1987;262:5592-5.
12. Hubbard, CJ. The effect of forskolin and LH on cAMP changes and maturation in the follicle-enclosed oocytes of hamsters. Acta Endocrinol 1985;110:413-20.
13. Whitman M, Cantley L. Phosphoinositide metabolism and the control of cell proliferation. Biochim Biophys Acta 1988;948:327-44.
14. Hubbard CJ, Oxberry BA, Savage R. EGF presence and effect on cAMP, steroids and oocyte maturation in hamster ovaries [Abstract]. 22nd Annual Meeting. Society for the Study of Reproduction, Columbia, MO, 1989.

58

Effects of TNF α and Prolactin: Increased hCG Binding in Human Granulosa Cells; Differential Interaction with hCG-Stimulated Progesterone Secretion

T.K. CLINTON, K.F. ROBY, R. LYLES, AND P.F. TERRANOVA

Tumor necrosis factor α (TNF α) has been localized within the granulosa and luteal compartments of the human ovary (1, 2). In addition, TNF α increases progesterone (PR) secretion and hCG binding of human granulosa/lutein cells in vitro (3). Prolactin has similar well-documented luteotropic effects on the rat corpus luteum. However, the role of prolactin in the regulation of human granulosa cell differentiation and early luteal development remains unclear. Depending on the concentration tested and the model used, prolactin has been shown to stimulate (4), inhibit (4, 5, 6, 7), and have no effect (5, 7) on the production of PR in human granulosa cells in vitro.

The objectives of this study were to *(a)* determine the effects of PRL on hCG binding and PR secretion of human granulosa/lutein cells and *(b)* compare and contrast the effects of PRL and TNF α on human granulosa/lutein cell steroidogenesis.

Materials and Methods

Human recombinant TNF α was supplied by Genentech, Inc. (San Francisco, CA): specific activity 4.03 U/mg and endotoxin <0.06 U/mg (Limulus Amoebocyte Lysate Assay). TNF α was tested at a concentration of 10 ng/mL, which is in the range of Kd (8). hCG was Chymodiactin from Ayerst, Canada. Previous experiments from this lab have indicated that a dose of 0.1-IU hCG stimulates progesterone production maximally (3). This concentration was used for all subsequent experiments. Human PRL (AFP 9042B) was supplied by the National Hormone and Pituitary Program (Baltimore, MD). PRL was tested at concentrations ranging from 10–1000 ng/mL. All dilutions were made with culture medium.

Human granulosa cells were obtained at the time of ova collection from women participating in an IVF/GIFT program. The women were treated with a combination of Lupron, Metrodin, and Pergonal to stimulate follicular development. hCG (10,000 IU) was administered 32 h prior to follicular aspiration. Follicular aspirates containing the granulosa cells were collected into Ham's F-12 and 1% heparin. The granulosa cells were then purified by centrifugation, using a 70% followed by a 35% Percoll gradient. After purification, the granulosa cells were washed 3 times with Dulbecco's Modified Eagle Medium/Ham's F-12 (1:1 v/v), supplemented with 20% fetal calf serum and 10% dimethyl sulfoxide. The cells were then frozen and stored in liquid nitrogen until needed. Immediately prior to culture, the cells were thawed quickly and washed 3 times with media.

The granulosa cells were cultured in Dulbecco's Modified Eagle Medium/Ham's F-12 (1:1 v/v), supplemented with 5% horse serum, 5% fetal calf serum, 20-nM selenium, 20-nM insulin, 50-U penicillin/mL, and 50-mg streptomycin/mL (9). Prior to cell culture, 24-well culture plates were coated with 0.3-µg collagen and 4-µg fibronectin in a total volume of 600 µL. After overnight incubation at 37°C, the collagen/fibronectin mixture was removed, and the wells were washed once with media. The granulosa cells were then plated at a density of 50,000 cells/well/mL media and cultured within a 100% humidified atmosphere of 5% CO_2 and air. After 24-h incubation, hormones and fresh media were added. The cells were then cultured for 10 days. Media were changed and fresh hormones added every 2 days. The spent media were frozen and stored at –20°C until progesterone determination by radioimmunoassay. At the end of the 10-day culture period, the cells were scraped from the plates for subsequent hCG binding determinations.

Concentrations of PR in the media were determined by radioimmunoassay, as previously described (10).

hCG was iodinated using the Iodogen method as described by Bolton and Hunter (11). At the end of the experiment period, the media were removed and the cells were washed twice and homogenized. The homogenates were centrifuged for 15 min at 3500 × g at 4°C. The supernates were discarded, and 100-µL [^{125}I]hCG (30,000 CPM) was added to the pellet. The mixtures were incubated overnight at room temperature, washed with ice cold buffer, and then centrifuged for 15 min at 3500 × g at 4°C. The supernates were aspirated, and pellets were counted. Specific binding was determined as cpm bound minus nonspecific cpm. Nonspecific binding was determined by incubating the homogenates with [^{125}I]hCG in the presence of 20-IU hCG.

Data were analyzed by either 1-way analysis of variance, followed by

Duncan's multiple range test, or 2-way analysis of variance, followed by the Scheffe' test. Values were considered significant when P ≤ 0.05.

Results

Effects of TNF α and hCG on Progesterone Secretion. TNF α alone increased PR production significantly, but not dramatically, above control cells in both patients (2-way ANOVA, treatment effect P < 0.006); the responses of 2 representative patients are shown in Figure 1. When TNF α and hCG (0.1 IU/mL) were administered together, PR levels increased to higher levels than hCG treatment alone on days 6–10, for patient *A* and days 4–10 for patient *B* (P < 0.001, Scheffe' test).

Effects of PRL and hCG on Progesterone Secretion. Ten ng/mL of PRL had no effect on PR secretion. When the concentration was increased to 50 ng/mL, PRL increased PR production significantly, but not dramatically, above controls (2-way ANOVA, treatment effect P < 0.0001); the responses of 2 representative patients are shown in Figure 2. When administered together, PRL (50 ng/mL) and hCG (0.1 IU/mL) did not increase PR production significantly on days 2–8 of culture over levels obtained with hCG alone. However, on day 10, PRL + hCG significantly increased PR levels above hCG-treated cells in both patients (P < 0.001, Scheffe' test). PRL + hCG increased PR secretion throughout the culture period when compared to nontreated cells (P < 0.001, Scheffe' test).

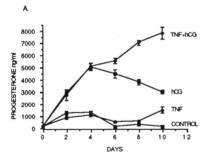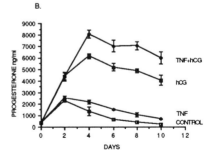

FIGURE 1. Effects of TNF α, hCG, and TNF α + hCG on granulosa/lutein cell PR production in 2 patients (*A* and *B*). Granulosa/lutein cells were cultured in the presence of TNF α (10 ng/mL), hCG (0.1 IU/mL), TNF α + hCG, or media alone (control) for 10 days. The media were changed, and PR in the media was determined every 2 days by RIA. (P < 0.006, 2-way ANOVA, treatment effect of TNF α vs. control; patients *A* and *B* are representative of 5 patients examined.)

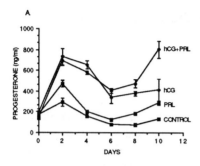
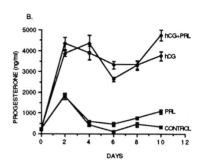

FIGURE 2. Effects of PRL, hCG, and PRL + hCG on granulosa/lutein cell PR production in 2 patients (*A* and *B*). Granulosa/lutein cells were cultured in the presence of PRL (50 ng/mL), hCG (0.1 IU/mL), PRL + hCG, or media alone (control) for 10 days. ($P < 0.0001$, 2-way ANOVA, for treatment effect of PRL vs. control; patients *A* and *B* are representative of 5 patients examined.)

Effects of TNF α on hCG Binding. On day 10 of culture, the specific binding of hCG to granulosa cells was significantly increased in hCG-treated cells compared to controls ($P < 0.05$, Duncan's). TNF α treatment increased hCG binding greater than either control or hCG treatment ($P < 0.01$; $P < 0.05$, respectively). When administered together, TNF α and hCG (0.1 IU/mL) significantly increased hCG binding when compared to hCG alone ($P < 0.01$, Duncan's). However, hCG binding in the TNF α + hCG group was not different from TNF α alone (Table 1).

Effects of PRL on hCG Binding. On day 10 of culture, PRL alone in concentrations ranging from 10–100 ng/mL increased the binding of hCG to granu-

TABLE 1. hCG binding to granulosa/lutein cells after 10 days of culture with TNF α (10 ng/mL), hCG (0.1 IU/mL), TNF α + hCG, or media alone (control).

Treatment	hCG Binding (% of Control)
TNF α	470[a]
hCG	202
TNF α + hCG	545[b]

Note: Results are expressed as percent of control ([experimental − control value/control value] × 100).

[a]$P < 0.05$ TNF α vs. hCG; [b]$P < 0.01$ TNF α + hCG vs. hCG. (Duncan's test).

TABLE 2. hCG binding to granulosa/lutein cells after 10 days of culture with PRL (50 ng/mL), hCG (0.1 IU/mL), PRL + hCG, or media alone (control).

Treatment	hCG Binding (% of Control)
hCG	80
PRL (ng/mL)	
10	202
100	276
1000	69
PRL + hCG	
10	113
100	78
1000	22

Note: Data are from 1 patient only.

losa cells when compared to controls and hCG alone. The hCG binding of cells treated with PRL (10–1000 ng/mL) and hCG was less than binding obtained with cells treated with only PRL (Table 2).

Discussion

TNF α and PRL each alone increased PR production and hCG binding in human granulosa/lutein cells in vitro. These findings indicate the possibility of luteotropic roles for TNF α and PRL. Another laboratory has also shown that TNF α stimulates granulosa/lutein PR secretion in vitro (2). Thus, it seems clear that TNF α and PRL can increase PR production, although the effect is not as great as with hCG (Figs. 1 and 2). Interestingly, the patterns of TNF α and PRL-stimulated PR production were very similar. This observation points to a possible relationship between TNF α and PRL. The possiblity exists that PRL induces TNF α production by the granulosa/lutein cells, which then increases P secretion. In addition, it may be possible that the increase in hCG binding induced by PRL may be mediated by the granulosal production of TNF α.

It was apparent that TNF α synergized with hCG in stimulating PR secretion and hCG binding. Since TNF α increased hCG binding, one possible explanation is that TNF α increased the number of hCG receptors, which, when in the presence of hCG, increased PR production above that of hCG alone. In contrast, PRL did not appear to synergize with hCG in increasing PR secretion or hCG binding. In fact, when compared to hCG binding obtained with PRL alone, the binding was reduced in the presence of both PRL and hCG. The mechanism of this reduced hCG binding remains unclear.

References

1. Roby KF, Terranova PF. Localization of immunoreactive tumor necrosis factor (I-TNF) in the human ovary. Biol Reprod [Suppl 1] 1989;40:171.
2. Zolti M, Meirom R, Shemesh M, et al. Granulosa cells as a source and target organ for tumor necrosis factor-α. FEBS 1990;261:253-5.
3. Roby KF, Lyles R, Terranova PF. Tumor necrosis factor-alpha increases progesterone secretion and chorionic gonadotropin binding in human granulosa-lutein cells. 72nd Annual Meeting. Endocrine Society, Atlanta, 1990.
4. McNatty KP, Sawyers RS, McNeilly AS. A possible role for prolactin in control of steroid secretion by the human Graffian follicle. Nature 1974;250:653-5.
5. Soto EA, Tureck RW, Strauss JF, III. Effects of prolactin on progestin secretion by human granulosa cells in culture. Biol Reprod 1985;32:541-5.
6. Cutie ER, Andino NA. Prolactin inhibits the steroidogenesis in midfollicular phase human granulosa cells cultured in a chemically defined medium. Fertil Steril 1988;49:632-7.
7. Lee MS, Ben-Rafael Z, Meloni F, Mastroianni L, Jr, Flickinger GL. Effects of prolactin on steroidogenesis by human luteinized granulosa cells. Fertil Steril 1986;46:32-6.
8. Le J, Vilcek J. Tumor necrosis factor and interleukin I: Cytokines with multiple overlapping biological activities. Lab Invest 1987;56:234-48.
9. McAllister JM, Kerin JP, Trant JM, et al. Regulation of cholesterol side-chain cleavage and 17α-hydroxylase activities in proliferating human theca interna cells in long term monolayer culture. Endocrinology 1989;125:1959-66.
10. Terranova PF, Garza F. Relationship between the preovulatory luteinizing hormone (LH) surge and androstenodione synthesis of preantral follicles in the cyclic hamster: Detection by in vitro responses to LH. Biol Reprod 1983;29:630-6.
11. Bolton AE, Humter WM. The labelling of proteins to high specific radioactivities by conjugation to a ^{125}I-containing acylating agent. Biochem J 1973;133:529-39.

59

Follicular Progesterone Production Stimulated by TNF α Is Modulated by PKC and Calcium

MARIA SANCHO-TELLO, KATHERINE F. ROBY, AND PAUL F. TERRANOVA

Tumor necrosis factor α (TNF α) stimulates progesterone (PR) production by preovulatory rat follicles in vitro (1, 2); however, TNF α-stimulated PR levels never reached those obtained after incubation with comparable doses of luteinizing hormone (LH), indicating the possibility of a different signal transduction mechanism. TNF α stimulates arachidonic acid release (3), involving cyclooxygenase and/or lipoxygenase pathways (4) and prostaglandin (PG) production (5), which ultimately may stimulate cAMP synthesis (6), or it may directly activate the cAMP-dependent pathway (7). Several studies revealed that protein kinase C (PKC) activators and/or inhibitors can alter TNF α action (8–10), while another study reported no relation between TNF α and PKC (7).

Since TNF α has been localized in the rat ovary (11) and has distinct effects on ovarian steroidogenesis (1, 2, 12, 13), it may be a physiologically important cytokine in the ovary. This study was designed to gain insight into the mechanism(s) by which TNF α stimulated follicular PR in the rat.

Materials and Methods

Human recombinant TNF α was supplied by Genentech, Inc., and by Amgen Biologicals (specific activity 4.03×10^7 and $>1 \times 10^7$ U/mg, respectively). Fifty units of TNF α (1.25–5.0 ng/mL) were used in all experiments (unless otherwise expressed); this is in the physiological range of Kd (14). Ovine LH-S25 was from NIDDK and the National Hormone and Pituitary Program. The protein kinase inhibitors, 1-(5-isoquinolinesulfonyl)-2-methylpiperazine

(H-7) and N-(2-guanidino-ethyl)-5-isoquinolinesulfonamide (HA1004), were dissolved in water; nordihydro-guaiaretic acid (NDGA) and indomethacin, in 5% sodium carbonate; phorbol 12-myristate 13-acetate (PMA) and calcium ionophore A23187, in ethanol; and EGTA, in incubation media.

Holtzman rats weighing ~220 g were monitored for estrous cycles by daily vaginal smears and were used after at least 3 consecutive 4- or 5-day cycles. Ovaries were removed at 0900 h on proestrus, and preovulatory follicles were dissected, cleaned, and placed in Medium 199 (Gibco) with 0.1% (w/v) bovine serum albumin (incubation medium). Eight to ten follicles per animal were obtained.

Follicles from 2–3 animals were pooled, randomly distributed in 24-well culture plates, and cultured (2 follicles/well) in 1 mL of incubation medium at 37°C (5% CO_2 and air), and at least 3 wells were used for each treatment. After 15 min of culture, hormones and/or drugs were added, and the follicles were further cultured for 24 h unless otherwise expressed. In time-course experiments, media were collected after 1 or 6 h of culture for steroid determinations; follicles were washed twice and incubated with fresh incubation media without TNF α until the 24-h period was completed. For cAMP and cGMP assays, follicles were incubated for 5–20 min or for 24 h, and an aliquot of media was taken at 6 and 12 h of culture. At the end of the culture periods, media and/or follicles were collected and frozen separately at –20°C until assayed.

Concentrations of PR were determined by RIA in unextracted media, as described elsewhere (15), as were PGE_2, $PGF_{2\alpha}$, and 6-keto-$PGF_{1\alpha}$ (16) and also cAMP and cGMP in media and in follicles (17).

Data were analyzed by two-way ANOVA, Duncan's multiple range test or Student's t-test.

Results and Discussion

The time-course of TNF α action is shown in Table 1. When follicles were exposed to TNF α for 1 or 6 h, PR levels were not different than the levels of controls at these times, or after 24 h of culture for 1 h of TNF α exposure. However, when exposed to TNF α for 6 or 24 h, PR levels were significantly higher at 24 h in the TNF α group than in the control group.

The cAMP levels in TNF α-stimulated follicles were never different than the levels in the control group (Table 2). Also, a higher amount of TNF α (500 U/mL) did not increase cAMP levels in follicles after 24 h of culture (0.14 ± 0.01 ng PR). However, when exposed to LH (5 ng or 5 μg/mL), cAMP levels in media and follicles were between 5 and 100 times higher than any other groups. Neither TNF α nor LH altered cGMP levels compared to controls (data not shown).

Although cAMP is the mediator that produces the highest gonadotropin-

TABLE 1. Progesterone levels (ng/mL/2 follicles), by time-course of TNF α action.

| Treatment | 1-h TNF α | | 6-h TNF α | | 24-h TNF α |
Group	1-h Culture	24-h Culture	6-h Culture	24-h Culture	24-h Culture
Control	0.26 ± 0.08	9.66 ± 3.52	0.78 ± 0.01	8.31 ± 1.77	6.61 ± 1.89
TNF α	0.22 ± 0.05	8.06 ± 1.54	1.29 ± 0.34	18.11 ± 3.04*	27.22 ± 5.47*

*$P < 0.05$ vs. control at the same time by Student's t-test.

stimulated steroidogenic response (18), other signaling systems, such as inositol phosphates (19), PKC (20), and calcium (19), also have a role in steroidogenesis. In different models, TNF α increased cAMP levels directly (7) or indirectly by increasing PG levels (6). We observed no increase of cAMP or cGMP in follicles or media, while the LH-increased cAMP in both follicles and media, strengthens our hypothesis that TNF α and LH utilize different mechanisms in stimulating PR secretion.

The results for TNF α, leukotrienes, and prostaglandins are as follows: TNF α-stimulated PR production was not affected by NDGA (1 µg/mL) or indomethacin (10 µM) (34.3 ± 9.2 ng PR/mL/24 h for TNF α culture versus 37.0 ± 18.0 for TNF α + NDGA and 48.2 ± 12.5 for TNF α + indomethacin). Also, PGE_2, $PGF_{2\alpha}$, and 6-keto-$PGF_{1\alpha}$ levels measured in media revealed both PGE_2 and $PGF_{2\alpha}$ levels as undetectable (<10 pg/mL), and 6-keto-$PGF_{1\alpha}$ levels were detectable but not different in TNF α and control groups (0.79 ± 0.12 ng/mL/24 h for control group versus 0.72 ± 0.06 for TNF α). Although in different cell types TNF α responses are related to cycloxygenase and/or lipoxygenase pathways (4) and are mediated by PG

TABLE 2. cAMP levels in follicles and media.

| Treatment | TNF α Exposure: ng cAMP/follicle | | | |
Group	5 min	10 min	20 min	24 h
Control	0.70 ± 0.17	0.59 ± 0.04	0.35 ± 0.07	0.09 ± 0.02
TNF α (50 U/mL)	0.67 ± 0.01	0.76 ± 0.11	0.34 ± 0.05	0.25 ± 0.05
LH (5 ng/mL)	ND	ND	ND	1.19 ± 0.08*

| Treatment | TNF α Exposure: ng cAMP/mL medium | | | | | |
Group	5 min	10 min	20 min	6 h	12 h	24 h
Control	0.15 ± 0.06	0.11 ± 0.02	0.09 ± 0.01	<0.08	<0.08	0.09 ± 0.01
TNF α	0.10 ± 0.02	0.12 ± 0.02	0.08 ± 0.01	0.11 ± 0.01	0.10 ± 0.01	0.10 ± 0.01
LH (5 ng/mL)	ND	ND	ND	ND	ND	1.95 ± 0.57*
(5 µg/mL)	ND	ND	ND	8.61 ± 1.11	11.29 ± 2.76*	3.14 ± 0.29*

*$P \leq 0.001$ vs. control and TNF α at the same time by Student's t-test; ND = not determined.

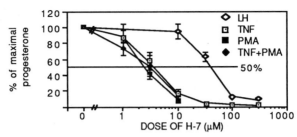

FIGURE 1. Effects of PKC inhibitor, H-7, on TNF α-, PMA- and LH-induced progesterone production. Two preovulatory rat follicles were incubated in 1 mL media for 24 h.

(5), it does not seem to be the pathway stimulated by TNF α to increase follicular PR production. It is known that granulosa cells are a major source of PG (21), whose synthesis can be increased by TNF α (13), but in our in vitro system, the follicles became atretic as evidenced by massive pyknosis in the granulosa layer (2), and thus, the cellular source of PG may be absent and therefore account for the failure to detect any increase in PG in response to TNF α. Theca can also be a source of follicular PG (21), and the site of action of TNF α in this in vitro system is the theca (2). Thus, the failure of TNF α to increase thecal production of PG is likely and indicates that the increase in PR may not be mediated by PG and/or leukotrienes.

The effects of the PKC inhibitor, H-7, on progesterone production are shown in Figure 1. TNF α-induced PR production was inhibited by H-7 (22) in a dose-dependent manner, with 50% inhibition corresponding to 5.2-μM H-7, determined by linear regression. LH-stimulated PR production was also inhibited by H-7 in a dose-dependent manner, but a higher concentration was needed (50% inhibition corresponded to 54.5-μM H-7). Since H-7 also blocks cAMP- and cGMP-dependent protein kinase, HA1004, a cAMP- and cGMP-dependent protein kinase inhibitor, with a very weak PKC inhibition (22) was tested. HA1004 did not decrease PR production (at 2.3 μM) after 24 h of culture (26.4 ± 6.1 ng PR/mL for TNF α culture versus 22.0 ± 6.1 for TNF α + HA1004). This correlates well with the failure to detect any increase in cAMP or cGMP in the media of TNF α-stimulated follicles.

The effects of PKC activators on TNF α are shown in Figure 2. PMA increased PR levels in media in a biphasic manner, with the maximum increase at 32-nM PMA (1 way ANOVA, P ≤ 0.03), which is a similar response to that previously reported for TNF α (1). When follicles were incubated with TNF α + PMA, PR was further increased above PMA alone in an additive manner (2-way ANOVA, P ≤ 0.001 for treatment effect), except for 320-nM PMA, when TNF α no longer increased PMA-stimulated PR levels (P > 0.2 by Student's t-test). H-7 also decreased PMA (8 nM) or PMA + TNF α-stimulated PR production, with a response identical to that observed for TNF α alone (Fig. 1; 50% decrease corresponded to 4.2- and

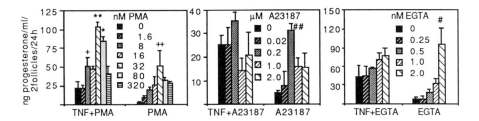

FIGURE 2. Effect of PMA, A23187, and EGTA on PR production. (+, P ≤ 0.05 vs. 0-
and 1.6-nM PMA + TNF α; **P ≤ 0.01 vs. 0-, 1.6-, 8-, 16-, and 320-nM PMA + TNF
α and 32-nM PMA; *P ≤ 0.05 vs. 8- and 16-nM PMA + TNF α and P ≤ 0.01 vs. 0-,
1.6-, and 320-nM PMA + TNF α and 80-nM PMA; ++P ≤ 0.05 vs. 8-nM PMA and P
≤ 0.01 vs. 0- and 1.6-nM PMA; ##P ≤ 0.05 vs. 0- and 0.02-μM A23187; #P ≤ 0.05 vs.
1- and 0.5-mM EGTA and P ≤ 0.01 vs. 0.25- and 0-mM EGTA, by Duncan's test.)

4.1-μM H-7 for PMA and PMA + TNF α, respectively). Collectively, these
results indicate that TNF α and PMA share a common pathway.

Previous studies reported that PMA stimulated basal PR production, but
inhibited gonadotropin-stimulated steroidogenesis, in granulosa (20, 23) and
luteal cells (24). Similarly, TNF α inhibited gonadotropin-stimulated steroidogenesis in granulosa cells (12). However, it has been shown that PKC
activators reduced the activity of TNF α in inducing cytolysis by reducing
the number of TNF α receptors, and the reduced TNF α binding was partially
recovered by PKC inhibitors (8). Thus, in some cell types, PKC activators
block TNF α effects by reducing TNF α binding.

Calcium ionophore, A23187, increases intracellular calcium, which is
necessary for PKC activation (25). When added to follicle cultures, a
biphasic response of PR accumulation in media was observed (1-way
ANOVA, P ≤ 0.014), with the highest values for 0.2-μM A23187. TNF α did
not increase PR levels in media in the presence of A23187 (2-way ANOVA,
P > 0.1 for treatment effect). Other studies reported that A23187 stimulated
PR production in a time- and concentration-dependent manner in granulosa
(26) and luteal cells, where it also enhanced LH-stimulated PR secretion
(27). However, in other models studied, A23187 has been found both to
enhance (10) or decrease TNF α action (8). When A23187 (0.2 μM) was
incubated in the presence of H-7 (300 μM, data not shown), with or without
TNF α, PR production was blocked, which indicates that A23187 stimulation of PR was probably mediated by PKC activation. Thus, although PKC is
a calcium- and phospholipid-dependent enzyme, it seems that both activators, PMA and A23187, work in a different manner in our model, since PMA
acts synergistically with TNF α while A23187 does not, as has been found
with another model (9) for some reason not yet well understood.

EGTA induced a dose-dependent increase of PR accumulation in media (1-way ANOVA, P ≤ 0.01). TNF α further increased PR in the presence of EGTA (2-way ANOVA, P ≤ 0.05); however at 1- and 2-mM EGTA, which would neutralize in excess the calcium in the media (Medium 199 has 1.8-mM calcium), TNF α was unable to further increase EGTA-stimulated PR production (P > 0.1 by Student's *t*-test). Other studies reported that EGTA reduced FSH-stimulated PR production in granulosa cells (26). Possibly, intracellular calcium is released when the extracellular is neutralized by the EGTA. Thus, it appears that calcium, which is involved in gonadotropin-stimulated steroidogenesis (19), may be important in regulating TNF α-induced steroidogenesis.

In summary, we report that TNF α-induced PR production by preovulatory rat follicles in vitro might be modulated by PKC, since PKC activators mimicked and a PKC inhibitor blocked TNF α action. To find that effect, which is not related to cAMP or cGMP increase, a period of at least 1 h of incubation with TNF α is needed.

Acknowledgments. The authors acknowledge support to MS-T in the form of a postdoctoral fellowship from CSIC, Spain.

References

1. Roby KF, Terranova PF. Tumor necrosis alpha alters follicular steroidogenesis in vitro. Endocrinology 1988;123:2952-4.
2. Roby KF, Terranova PF. Effects of tumor necrosis factor-α in vitro on steroidogenesis of healthy and atretic follicles of the rat: Theca as a target. Endocrinology 1990;126:2711-8.
3. Hepburn A, Boeynaems JM, Fiers W, Dumont JE. Modulation of tumor necrosis factor-α cytotoxicity in L929 cells by bacterial toxins, hydrocortisone and inhibitors of arachidonic acid metabolism. Biochem Biophys Res Commun 1987; 149:815-22.
4. Kettelhut IC, Fiers W, Goldberg AL. The toxic effects of tumor necrosis factor and their prevention with cyclooxygenase inhibitors [Abstract]. Fed Proc 1987; 46:1429A.
5. Antonipillai I, Wang Y, Horton R. Tumor necrosis factor and interleukin-1 may regulate renin secretion. Endocrinology 1990;126:273-8.
6. Lehmann V, Benninghoff B, Droge W. Tumor necrosis factor-induced activation of peritoneal macrophages is regulated by prostaglandin E₂ and cAMP. J Immunol 1988;141:587-91.
7. Zhang Y, Lin JX, Vilcek J. Synthesis of interleukin 6 (interferon-β₂/B cell stimulatory factor 2) in human fibroblasts is triggered by an increase in intracellular cyclic AMP. J Biol Chem 1988;263:6177-82.
8. Johnson SE, Baglioni C. Tumor necrosis factor receptors and cytocidal activity

are down-regulated by activators of protein kinase C. J Biol Chem 1988; 263:5686-92.

9. Munoz-Fernandez MA, Pimentel-Muinos FX, Alonso MA, et al. Synergy of tumor necrosis factor with protein kinase C activators on T cell activation. Eur J Immunol 1990;20:605-10.

10. Sehgal PB, Walther Z, Tamm I. Rapid enhancement of β_2-interferon/B-cell differentiation factor BSF-2 gene expression in human fibroblasts by diacylglycerols and the calcium ionophore A23187. Proc Natl Acad Sci USA 1987;84:3663-7.

11. Roby KF, Terranova PF. Localization of tumor necrosis factor (TNF α) in the rat and bovine ovary using immunocytochemistry and cell blot: Evidence for granulosal production. In: Hirshfield AN, ed. Growth Factors and the Ovary. New York: Plenum Press, 1989:273-8.

12. Adashi EY, Resnick CE, Croft CS, Payne DW. Tumor necrosis factor α inhibits gonadotrophin hormonal action in nontransformed ovarian granulosa cells. J Biol Chem 1989;264:11591-7.

13. Zolti M, Meirom R, Shemesh M, et al. Granulosa cells as a source and target organ for tumor necrosis factor-α. FEBS Lett 1990;261:253-5.

14. Le J, Vilcek J. Tumor necrosis factor and interleukin 1: Cytokines with multiple overlapping biological activities. Lab Invest 1987;56:234-48.

15. Terranova PF, Garza F. Relationship between the preovulatory luteinizing hormone (LH) surge and androstenedione synthesis of preantral follicles in the cyclic hamster: Detection by in vitro responses to LH. Biol Reprod 1983;29: 630-6.

16. Brannian JD, Terranova PF. Exogenous progesterone reduces follicular prostaglandin E and 6-keto prostaglandin F-1α in the cyclic hamster. J Reprod Fertil 1990;89:223-30.

17. Krishna A, Terranova PF. Relationships between LH stimulation in vitro and progesterone, androstenedione and cyclic AMP synthesis in preantral follicles of the cyclic hamster. J Endocrinol 1987;114:55-63.

18. Marsh JM. The role of cyclic AMP in gonadal steroidogenesis. Biol Reprod 1976;14:30-53.

19. Davis JS, Weakland LL, Farese RV, West LA. Luteinizing hormone increases inositol triphosphate and cytosolic free Ca^{2+} in isolated bovine luteal cells. J Biol Chem 1987;262:8515-21.

20. Shinohara O, Knecht M, Feng P, Catt KJ. Activation of protein kinase C potentiates cyclic AMP production and stimulates steroidogenesis in differentiated ovarian granulosa cells. J Steroid Biochem 1986;24:161-8.

21. Armstrong DT. Prostaglandins and follicular functions. J Reprod Fertil 1981; 62:283-91.

22. Hidaka H, Inagaki M, Kawamoto S, Sasaki Y. Isoquinolinesulfonamides, novel and potent inhibitors of cyclic nucleotide dependent protein kinase and protein kinase C. Biochemistry 1984;23:5036-41.

23. Welsh TH, Jones PBC, Hsueh AJW. Phorbol ester inhibition of ovarian and testicular steroidogenesis in vitro. Cancer Res 1984;44:885-92.

24. Baum MS, Rosberg S. A phorbol ester, phorbol 12-myristate 13-acetate, and a

calcium ionophore, A23187, can mimic the luteolytic effect of prostaglandin $F_{2\alpha}$ in isolated rat luteal cells. Endocrinology 1987;120:1019-26.

25. Nishizuka Y. Studies and perspectives of protein kinase C. Science 1986;233:305-12.

26. Tsang BK, Carnegie JA. Calcium requirement in the gonadotropic regulation of rat granulosa cell progesterone production. Endocrinology 1983;113:763-9.

27. Sawyer HR, Abel JH, McClellan MC, Schmitz M, Niswender GD. Secretory granules and progesterone secretion by ovine corpora lutea in vitro. Endocrinology 1979;104:476-86.

60

Flow Cytometric Analysis of Class I and II MHC Antigens on Ovine Luteal Cell Types

NICHOLAS KENNY, JAMES R. HERMAN, B. GEORGE BARISAS, AND DEBORAH A. ROESS

Secretion of progesterone by the corpus luteum (CL) is essential for the maintenance of early pregnancy in many species (1). The identification and characterization of two functionally and morphologically distinct types of steroidogenic luteal cells has provided several insights into the control of CL function (2). However, cells of the immune system may also play significant roles in the function and control of this ephemeral endocrine gland. Macrophages, lymphocytes, mast cells, monocytes, and eosinophils are found in CL of a variety of species (3). Their presence may indicate some role for the immune system in CL function.

Major histocompatibility complex antigens (MHC) are molecules pivotal to any immune response. MHC I is present on virtually all cell types and allows surveillance of cellular antigens for abnormalities (4). MHC I may have additional functions including involvement in the function of receptors for certain hormones (5). MHC II is normally restricted to specific, specialized antigen-presenting cells (macrophages, B-lymphocytes, and dendritic cells) but is expressed ectopically in some nonlymphoid tissues and is more widespread than was originally thought (6). MHC II is expressed aberrantly on target tissues in several autoimmune diseases, e.g., on β-cells of the pancreas in type I diabetes (7) and on thyroid epithelium in Graves' disease (8). This expression may allow cells to present autoantigen previously unavailable for immunological surveillance and give rise to chronic inflammatory reactions typical of autoimmune disease. These cell surface proteins may also function in conjunction with lymphoid cells in luteolysis.

Luteolysis in ruminants is initiated by prostaglandin $F_{2\alpha}$ ($PGF_{2\alpha}$) released from the uterus, and there is good evidence that $PGF_{2\alpha}$ of intra-luteal origin is luteolytic in nonhuman primates and women (1). However, the complete luteolytic mechanism, and the way in which this is brought about by $PGF_{2\alpha}$, remains elusive. Infiltration, or proliferation, of lymphocytes and macrophages into the corpus luteum at the onset of luteolysis occurs in the cow (9), mouse (10), human (11), guinea-pig (12), and rabbit (13). Together with the associated eosinophilia (14), these events suggest immune system involvement in luteolysis. Eosinophilia and macrophage infiltration associated with CL regression are typical of the inflammatory reaction associated with autoimmune endocrine disease; one component of luteolysis may involve a form of autoimmune rejection. γ-interferon (normally secreted by activated T-cells) will induce MHC II expression on bovine luteal cells (15). MHC II is present on human endometrial epithelial cells, both during the menstrual cycle and in diseased states such as endometritis (16), and is also inducible by γ-interferon (17). Induction of MHC II by γ-interferon has also been demonstrated for thyroid epithelium (18), and such in vitro-induced MHC II-positive cells are competent to present antigen to specific T-cells (19). MHC II is expressed by bovine luteal cells toward the end of the estrous cycle (20) and may have physiological relevance in the CL. A cyclic pattern of tissue growth and destruction is characteristic of both the CL and the endometrium; it is intriguing that MHC II may also be expressed cyclically in both tissues. Examination of the expression and physiological function of MHC in the CL may reveal a novel role for MHC and shed new light on interactions between the immune and endocrine systems.

Methods and Results

Since MHC participation is central to immunologic responses, we characterized its expression on ovine luteal cells obtained at defined stages of the estrous cycle and early pregnancy. Flow cytometry of cells immunofluorescently labeled with antibodies specific for MHC I and II allows rapid, accurate, and quantitative assessment of the amount of fluorescent label present on an individual cell. In a series of 3 preliminary experiments, small and large ovine luteal cell fractions were prepared (21) from luteal tissue obtained on days 10 (mid-luteal) and 14 (late luteal) of the estrous cycle and day 14 of early pregnancy on 3 separate occasions (n = 3–4 animals/day). Collagenase-dispersed luteal cells sustain damage to surface receptors, and therefore, cells were stored in sterile culture medium (M-199 containing antibiotics and 0.1% BSA) at 4°C for 18–24 h to allow regeneration of surface antigens. Cells were then washed twice in balanced salt solution containing 0.1% azide (BSS) to prevent antibody-induced capping and internalization of cell-surface antigens during immunofluorescent labeling.

Monoclonal antibodies against ovine MHC I (SBU I 41-19; 22) and MHC II (SBU II 28-01; 23) were obtained from Dr. M. Brandon, University of Melbourne, Australia. Procedures employed in the characterization of these antibodies (22, 23) were adapted for indirect immunofluorescent staining of luteal cells. Cells ($3–5 \times 10^6$ cells/mL) were resuspended in BSS containing 2.5% fetal bovine serum (BSS-FBS) to reduce nonspecific labeling. Primary unlabeled antibody (10–25 µg) was added to 1 mL of cells and incubated at 4°C for 1 h, after which the cells were washed twice with BSS-FBS. FITC-anti mouse IgG was added, cells were incubated for a further hour at 4°C, and they were then washed twice in BSS-FBS to remove free FITC-anti-mIgG. Nonspecific labeling was assessed in parallel incubations in which nonspecific mIgG replaced the primary antibody or the primary antibody was omitted. Cell auto-fluorescence was assessed in the absence of FITC-label.

Immunofluorescently labeled cells, resuspended at 1×10^6 /mL with a fine-bore pipette, were filtered through 44-µm mesh nylon to remove cell clumps and any cellular debris, yielding a suspension of single cells. Cell samples were introduced at a flow rate of 100–1000 cells/sec into a 2-laser, 4-channel custom flow cytometer (24). Data for forward angle and right angle light scatter and for fluorescence emission were collected by a photodiode and two photomultipliers in 3 channels. Data were collected from a minimum of 3 sets of 10,000 cells and were analyzed with multi-parameter scatter plots and single-parameter histograms incorporating interactive statistics developed within our laboratory (24). The number of specifically labeled cells was calculated by subtracting signals due to nonspecifically labeled cells. Qualitative confirmation of these observations was obtained by fluorescence microscopy.

Expression of MHC I and II in large and small luteal cell fractions is summarized in Table 1. Essentially all cells in both fractions were positive for MHC I; this is expected since the absence of MHC I is a lethal deletion leading to tissue rejection. MHC II expression also occurred in both cell fractions. Interpretation of MHC II expression in the small luteal cell fraction is complex; although this fraction is enriched in small steroidogenic luteal

TABLE 1. Expression of MHC I and II in large and small luteal cell fractions.

Day	(% Positive Cells)			
	MHC I		MHC II	
	Small	Large	Small	Large
10	85.1 ± 3.6	75.9 ± 3.2	16.6 ± 1.2	13.6 ± 1.2
14	88.9 ± 3.8	ND	25.2 ± 1.6	25.8 ± 1.6
14 P	87.4 ± 3.6	79.2 ± 3.4	19.9 ± 1.4	7.5 ± 0.8

cells and is essentially free of large luteal cells, this fraction also contains significant numbers of cell types of a similar size, probably including T-cells, macrophages, fibroblasts, and endothelial cells. In contrast, the large luteal cell fraction is primarily composed of large steroidogenic luteal cells to which MHC II expression is attributable per se. This was confirmed by MHC II co-localization with large cells on fluorescence versus cell-size scatter plots. MHC II expression on this cell population increased between days 10 and 14, but was suppressed in cells from pregnant animals.

Discussion

MHC II expression on large luteal cells raises the intriguing possibility that these cells may present autoantigen to T-cells during luteolysis, perhaps in a manner analogous to that proposed for the presentation of antigen in autoimmune endocrine disease (8). Further, the reduced expression of MHC II on cells from pregnant animals indicates suppression of MHC compared to regressing tissue, supporting the notion that a specific immunoregulatory function is involved in the luteolytic process. The physiologic function of MHC II on large luteal cells is unknown, but it is interesting to speculate that these cells may be competent to present antigen to T-cells, as is the case in γ-interferon-induced MHC II positive thyroid epithelial cells (19).

How this expression arises is again unclear; possibly γ-interferon release from activated T-cells infiltrating the regressing CL stimulates large cells to express MHC II, a phenomenon known to occur on bovine luteal cells in vitro (15). Interpretation of the observed MHC II expression in the small luteal cell fraction is more complex. Co-purification of macrophages and T-cells with this fraction allows for several scenarios to account for the presence of MHC II. We propose to address this question in experiments using luteal cells depleted of macrophages and/or lymphocytes and to identify the populations of macrophages and T-cells in the CL using the techniques described above.

These preliminary data are encouraging, and we plan to adopt several complimentary approaches to investigate the role of MHC molecules and the immune system in CL function. Our working model is that $PGF_{2\alpha}$-induced luteal cell damage initiates both eosinophilia and macrophage infiltration akin to an inflammatory response. Ensuing infiltration and activation of T-cells leads to γ-interferon release and induction of MHC II expression. A number of events may now operate in concert to promote luteolysis. First, eosinophils and macrophages interact to promote further cell damage and/or lysis. Second, activated T-cells amplify this initial immune response. Third, MHC II expression on luteal cells makes possible presentation of autoantigen leading to further T-cell activation. The sum of these events would ensure the progression of rapid structural luteolysis. This could be averted in the pregnant state due to the altered pattern of $PGF_{2\alpha}$ secretion and the immunosuppressive actions of PGE_2. While this model is surely an oversimplification of a complex process, it provides a basis for testable hypotheses.

Acknowledgments. This research was supported in part by NIH Grants AI-26621 and AI-21873 (BGB) and HD-23236 (DAR) and by a Lutheran Brotherhood Scholarship (JRH).

References

1. Auletta FJ, Flint APF. Mechanisms controlling corpus luteum function in sheep, cows, nonhuman primates, and women especially in relation to the time of luteolysis. Endocr Rev 1988;9:88-105.
2. Niswender GD, Schwall RH, Fitz TA, Farin CE, Sawyer HR. Regulation of luteal function in domestic ruminants: New concepts. Recent Prog Horm Res 1985; 41:101-51.
3. Adashi EY. Editorial: Cytokine-mediated regulation of ovarian function: Encounters of a third kind. Endocrinology 1989;124:2043-4.
4. Guillet J-G, Lai M-Z, Briner TJ, Buus S, Sette A, Grey HM, Smith JA, Gefter ML. Immunological self, nonself discrimination. Science 1987;235:865-70.
5. Edidin M. Function by association? MHC antigens and membrane receptor complexes. Immunol Today 1988;9:218-9.
6. Daar AS, Fuggle SV, Fabre JW, Ting A, Morris PJ. The detailed distribution of MHC class II antigens in normal human organs. Transplantation 1984;38:293-8.
7. Zauderer M. Origin and significance of autoreactive T cells. Adv Immunol 1989; 45:417-37.
8. Bottazzo GF, Pujol-Borrel R, Hanafusa T, Feldman R. Role of aberrant HLA-DR expression and antigen presentation in induction of endocrine autoimmunity. Lancet 1983;ii:1115-8.
9. Lobel BL, Levy E. Enzymatic correlates of development, secretory function and regression of follicles and corpora lutea in the bovine ovary, II. Formation, development, and involution of corpora lutea. Acta Endocrinol 1968;59(suppl 132):35-51.
10. Hume DA, Halpan D, Charlton H, Gordon S. The mononuclear phagocyte system of the mouse defined by immunohistochemical localization of antigen F4/80: Macrophages of endocrine organs. Proc Natl Acad Sci USA 1984;81:4174-7.
11. Adams EC, Hertig AT. Studies on the human corpus luteum, I. Observations on the ultrastructure of development and regression of the luteal cells during the menstrual cycle. J Cell Biol 1969;41:696-715.
12. Paavola LG. The corpus luteum of the guinea pig, IV. Fine structure of macrophages during pregnancy and postpartum luteolysis, and the phagocytosis of luteal cells. Am J Anat 1979;154:337-64.

13. Bagavandoss P, Wiggins RC, Kunkel L, Remick DG, Keyes PL. Tumor necrosis factor production and accumulation of inflammatory cells in the corpus luteum of pseudopregnancy and pregnancy in rabbits. Biol Reprod 1990;42:367-76.

14. Nett TM, McClellan MC, Niswender GD. Effects of prostaglandins on the ovine corpus luteum: Blood flow, secretion of progesterone and morphology. Biol Reprod 1976;15:66-78.

15. Fairchild DL, Pate JL. Interferon-γ induction of major histocompatibility complex antigens on cultured bovine luteal cells. Biol Reprod 1989;40:453-7.

16. Tabibzadeh SS, Bettica A, Gerber MA. Variable expression of Ia antigens in human endometrium and in chronic endometritis. Am J Clin Pathol 1986;86: 153-60.

17. Tabibzadeh SS, Gerber MA, Satyaswaroop PG. Induction of HLA-DR antigen expression in human endometrial epithelial cells in vitro by recombinant γ-interferon. Am J Pathol 1986;125:90-6.

18. Charriere J. Immune mechanisms in autoimmune thyroiditis. Adv Immunol 1989;46:263-334.

19. Londei M, Lamb JR, Bottazzo GF, Feldmann M. Epithelial cells expressing aberrant MHC class II determinants can present antigen to cloned human T-cells. Nature 1984;312:639-41.

20. Fairchild DL, Pate JL. MHC antigen expression on bovine luteal cells varies during the estrous cycle. Biol Reprod 1989;40 (suppl 1):236a.

21. Harrison LM, Kenny N, Niswender GD. Progesterone production, LH receptors, and oxytocin secretion by ovine luteal cell types on days 6, 10, and 15 of the estrous cycle and day 25 of pregnancy. J Reprod Fertil 1987;79:539-48.

22. Gogolin-Ewens KJ, Mackay CR, Mercer WR, Brandon MR. Sheep lymphocyte antigens (OLA), I. Major histocompatibility complex class I molecules. Immunology 1985;56:717-22.

23. Puri N, Mackay CR, Brandon MR. Sheep lymphocyte antigens (OLA), II. MHC class two molecules. Immunology 1985;56:725-33.

24. Herman JR, Boullier JA, Roess DA, Parr RO, Barisas BG. Examination of cytokinetics and ploidy obtained from paraffin-embedded prostatic tissue. Cytometry, 1990.

61

Thymulin (Serum Thymic Factor) Modulation of Porcine Granulosa Cell Responsiveness to Gonadotropins In Vitro

F. LEDWITZ-RIGBY AND P.G. SCHEID

The ovaries of several species contain macrophages and mast cells (1). These immune system cells have been associated with ovarian processes, such as follicular atresia and luteolysis. Substantial evidence has been gathered to demonstrate direct actions of a number of molecules of the immune system in altering granulosa cell functions. Tumor necrosis factor α inhibits follicle stimulating hormone (FSH) induction of aromatase activity (2) and stimulation of adenyl cyclase activity (3). Interleukin-I inhibits porcine granulosa cell progesterone secretion and adenyl cyclase activity with a time-course and mode of action (4, 5) remarkably similar to that of inhibitory porcine follicular fluid (luteinization inhibitor activity) (6, 7, 8). Immune system molecules such as thymosin $\alpha 1$ and thymosin β have been detected in follicular fluid in concentrations greater than those found in blood (9, 10). In addition, products of macrophages, which have not yet been identified, have been shown to stimulate granulosa cell progesterone production in vitro (11).

The studies mentioned above suggest that the story of local regulation of follicular development includes an interaction between ovarian and immune system cells. In addition, it is possible that the granulosa cells are themselves sources of at least some of the molecules previously identified as immune system products (12, 13). These observations led us to examine whether another immune system product, serum thymic factor (STF) recently renamed thymulin, might influence porcine granulosa cell function. Thymulin is a nonpeptide with the structure: pGlu, Ala, Lys, Ser, Glyn, Gly, Gly, Ser, Arg. It is produced by thymic epithelial cells and stimulates differentiation of T-cells (9, 14).

We chose to examine the effects of thymulin on porcine granulosa cells collected from small, immature antral follicles (1–3 mm in diameter) in order to see if thymulin could stimulate granulosa cell-specific maturational changes in immature cells. Such cells typically exhibit only low levels of steroid hormone production and respond more to FSH than to luteinizing hormone (LH). During maturation in vivo or artificially stimulated maturation in vitro, they first develop increased aromatase activity, followed by an increased ability to respond to gonadotropins with progesterone secretion. While these steroidogenic changes are occurring, the cells also shift from being predominantly dependent on FSH to becoming dependent on LH. The shift in gonadotropin dependency is accompanied by a decrease in FSH receptors and an increase in LH receptors (15).

Methods

Granulosa cells were collected from ovaries obtained at a local slaughterhouse, as previously described (16). Initial inocula of 5×10^5 viable cells were incubated in monolayer for 2–6 days in Medium 199 supplemented with 10% porcine serum, insulin, transferrin, selenium, cortisol, thyroxine, and L-glutamine as previously published (17). STF (Sigma, St. Louis, MO) and gonadotropins (NIH-LH-S22 and NIH-FSH-S12) were initially dissolved in sterile water and diluted just before adding to the cultures in sterile Medium 199. Aromatase assays contained 5 or 6 replicates per treatment per experiment, while radioimmunoassays (RIA) of progesterone secreted into the media were performed for 3 or 4 cultures per treatment per experiment. Aromatase activity was determined by incubating granulosa cells with ^{3}H (1, 2) testosterone and measuring the radioactivity released into the media as ^{3}H water, as previously described (17). Radioactivity, which remained in the media following charcoal precipitation of "cultures" containing no cells, was subtracted as background from all determinations. All data were subjected to analysis of variance and Duncan's test.

Results

Two-day preincubations with thymulin (25 to 100 ng/mL) stimulated basal aromatase activity in a dose-related manner during 3- or 4-h assays of aromatase activity performed in the absence of thymulin (Fig. 1). If FSH (200 ng/mL) was present during the preincubation, thymulin had no significant effect on aromatase activity. Preincubations with thymulin, lasting 3 or 4 days, did not significantly alter aromatase activity in the presence or absence of FSH.

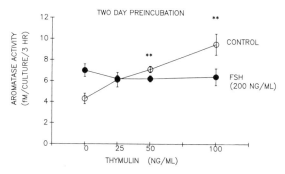

FIGURE 1. Effects of thymulin on basal aromatase activity. Porcine granulosa cells were preincubated for 2 days in the presence or absence of thymulin and/or FSH. Aromatase activity was assayed during a 3-h incubation in the absence of either hormone. P lot compares cells incubated with/without thymulin at the same concentration of FSH (**P < 0.01). FSH alone also significantly enhanced aromatase activity (P < 0.05).

In contrast to the effects of thymulin on aromatase activity, thymulin had a continued effect in stimulating progesterone secretion over 6 days of incubation. Thymulin had no significant effect on basal progesterone secretion, but enhanced both FSH- and LH-stimulated progesterone secretion (Figs. 2 and 3). FSH-stimulated progesterone secretion was enhanced to the greatest extent over the first 2 days in culture and declined in magnitude with longer incubations. Thymulin enhancement of LH-stimulated progesterone, however, increased with time in culture.

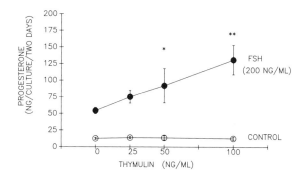

FIGURE 2. Effects of thymulin on FSH-stimulated progesterone secretion. Progesterone secreted into the media during a 2-day incubation with thymulin was greater than that secreted in its absence at the same concentration of FSH (*P = 0.05; **P = 0.07). FSH alone also significantly stimulated progesterone secretion (P < 0.05).

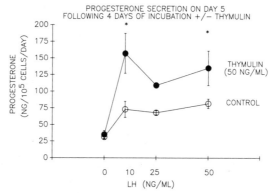

FIGURE 3. Effects of thymulin on LH-stimulated progesterone secretion. Granulosa cells were preincubated with or without thymulin for 4 days and tested for their responsiveness to LH on the fifth day. Progesterone secreted following a preincubation with thymulin was greater than that secreted by cells not exposed to thymulin in response to the same concentration of LH (*P < 0.05).

Thymulin did not alter either the plating efficiency or the cell doubling rate in culture as compared to cells incubated in its absence in either control media or with 500-ng LH/mL (Fig. 4).

Discussion

These observations suggest that thymulin could have a role in enhancing porcine granulosa cell maturation. The effects of thymulin are unlike those reported for any of the other immune system products that influence granu-

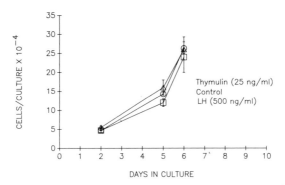

FIGURE 4. Effects of thymulin on plating efficiency or doubling rate of granulosa cells. Cultures were inoculated with 500,000 cells in the presence or absence of thymulin or LH. On days 2, 5, and 6, three cultures per treatment group day were ended and attached cell numbers determined. Efficiency and doubling rate were not altered.

losa cell function. The three changes we have observed: increased aromatase activity, increased responsiveness of the progesterone-producing enzymes to gonadotropin stimulation, and the changeover from being an FSH-responsive to LH-responsive cell resemble the normal maturational changes these cells experience with follicular enlargement and maturation. If thymulin is present within the maturing follicle, it could contribute to the maturation-stimulating activity reported in follicular fluid (18, 19). Neonatal thymectomy produces defects in reproductive function in rodents including increased follicular atresia, premature ovarian failure, and increased ovarian dysgenesis (12). While many of these alterations have been attributed to an immune attack on the ovary and decreased gonadotropin secretion, it is also possible that immune cells must invade the ovary and produce a maturation stimulating molecule to enhance follicular development.

References

1. Bulmer D. The histochemistry of ovarian macrophages in the rat. J Anat 1964; 98:313-9.
2. Emoto N, Baird A. The effect of tumor necrosis factor/cachectin on follicle stimulating hormone induced aromatase activity in cultured rat granulosa cells. Biochem Biophys Res Commun 1988;153:792-8.
3. Adashi EY, Resnick CE, Croft CS, Payne DW. Tumor necrosis factor alpha inhibits gonadotropin hormonal action in nontransformed ovarian granulosa cells. J Biol Chem 1989;264:11591-7.
4. Fukuoka M, Mori T, Taii S, Yasuda K. Interleukin-1 inhibits luteinization of porcine granulosa cells in culture. Endocrinology 1988;122:367-9.
5. Fukuoka M, Yasuda K, Taii S, Takakura K, Mori T. Interleukin-1 stimulates growth and inhibits progesterone secretion in cultures of porcine granulosa cells. Endocrinology 1989;124:884-90.
6. Ledwitz-Rigby F, Rigby BW, Gay VL, Stetson M, Young J, Channing CP. Follicular fluid inhibition of luteinization of porcine granulosa cells in vitro: Assay and influence of maturation. J Endocrinol 1977;74:175-84.
7. Rigby BW, Ledwitz-Rigby F, Hunzicker-Dunn M. Follicular fluid depression of ovarian granulosa cell adenylyl cyclase. Mol Cell Endocrinol 1980;17:17-28.
8. Ledwitz-Rigby F. Reversal of follicular fluid inhibition of granulosa cell progesterone secretion by manipulation of intracellular cyclic AMP. Biol Reprod 1980;23:324-30.
9. Wise TH. The thymus: Old gland, new perspectives. Dom Anim Endocrinol 1988;5:109-28.
10. Naz RK, Naylor PH, Goldstein AL. Thymosin-alpha 1 levels in human seminal plasma and follicular fluid: Implication in germ cell function. Int J Fertil 1987;32:375-9.
11. Halme J, Hammond MG, Syrop CH, Talbert LM. Peritoneal macrophages modulate human granulosa-luteal cell progesterone production. J Clin Endocrinol Metab 1985;61:912-6.

12. Vakharia DD, Kinder JE, Wise TH. Thymosin-alpha 1 in the ovary and the levels of thymosin-alpha 1 and t lymphocytes during estrous cycle in swine. In: Tumbleson ME, ed. Swine in biomedical research, vol 1. New York: Plenum Press, 1986:1925-36.

13. Roby KF, Terranova PF. Localization of tumor necrosis factor in the rat and bovine ovary using immunocytochemistry and cell blot: Evidence for granulosal production. In: Hirshfield AN, ed. Growth factors and the ovary. New York, Plenum Press, 1989:273-8.

14. Bach JF, Dardenne M. Thymulin. A zinc-dependent hormone. Med Oncol Tumor Pharmacother 1989;6:25-9.

15. Channing CP, Kammerman S. Characterization of gonadotropin receptors of porcine granulosa cells during follicular maturation. Endocrinology 1973;92:531-40.

16. Channing CP, Ledwitz-Rigby F. Methods for assessing hormone mediated differentiation of ovarian cells in culture and in short term incubations. In: Hardman J, O'Malley BW, eds. Methods in enzymology. New York: Academic Press, 1975;39:183-230.

17. Ledwitz-Rigby F, Gross TM, Schjeide OA, Rigby BW. The glycosaminoglycan chondroitin-4-sulfate alters progesterone secretion by porcine granulosa cells. Biol Reprod 1987;36:320-7.

18. Ledwitz-Rigby F, Rigby BW. Follicular fluid stimulation of steroidogenesis in immature granulosa cells in vitro. Mol Cell Endocrinol 1979;14:73-9.

19. Ledwitz-Rigby F. Follicular fluid stimulation of estrogen secretion by immature porcine granulosa cells. Mol Cell Endocrinol 1983;29:213-22.

Author Index

Subject Index